# END-OF-LIFE CARE
## Clinical Practice Guidelines

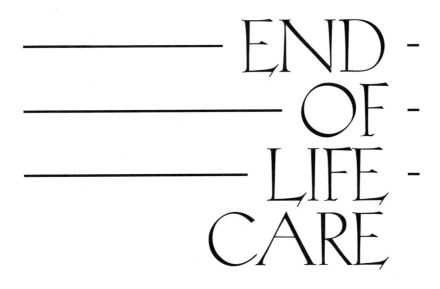

# END - OF - LIFE - CARE

## Clinical Practice Guidelines

**Kim K. Kuebler, MN, RN, ANP-CS**
Primary/Oncology/Palliative Care
Private Practice
Adjuvant Therapies, Inc.
Lake, Michigan

**Patricia H. Berry, PhD, RN, CHPN, CS**
Assistant Professor
University of Utah College of Nursing
Salt Lake City, Utah

**Debra E. Heidrich, MSN, RN, CHPN, AOCN**
Nursing Consultant
West Chester, Ohio

## W.B. SAUNDERS COMPANY
Philadelphia London New York St. Louis Sydney Toronto

**W.B. Saunders Company**

The Curtis Center
Independence Square West
Philadelphia, PA 19106

**Vice President and Publishing Director, Nursing:** Sally Schrefer
**Executive Editor:** Barbara Nelson Cullen
**Managing Editor:** Sandra Clark Brown
**Publishing Services Manager:** Catherine Jackson
**Project Manager:** Marc P. Syp
**Designer:** Amy Buxton
**Cover Designer:** Elizabeth Rudder

End-of-life care: clinical practice guidelines/ [edited by] Kim K. Kuebler, Patricia H. Berry, Debra E. Heidrich.
 p. ; cm.
 Includes bibliographical references and index.
 ISBN 0-7216-8452-1
 1. Terminally ill. 2. Terminal care. 3. Nurse practitioners. I. Kuebler, Kim K. II. Berry, Patricia H. III. Heidrich, Debra E.
 [DNLM: 1. Nursing Care--methods. 2. Terminal Care--methods. 3. Nurse Practitioners. 4. Palliative Care--methods. WY 152 E555 2002]
 R726.8 .E535 2002
 616'.029--dc21
                2001049607

# Contributors

**Patricia H. Berry, PhD, RN, CHPN, CS**
Assistant Professor
University of Utah College
  of Nursing
Salt Lake City, Utah
*Chapter 1* The Advanced Practice Nurse
  in End-of-Life Care
*Chapter 2* Clinical Practice Guidelines
  for Advanced Practice Nursing
*Chapter 3* End-of-Life Care
*Chapter 4* The Dying Process
*Chapter 5* Grief and Bereavement
*Chapter 9* Pulmonary Disease
*Chapter 19* Cough
*Chapter 26* Hiccup
*Chapter 28* Pain

**James M. Deshotels, SJ, APRN, MPH**
Mission Development Director
Daughters of Charity Services
  of New Orleans
New Orleans, Louisiana
*Chapter 14* HIV- and AIDS-Related
  Disease

**Nancy K. English, PhD, APN, CS**
Coordinator, Palliative Care
The Children's Hospital
Staff Nurse
Hospice of Metro Denver
Denver, Colorado
*Chapter 6* Complementary Therapies

**Julie Griffie, RN, MSN, CS**
Clinical Nurse Specialist
Palliative Care
Medical College of Wisconsin
Milwaukee, Wisconsin
*Chapter 4* The Dying Process
*Chapter 27* Nausea and Vomiting
*Chapter 28* Pain

**Debra E. Heidrich, MSN, RN, CHPN, AOCN**
Nursing Consultant
West Chester, Ohio
*Chapter 4* The Dying Process
*Chapter 12* Neurologic Disease
*Chapter 13* Malignancies
*Chapter 15* Ascites
*Chapter 16* Anxiety
*Chapter 18* Constipation
*Chapter 21* Delirium/Acute Confusion
*Chapter 23* Diarrhea
*Chapter 28* Pain
*Chapter 29* Palliative Care Emergencies
*Chapter 31* Ulcerative Lesions

**Kim K. Kuebler, MN, RN, ANP-CS**
Primary/Oncology/Palliative Care
Private Practice
Adjuvant Therapies, Inc.
Lake, Michigan
*Chapter 1* The Advanced Practice Nurse
  in End-of-Life Care
*Chapter 2* Clinical Practice Guidelines
  for Advanced Practice Nursing

*Chapter 3* End-of-Life Care
*Chapter 11* Renal Disease
*Chapter 14* HIV- and AIDS-Related
    Disease
*Chapter 16* Anxiety
*Chapter 17* Cachexia and Anorexia
*Chapter 20* Dehydration
*Chapter 21* Delirium/Acute Confusion
*Chapter 22* Depression
*Chapter 24* Dyspnea

**Diane B. Loseth, RN, MSN, OCN**
Clinical Nurse Specialist
Pain and Palliative Care Service
Memorial Sloan-Kettering Cancer
    Center
New York, New York
*Chapter 7* Psychosocial and Spiritual
    Care

**†Sandy McKinnon, RN, MN**
Manager, Acute Palliative Care Unit
Grey Nuns Community Hospital
    and Health Centre
Regional Palliative Care Program
Capital Health Authority
Edmonton, Alberta, Canada
*Chapter 17* Cachexia and Anorexia
*Chapter 20* Dehydration
*Chapter 25* Fatigue
*Chapter 27* Nausea and Vomiting
*Chapter 28* Pain
*Chapter 29* Palliative Care Emergencies

**Kate Ford Roberts, RN, MA**
Clinical Nurse Specialist,
    Palliative Care
Department of Nursing
University of Wisconsin Hospital
    and Clinics
Madison, Wisconsin
*Chapter 5* Grief and Bereavement

**Carol L. Scot, MD**
Provider, Adjuvant Therapies, Inc.
Medical Director
Hospice of Central Michigan
Mt. Pleasant, Michigan
Associate Medical Director
Sparrow Hospice Services
Lansing, Michigan
*Chapter 8* Cardiovascular Disease
*Chapter 30* Pruritus

**Pamela Sue Spencer, BA, RN,
    BSN, FNP**
Family Nurse Practitioner,
    Primary Care
Saginaw Veterans Administration
Saginaw, Michigan
*Chapter 10* Gastrointestinal Disease

---

† deceased

# Reviewers

**Lynn Borstelmann, RN, MN, AOCN, CHPN**
Director, Continuum of Care
University Hospital
SUNY Upstate Medical University
Syracuse, New York

**James F. Cleary, MD, FRACP, FAChPM**
Assistant Professor of Medicine
Director of Palliative Care Medicine Program
University of Wisconsin
Madison, Wisconsin

**Susan Duke, MSc, BSc, RGN, RNT, PGDE, ONC**
Consultant
Royal Berkshire and Battle Hospitals NHS Trust
Reaching, United Kingdom

**Michael E. Frederich, MD**
Medical Director
San Diego Palliative Home Healthcare
San Diego, California

**Kathleen Murphy-Ende, PhD, RN, AOCN**
Nurse Practitioner
University of Wisconsin School of Nursing and Hospital and Clinics
Madison, Wisconsin

**Judith A. Paice, PhD, RN, FAAN**
Research Professor of Medicine
Northwestern University Medical School
Northwestern Memorial Hospital
Chicago, Illinois

This textbook is dedicated to
the memory of my son,
Jacob James, whose spirit continues
to live. . .

K. Kuebler

# Foreword

It was just about 20 years ago that I devised and implemented a curriculum for staff and volunteers of a new hospice. As I cobbled concepts from the philosophy, sociology, psychiatry, cancer, community health, and rehabilitation literature to supplement the very few hospice-specific articles and monographs then available, I thought about developing a nursing text for what seemed to me ought to become a discrete specialty. In 1982, when the hospice option to the Medicare benefit was passed, thus assuring reimbursement from a major source, my intuition was confirmed. I found a collaborator and we got to work.

That book,[1] published in 1986, was at the time reviewed enthusiastically and regarded as state-of-the-art. Most gratifyingly, it proved useful in practice. In 1988, it received a commendation from the *American Journal of Nursing* as the only hospice text cited by a nationwide survey of 100 independent nurse practitioners as essential for their professional libraries. The book covered ten categories of symptom control in one 17-page chapter that listed 16 references. It dealt with treatment of pain in another 11-page chapter using a total of 29 sources.

What a difference two decades can make! This new text covers 17 symptoms, each commanding a technically detailed chapter of its own; each arrayed with clinical practice guidelines appropriate for both standard and advanced practice nurses; and many providing case examples. An encyclopedic section on the treatment of pain incorporates 64 references. In addition, there is an extensive review of end-stage processes for cardiovascular, pulmonary, gastrointestinal, renal, neurologic, and endocrine diseases, as well as malignancies and acquired immune deficiency syndrome (AIDS). The book also deals with complementary therapies, psychosocial and spiritual issues, and uncomplicated and complicated grief and mourning. Indeed, end-of-life care has become a unique specialty, commanding end-of-life care credentials in both medicine and nursing.

The appearance of this book also addresses another highly significant and relatively recent development in health care services in the United States—that of the proliferation of advanced practice nurses (APNs). Over the past 15 years, various research projects have documented the clinical and fiscal value of APNs. Patient and family satisfaction with their care is legendary. As direct reimbursement mechanisms for APN services expand, their number increases dramatically.

---

[1] Amenta, M. O., & Bohnet, N. L. (1986). *Nursing care of the terminally ill.* Boston: Little, Brown & Company.

A future is being laid with the guidelines presented in this text, which serve not only as blueprints for clinical care in any setting but also as bases for collaborative practice arrangements for APNs. That future will provide, through advanced practice end-of-life care, the epitome of professional nursing's potential.

Madalon O'Rawe Amenta RN, DrPH
Founding Executive Director of the Hospice
and Palliative Nurses Association

# Preface

The purpose of *End-of-Life Care: Clinical Practice Guidelines* is to provide advanced practice nurses (APNs) the guidelines and tools to provide comprehensive end-of-life care. Specifically, *End-of-Life Care: Clinical Practice Guidelines* aims to:

1. Suggest a theoretical framework to guide your care of patients and their families at the end of life.
2. Encourage you to identify interdisciplinary resources in your area to help with the care of patients and their families at the end of life. We find that end-of-life care demands an interdisciplinary team approach. Few of us, unless specifically prepared to do so, can, for example, manage complicated grief or the patient dually diagnosed with a terminal and mental illness or current or past substance abuse. Some symptoms in end-of-life care require physician collaboration; others may require referral to a specialist for further evaluation and treatment.
3. Review the use of collaborative practice agreements and clinical practice guidelines in a physician collaborative practice agreement and relationship.
4. Review the historical underpinnings of the hospice and palliative care movements.
5. Propose an approach to measuring outcomes in the end-of-life care you provide, thereby justifying the value of the care to colleagues, organizations, and third-party payers.
6. Review the advanced and end-stage disease processes for cardiovascular, pulmonary, gastrointestinal, renal, neurologic, and endocrine diseases, as well as malignancies and acquired immune deficiency syndrome (AIDS).
7. Provide extensive evidenced-based clinical practice guidelines for 17 symptoms encountered in end-of-life care. Our hope is that you can utilize these guidelines as a collaborative practice agreement with a physician. We believe including these practice guidelines within a collaborative practice agreement and relationship both facilitates improved outcomes for patients with advanced disease and their families.
8. Present extensive information about the use of complementary therapies in end-of-life care, including the research evidence of their effectiveness and resources useful for your own practice.
9. Describe some of the psychosocial issues faced by patients and their families at the end of life.
10. Review uncomplicated and complicated grief and mourning, providing suggestions on supporting families after the patient's death.
11. Describe the dying process, allowing you to anticipate and "normalize" these inevitable changes for the patient and family.

Most of all, however, we hope *End-of-Life Care: Clinical Practice Guidelines* will provide you with a framework for reflecting on your scope of practice and empower you to include end-of-life care in your day-to-day care of patients and families. As you well know, APNs often develop long-term relationships with the patients and families they care for, and maintaining that care until the end of life is fundamental to basic and advanced practice nursing.

### Definitions of Terms

We have defined the following terms used throughout *End-of-Life Care: Clinical Practice Guidelines:*

**Family:** Persons within the patient's supportive system of the patient's own choosing. These significant others may be relatives, friends, partners, neighbors, or anyone providing support to the patient.

**Advanced practice nurse (APN):** A registered nurse who has completed a master's or doctoral program in a clinical nurse specialist or nurse practitioner program. The clinical nurse specialist or nurse practitioner is certified by the American Nurses Credentialing Center in his or her specialty.

**End-of-life care:** Aspects of both palliative and hospice care—the area of health care that supports the multidimensional aspects of both the patient and family, promoting the quality of life until death.

**Disease trajectory:** The predicted course of a disease. Most diseases have predictable courses. Some interventions, like those directed at control of disease or treating the underlying cause of a symptom, may be more appropriate earlier in the course of the disease. As the disease progresses, aggressive interventions like surgery or several weeks of radiation may not be appropriate given the status of the disease or the wishes of the patient and family. Therefore, it is essential that the APN combine knowledge of the disease process and the goals of care to best assist the patient and family. This requires continuous and ongoing assessment and evaluation.

**Terminally ill, postcurative dying persons or patients:** Patients diagnosed with an advanced chronic or end-stage illness for which there is no cure and patients for which curative efforts have been exhausted. The treatment and goals of care are primarily directed at control of symptoms.

**Palliative care:** The active total care of patients whose disease is not responsive to curative treatment. Control of pain; other symptoms; and psychologic, social, and spiritual problems is paramount. The goal of palliative care is to achieve the best quality of life for patients and their families (World Health Organization, 1990).

As nurses experienced in assisting dying persons and their families at their most vulnerable times, we know it is an honor and privilege. Nowhere else in the practice of nursing are we invited to be companions on such a remarkable journey. Nowhere else in the practice of nursing are we better able to use our nursing skills to the fullest. Caring for dying persons and their families at the end of life with skilled and compassionate care will leave memorable and intimate moments for those patients and families you care for.

## References

WORLD Health Organization. (1990). *Cancer Pain Relief and Palliative Care* (Technical report series 804). Geneva: Author.

Kim K. Kuebler
Patricia H. Berry
Debra E. Heidrich

# Acknowledgements

The support, guidance, and friendship of many are indispensable to the completion of a work such as this. While we cannot possibly thank everyone, there are several persons deserving of special recognition.

We are grateful to our editors at W. B. Saunders, Thomas Eoyang and Sandra Brown, who provided guidance and encouragement throughout this often challenging process. We also acknowledge the many patients and families we have cared for. Thank you for allowing us to walk alongside on each of your journeys and for teaching us what is really important at life's end.

We, with gratitude and sadness, recognize Sandy McKinnon, MN, RN, a contributor, colleague, and friend, who died before this book was completed. Sandy, formerly the Manager of the Acute Palliative Care Unit at Grey Nuns Community Hospital in Edmonton, Alberta, Canada, was a remarkable palliative care nurse. She brought tremendous insight and expertise to this book and will be greatly missed.

We wish to recognize Madalon Amenta with admiration and gratitude for her work in defining the role of the hospice nurse in the United States. She is a friend, mentor, and colleague to all of us. We would not be able to complete a work such as this had it not been for Madalon's vision, energy, and commitment to hospice nursing.

A special thanks to our coworkers, friends, and families who contributed, even without realizing—the ability to bounce ideas off you for a reality check has been of priceless value. You know who you are!

**KKK, PHB, DEH**

I acknowledge Dr. Robert Twycross from Sir Michael Sobell House, Oxford, England for sharing his palliative care expertise and allowing us to reproduce his tables throughout the text and Sue Duke, RGN, RNT, PGDE Lecturer Practitioner in Palliative Care from Sir Michael Sobell House, Oxford and Oxford Brookes University for sharing her palliative care expertise and British hospitality. I also recognize my two children, Kayne Lucas and Kendal Kathleen, for their patience, acceptance, and unconditional love.
KKK

Special recognition goes to my daughter, Amelia Emery. Thanks for being my cheerleader and biggest supporter. Being your mom is the greatest joy I've ever known. I also wish to gratefully acknowledge my husband Merle for his unwavering support, perspective, and editing expertise. I know it sounds cliché, but I could never have done this without you! I dearly love you both.
PHB

I wish to acknowledge my husband, Bill, for his encouragement and support and my children, Bill and Emily, for their patience and understanding near deadlines. I also thank Pat and Kim for inviting me to be a part of this work.
DEH

# Contents

**PART FOUR**

# Clinical Practice Guidelines, *187*

# END-OF-LIFE CARE
## Clinical Practice Guidelines

# PART ONE

# General Principles
# of End-of-Life Care

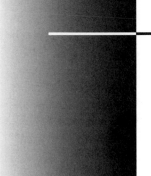

C H A P T E R **1**

# The Advanced Practice Nurse in End-of-Life Care

PATRICIA H. BERRY, KIM K. KUEBLER

The United States is facing an impending crisis in end-of-life health care delivery, prompted by an aging and increasingly culturally diverse population. Other relevant factors include increased public concern regarding suffering (as evidenced by the demand for physician-assisted suicide), recognition of the limits of technology, increased emphasis on pain management by health care accreditation organizations, and renewed interest in end-of-life care (AACN, 1999). The American Association of Colleges of Nursing (AACN), in recognition of the important role of nursing in the care of dying persons and their families, recently issued the position statement, *Peaceful Death: Recommended Competencies and Curricular Guidelines for End-of-Life Nursing Care* (AACN, 1999).

Nursing in end-of-life care, exemplified by the advanced practice nurse (APN), is gaining increased recognition. APNs consistently demonstrate an ongoing commitment to the care of the frail elderly, poor, culturally diverse, nursing home, and rural populations—areas where end-of-life care, including hospice and palliative care, is often unavailable (Ryan, 1999; Schulz, Cukr, & Ludwick, 1999; Shi & Samuels, 1997). An estimate suggests the underutilization of nurse practitioners, because of practice restrictions in state laws and denied access for consumers, costs the United States nearly $9 billion a year, inflating the cost of health care (Nichols, 1992). The estimation of the positive value of advanced practice nursing in end-of-life care can only be imagined.

Nurse practitioners (NPs) are the largest group of nonphysician clinicians, having doubled their numbers from 1990 to 1996. From 1996 to 2005, the nurse practitioner workforce is projected to increase from 55,000 to approximately 106,500, while the increase in primary care physicians is estimated at 10% (Cooper, Laud, & Dietrich, 1998). By the year 2015, 151,000 nurse practitioners are expected to be practicing (Herrick, 1998).

Compelling evidence is mounting that suggests nurse practitioner care rivals the effectiveness of medical care, often at decreased cost (Mundinger et al., 2000; Naylor et al., 1999).

Two studies demonstrate that outcomes of NP care compare favorably with those of medical care, often at lower cost. The first describes the success of NPs treating patients with chronic illnesses such as asthma, diabetes, and hypertension. NPs and physicians prescribed, consulted, referred, and admitted patients using the same referral source of specialists, inpatient settings, and emergency rooms, and the result was a remarkable parity in outcomes that has gained national attention and is viewed as a major breakthrough for the profession (Mundinger et al., 2000). The second study examined the effect of APN management on survival rates for older patients with cancer discharged home from postsurgical interventions. This study credits the APN with earlier assessment and treatment of physical problems, often relieving patients of psychologic concerns. Using standardized protocols, the APN provides direct physical care, information/education, ongoing psychosocial support, and management of surgical complications, which results in increased length of survival compared with usual ambulatory follow-up care (McCorkle et al., 2000).

The decrease in cost is accounted for, in part, by an increase in adherence to medications and outpatient treatments and a reduction in hospital admissions, emergency room visits, use of support services, and referrals to medical specialists. Additionally, patient satisfaction with nurse practitioner care equals or surpasses that of their physician colleagues (Brown & Grimes, 1995; Perry, 1995).

End-of-life care is maturing as a unique nursing specialty. Medicare regulations, and thus Medicare reimbursement, requires a collaborative agreement with a physician, and while much of end-of-life care can be done independently, it is best provided with access to an interdisciplinary team, including a physician. Patients and families at the end of life have unique and often complex needs.

## ■ THEORIES AND MODELS GUIDING END-OF-LIFE CARE

Some of the theories guiding end-of-life care are presented in this section. When reviewing these theories, it is important to consider the individual practice setting in which they are to be applied. End-of-life care is an essential part of the care of any patient and family. Unlike with other health care situations, end-of-life care requires competent, compassionate, and skilled attention because there is often only one chance to "get it right." In other words, there are no "dress rehearsals" for end-of-life care. The following four theories and models are presented for consideration: physical care as first priority (Maslow's hierarchy of needs), helping relationships, the Macmillan nurse model, and the interdisciplinary model of care.

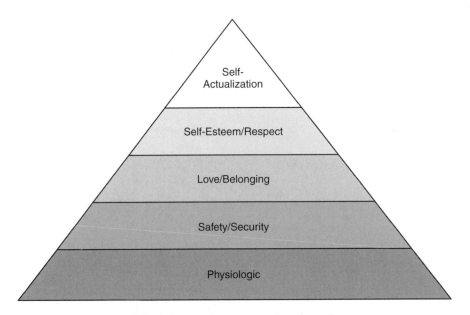

**FIG. 1-1**   Maslow's Hierarchy of Needs.

## ■ PHYSICAL CARE AS FIRST PRIORITY (MASLOW'S HIERARCHY OF NEEDS)

Maslow's hierarchy of needs (Maslow, 1954), a theory of motivation, is familiar to most who have taken an introductory psychology course. It represents human needs on a continuum, with physical needs taking priority as depicted in Figure 1-1. Those needs that are unmet and have the highest priority dominate behavior and demand satisfaction (Maslow, 1954). Implicitly, if one does not meet physical needs first then those needs higher on the hierarchy will go unmet or be distorted or ignored. It is difficult, for instance, for a person who is unable to breathe to contemplate the nature of existence. It is imperative to address physical symptoms before any other issue—such as quality of life, feelings about impending death, or even the consideration of ethically disturbing issues such as assisted suicide—is addressed in any terminal care situation. This priority of physical care and comfort is often ignored by nurses at all levels—even among some APNs.

It is extremely important to consider physical care as a priority in the care of patients and families at the end of life. If a patient's pain is not controlled and sleep is disrupted, the family caregiver's sleep is disrupted as well. Controlling the physical symptoms of the disease helps not only the patient but the family members as well. The patient and family can discuss and consider the goals of care and, most importantly, choose what they want to do as the patient's life draws to a close.

## ■ HELPING RELATIONSHIPS

Many theories and models serve as a basis for establishing and maintaining meaningful, helpful, and therapeutic relationships with patients and their families. The value of establishing a therapeutic nurse-patient and family relationship is not new. However, the actual manner in which a philosophy is implemented is the heart of the matter (Paulen & Rapp, 1981). One of the most helpful and applicable models of establishing a therapeutic relationship in end-of-life care is Carl Roger's theory of helping relationships. He suggests that the characteristics of a helping relationship are empathy, unconditional positive regard, and genuineness (Rogers, 1961). These characteristics, defined below as part of the nurses' approach to patients and families, are essential in facilitating care at the end of life. "Attention to detail" is added because it is recognized that this additional characteristic is also essential for quality end-of-life care (Du Boulay, 1984; Twycross, 1997). Consider these characteristics of helping relationships in the context of your own practice. Ask yourself, how easy or difficult would it be to follow these characteristics? How can these characteristics facilitate your interactions with patients and families, and thus, improve the quality of the care you provide? While especially applicable to end-of-life care, these characteristics are really pertinent to any helping relationship.

- Empathy—The ability to put oneself in another person's place and understand the patient/client from his or her own frame of reference; this requires the deliberate setting aside of one's own frame of reference, beliefs, values, and bias.
- Unconditional positive regard—A warm feeling towards others with a nonjudgmental acceptance of all they reveal themselves to be; the ability to convey a sense of respect and esteem at a time and place at which it is particularly important to do so.
- Genuineness—The ability to convey trustworthiness and openness that is real, rather than a professional facade; also, the ability to admit that one has limitations, makes mistakes, and does not have all the answers.
- Attention to detail—The learned and practiced ability to think critically about a situation and not make assumptions. The APN, for example, discusses challenging patient and family concerns with colleagues and other members of the interdisciplinary team. He or she considers every "what if" before making a decision and, in particular, any judgment. Finally, the APN is constantly aware of how his or her actions, attitudes, and words may be interpreted—and even misinterpreted—by others (Twycross, 1997; Berry & Griffie, 2000; Rogers, 1961).

The interactions with health care providers, control of symptoms, and the overall care—positive and negative—set an important and sometimes permanent climate for the patient's care and form lasting memories for family members. Indeed, the care received by both the terminally ill person and his/her family members are predominant aspects of the survivor's memory and the bereavement process (Berns & Colvin, 1998). Genuine openness, characterized by empathy and positive regard, in the approach to patients and families at the end of life goes a long way toward creating a meaningful, individualized, deeply profound, and memorable experience.

## ■ THE MACMILLAN NURSE MODEL OF PRACTICE

The Macmillan nurse model originated in the United Kingdom, and provides yet another theory or model for end-of-life care nursing practice. The Macmillan nurse is typically a clinical nurse specialist having undergone advanced palliative care training and is considered the expert clinician within British communities (Bullen, 1994; Webber, 1994). In fact, a unique part of the Macmillan model of practice is that the nurse is also a nurse to the community he or she serves. The Macmillan nurse model embraces a multiplicity of specialties, including, but certainly not limited to end-of-life care. Components of the Macmillan model—expert practitioner, consultant, educator, researcher, and leader—can easily be incorporated into the APN's palliative care practice. In many ways, the Macmillan nurse model is similar to that of the clinical nurse specialist and other advanced practice nursing roles in the United States.

### Expert Practitioner

The Macmillan nurse is a specialized practitioner, accepted in the British medical communities as a product of formal education and ongoing clinical experiences lending to expertise in a specific area. Generally, the model of practice includes both physical and psychologic assessments of the patient and family. The Macmillan nurse is able to assess and plan care for patients and families with complex symptoms or psychologic distress that can be managed effectively by established practice guidelines (Bullen, 1994; Webber, 1994).

### Consultant

Other members of the health care team may consult with the Macmillan nurse for information, advice, and guidance in offering state-of-the-art palliative care, eventually extending their own practice knowledge and skills (Webber, 1994). The Macmillan nurse may also consult with others on the health care team as well, providing continuity and coordination.

### Educator

Educating other health care professionals, including nurses, is a major part of the Macmillan nurse's role. Whether on a one-to-one basis in the clinical setting or as formal, didactic instruction, the Macmillan nurse's role ensures that clinical education is sound and reflects current research and practice. The Macmillan nurse also functions within the community as a whole, identifying educational needs for the general public, patients and families, colleges of nursing, and other institutional settings.

## Researcher

Macmillan nurses not only use clinical evidence to support their practice but also disseminate these results and contribute to data collection critical to improving the care of patients and families at the end of life. Because of their involvement in their communities, they also advise on areas of clinical practice that may require further evaluation and research.

## Leader

With a strong commitment and responsibility to the community in which he or she works, the Macmillan nurse works to identify and act in areas where improving the care of those with end-stage illness is needed. The British medical community encourages the development of new approaches and services and changes in practice—the Macmillan nurses play a key role in this innovation. The Macmillan nurse may influence policies that affect patient care and their families and serve on committees, as well as provide a forum for the collection of data and appropriate information to be used by groups that decide upon policy (Webber, 1994).

For example, the Macmillan model of practice lends itself well to a rural practice setting. The APN, using the Macmillan model of practice, may serve as the only palliative care expert in the area, providing both direct care and acting as a consultant to other providers, including joint home visits with the local hospice program staff. He or she may also serve as an educator for undergraduate and graduate students and the community as a whole. The APN may also be asked to take leadership roles in research and advocacy at state and local levels.

## ■ THE INTERDISCIPLINARY MODEL OF CARE

The need for the interdisciplinary team approach in hospice and palliative care is based on, in large part, meeting the varied and complex needs of the patient and family. Human beings, alone and in families, have needs that transcend the physical, including emotional, spiritual, and social needs among many others. In addition, the work of caring for dying persons and their families is often difficult and exhausting; indeed, many feel that for a while the interdisciplinary team takes up part of the burden for the patient and family; no one person can do this work alone. The team works together so that patients and families receive the best care—care with realistic goals and expectations that is planned and delivered based on individual needs.

Think of the last time you saw a quilt, first from a distance, and then close-up. From a distance the different patterns and colors blend; closer, one can see and appreciate each piece's individual contribution to the whole quilt. Such is the interdisciplinary team and its approach to dying patients and their families (Eng, 1993). Just as no two quilts are the same, no two people live or die the same way or have the same needs or concerns. The interdisciplinary team, through ongoing interactions with the patient and family, as well as with each other, develops a plan of care unique to the needs and concerns of the hospice patient and family. The plan of care becomes as a quilt; each individual part ultimately affects the beauty of the whole.

There is a subtle difference between interdisciplinary and multidisciplinary, but the most distinguishing characteristic lies in the relationship between team members. Multidisciplinary team members each follow their own piece of the care plan, do the interventions, and record them in the patient's medical record. Interdisciplinary team members are more aware of the overall plan, work collaboratively with each other, and thus often experience significant "role blurring." It is within those blurred or overlapped edges where team members are able to work together to ease the suffering of the patient and family. That's the beauty of the interdisciplinary team (the preferred type of team in palliative care)—the distinct disciplines of medicine, nursing, social work, clergy or counseling, volunteer, and others—working together with the patient and family so that their needs are met.

Expecting persons from diverse perspectives to work together is not always an easy task, however. Teamwork is not easy. As one hospice and palliative care professional put it, when enthusiasts report acting as a team they should be asked to show their scars: "If they don't have any scars, they haven't worked as a team. Teams don't just happen. They slowly and painfully evolve. The process is never complete" (Vachon, 1987).

The following section highlights the roles of the interdisciplinary team members, relying on the lessons learned from the hospice interdisciplinary team (Berry & Zeri, 1999; National Hospice and Palliative Care Organization, 1996). As you consider each role, consider that for each member of the team two key components are necessary for effective individual and team functioning: competence in their specific discipline and the ability to educate and teach others (Eng, 1993). An interdisciplinary team is functioning well when the members can educate each other, the patient, and the family freely. This ability is called *integrative power* and is essential in the function of an interdisciplinary team (Eng, 1993). For example, the physician's contribution to the plan of care is as important as that of the volunteer or nursing assistant.

## The Patient and Family

The interdisciplinary team would be incomplete without the inclusion of the patient and family. The patient and family are the final authority for establishing the goals of their care. The interdisciplinary team helps to identify which problems can be solved and consults with the family about their expectations. The team then gives of its knowledge and support to help the patient and family make the best choices for themselves.

## Nursing

Hospice and palliative nursing is the provision of palliative nursing care for the terminally ill and their families with an emphasis on their physical, psychologic, emotional, and spiritual needs. This care is accomplished in collaboration with the interdisciplinary team. Hospice and palliative nursing, then, is holistic practice conducted within an affiliative matrix. The hospice nurse, in developing and maintaining collaborative relationships with other members of the interdisciplinary team, must be flexible in dealing with the inevitable role blending that takes place (Hospice Nurses Association, 1994).

## Social Services

The role of the social worker in hospice differs from the "traditional" medical social work role. The social worker plays an important part in bridging the gap between physical and psychosocial care of the patient and family. The social worker, in conjunction with other members of the team, works to identify the patient and family experience of suffering, and then develops strategies to ease it.

## Physician and APN Services

Physician and APN services on an interdisciplinary team are crucial for the provision of quality pain and symptom management. In addition to overseeing the care of the patient and family, the physician or APN also can provide and interpret disease-related information to other team members.

## Spiritual Care Services

Available spiritual counseling and support for patients and families facing end-stage disease is essential, as spiritual suffering is often a component in the suffering in end-stage illness. Spiritual care services must be consistent with the patient's and family's beliefs and desires. We urge you to identify the spiritual care resources available to you in your community.

## Other Team Members

Based on the setting and goals of care, there may be other members on the interdisciplinary team, including volunteers, nursing assistants or home health aides, physical and occupational therapists, art and music therapists, or pharmacists, among others. Finally, given that the patient and family are the unit of care in hospice, care does not end with the death of the patient; the provision of bereavement support is an important part of both hospice and palliative care.

# ■ PIECING THE QUILT TOGETHER—THE FUNCTION OF THE INTERDISCIPLINARY TEAM

The interdisciplinary team works together to meet the physiologic, psychologic, social, spiritual, and economic needs of patients and families facing terminal illness and bereavement. This is accomplished through the development and maintenance of an integrated, individualized plan of care. This plan of care is based on assessments of the patient and family by interdisciplinary team members. From these assessments the patient's and family's needs and concerns are identified. The plan of care is then implemented by the team.

Interdisciplinary team members must be accomplished and comfortable in all aspects of their roles in order to gain the trust and respect of the patient and family as well as other team members. They must not underestimate or overestimate the importance of their own roles on the team. Indeed, they must be comfortable enough with themselves as professionals to tolerate—and even welcome—the blurring of roles innate in the hospice approach to care. Likewise, interdisciplinary team members must be able to "give their skills away" through teaching patients, families, other health care professionals, and even fellow team members. This gift should be given without expected return, recognition, or reward.

When interdisciplinary team members can integrate competent caregiving and teaching into their day-to-day work, it is possible to achieve a sharing of power or "integrative power" (Eng, 1993). In a patient care situation, integrative power is essential to empowering families with confidence in their own judgments and abilities to care for an ill family member. Empowerment also enables families to reflect on their experience with the satisfaction that they accomplished their goals in the best way possible—a way that was uniquely theirs. A cohesive, well-functioning, and healthy interdisciplinary team is a perfect example of the old saying: "The sum of the whole is greater than the sum of the parts." Integrative power at work within an interdisciplinary team is equally influential in the team's health and overall functioning (Berry & Zeri, 1999).

# ■ THE APN

The presence of APNs in any health care arena, especially end-of-life care, fosters improved care for dying patients and their families. The APN is also prepared, by virtue of education and experience, to provide specific interventions based on the whole and multidimensional person (e.g., physical, emotional, spiritual, cognitive, familial, and social aspects) and thus provide individual and unique intervention. Identifying not only physical needs but also how the patient's emotional and spiritual dimensions interface with his or her quality of life is an important component of the APN's role. We are able to meet patients and their families along the continuum of their disease process—from the initial diagnosis to death and beyond—promoting improved outcomes (Kuebler, 1997).

# ■ THE APN IN HOSPICE CARE

The Medicare hospice benefit, reimbursed under Medicare Part A, does not provide for direct reimbursement for APN services (APNs can only seek reimbursement under Medicare part B [Buppert, 1998]). Meanwhile, many hospice programs across the country are struggling from the financial restraints related to a decreasing average length of stay (LOS) and thus the provision of more time-intensive and costly service. More research is needed to establish the positive contributions of APNs hospice settings. The resulting data will support lobbying efforts aimed at modifying the Medicare Hospice Benefit to allow direct reimbursement to hospices for the services of APNs. Many hospice programs, however, use APNs despite a lack of direct reimbursement. Their roles vary widely.

# ■ PALLIATIVE CARE AND THE APN

There is a well-documented need to improve the care of persons living with advanced illness. In response to this need in the United States, palliative care programs are beginning to establish with greater regularity—but almost two decades behind those of Canada and Western Europe, where palliative care is a medical specialty (Walsh, 1998). The APN, largely because of the reimbursement structure, fits into these settings of care much more readily. In response to these needs, several graduate nursing programs now offer a specialty in palliative care, and nationally, substantial efforts exist to ensure the inclusion of end-of-life care in nursing education. Hopefully, offering palliative care APN education will provide more opportunities for the APN to specialize in the care of patients and families at the end of life.

We believe the APN's role in palliative care can help bridge the gap in a fragmented care system and help promote continuity and coordination of care. We also acknowledge the current paradigm shift in both nursing and end-of-life care. In order to achieve credibility as APNs, as well as positive care outcomes for patients and families at the end of life, we must add to the body of knowledge in end-of-life care. We are hopeful that the comprehensive review of the literature used to develop these practice guidelines can be used by you to improve the care of your dying patients and their families, a unique and rewarding experience.

## References

American Association of Colleges of Nursing (AACN). (1999). *Peaceful death: Recommended competencies and curricular guidelines for end-of-life nursing care.* Washington, DC: Author.

Berns, R., & Colvin, E. R. (1998). The final story: Events at the bedside of dying patients as told by survivors. *ANNA Journal, 25,* 583-7.

Berry, P. H., & Griffie, J. (2000). Planning for the actual death. In B. R. Ferrell & N. Coyle (Eds.). *Textbook of palliative nursing* (pp. 382-394). New York: Oxford University Press.

BERRY, P. H., & Zeri, K. (1999). *Hospice-I: Basic hospice computer-assisted instruction system.* Manchester, MO: ASK Data Systems.

BROWN, S. A., & Grimes, D. E. (1995). A metaanalysis of nurse practitioners and nurse midwives in primary care. *Nursing Research, 44,* 336-7.

BULLEN, M. (1994). Macmillan nurses: fighting cancer with more than medicine. *RCN Nursing Update, 3*(21), 3-13.

BUPPERT, C. (1998). HCFA releases final rules on PA and NP Medicare reimbursement. *Clinician News, 2*(6), 1-27.

COOPER, R. A., Laud, P., & Dietrich, C. L. (1998). Current and projected workforce of nonphysician clinicians. *Journal of the American Medical Association, 280,* 788-94.

DU BOULAY, S. (1984). *Cicely Saunders: Founder of the modern hospice movement.* London: Hodder & Stoughton.

ENG, M. A. (1993). The hospice interdisciplinary team: A synergistic approach to the care of dying patients and their families. *Holistic Nursing Practice, 7*(4), 49-56.

HERRICK, T. (1998). MDs put PAs/NPs under microscope: Docs scrutinize how NPCs influence supply and demand. *Clinician News, 2*(6), 1.

HOSPICE Nurses Association. (1994). *Standards of hospice nursing practice and professional performance.* Pittsburgh: Hospice Nurses Association.

KUEBLER, K. (1997). Signs of a change in seasons: The hospice and palliative care nurse practitioner. *Fanfare, 11*(2), 1-8.

MASLOW, A. (1954). *Motivation and personality.* New York: Harper.

McCORKLE, R., Strumpf, N. E., Nuamah, I. F., Adler, D. C., Cooley, M. E., Jepson, C., Lusk, E. J., & Torosian, M. (2000). A specialized home care intervention improves survival among older post-surgical cancer patients. *Journal of the American Geriatrics Society, 48*(12), 1707-13.

MUNDINGER, M. O., Kane, R. L., Lenz, E. R., Tottne, A. M., Tsai, W. Y., Cleary, P. D., Friedewald, W. T., Siu, A. L., & Shelanski, M. L. (2000). Primary care outcomes in patients treated by nurse practitioners or physicians. *Journal of the American Medical Association, 283,* 59-68.

NATIONAL Hospice Organization. (1996). *Hospice operations manual.* Arlington, VA: National Hospice Organization.

NAYLOR, M. D., Brooten, D., Cambell, R., Jacobsen, B. S., Mezey, M. D., Pauly, M. V., & Schwartz, J. S. (1999). Comprehensive discharge planning and home follow-up of hospitalized elders: A randomized clinical trial. *Journal of the American Medical Association, 281,* 613-20.

NICHOLS, L. M. (1992). Estimating cost of underusing advanced practice nurses. *Nursing Economics, 10*(5), 343-51.

PAULEN A., & Rapp, C. (1981). Person-centered caring. *Nursing Management, 12*(9), 17-21.

PERRY, K. (1995). Why patients love physician extenders. *Medical Economics,* August 21, 58-67.

ROGERS C. (1961). *On becoming a person: A therapist's view of psychology.* Boston: Houghton Mifflin.

RYAN, J. W. (1999). Collaboration of the nurse practitioner and physician in long-term care. *Lippincott's Primary Care Practice, 3*(2), 127-34.

SCHULZ, M., Cukr, P., & Ludwick, R. (1999). Developing a community-based screening program: Commitment to the underserved. *Journal of the American Academy of Nurse Practitioners, 11*(6), 249-52.

SHI, L., & Samuels, M. E. (1997). Practice environment and the employment of nurse practitioners, physician assistants, and certified nurse midwives by community health centers. *Journal of Allied Health, 26*(3), 105-11.

TWYCROSS, R. (1997). *Symptom management in advanced cancer* (2nd ed.). Oxon, UK: Radcliffe Medical Press.

VACHON, M. L. S. (1987). Team stress in palliative/hospice care. *Hospice Journal, 3*(2/3), 75-103.

WALSH, D. (1998). The Medicare hospice benefit: A critique from palliative medicine. *Palliative Medicine, 1*(2), 147-49.

WEBBER, J. (1994). A model response. *Nursing Times, 90*(25), 66-68.

# CHAPTER 2

# Clinical Practice Guidelines for Advanced Practice Nursing

KIM K. KUEBLER, PATRICIA H. BERRY

I nitially, the authors of this textbook agreed on the term "practice protocols" as the primary goal for publication, but after several conversations and much research about the differences between "guidelines" vs. "protocols" we decided to focus primarily on guidelines. We recognize that the various state practice acts do require advanced practice nurses (APNs) to use practice protocols to govern their clinical decision-making. We believe this publication can easily be used as a clinical practice contract between the advanced practice nurse and his or her collaborative physician regardless of state-specific practice mandates. In this chapter we also discuss guidelines and protocols, collaborative practice agreements, Medicare reimbursement, a consideration of state nurse practice rules and regulations, and where to obtain additional information.

## ■ DEFINITION OF GUIDELINES

*Guidelines* are developed to provide the APN with usable, overarching recommendations and expected clinical outcomes for the patient and his or her family (Eddy, 1990). The American Nurses Association (ANA) *Social Policy Statement,* revised in 1996, defined these four essential features of nursing practice (ANA, 1996a):
- Attending to the full range of human experiences and responses to health and illness, without restriction—differing from the problem-focused approach
- Integrating objective data with knowledge gained from an understanding of the patient's or group's subjective experience
- Applying scientific knowledge to the processes of diagnosis and treatment
- Providing a caring relationship that facilitates health and healing

The American Nurses Association's *Scope and Standards of Advanced Nursing Practice* defines the *APN* as follows:

*Advanced practice registered nurses manifest a high level of expertise in the assessment, diagnosis, and treatment of the complex responses of individuals, families, or communities to actual or potential health problems, prevention of illness and injury, maintenance of wellness, and provision of comfort. The APN has a master's or doctoral education in a specific area of advanced nursing practice, supervised practice during graduate education, and ongoing clinical experiences. Advanced practice registered nurses continue to perform many of the same interventions used in basic nursing practice. The difference in this practice relates to a greater depth and breadth of knowledge, a greater degree of synthesis of data, and complexity of skills and intervention (ANA, 1996b).*

The ANA also maintains that "advanced practice registered nurses integrate education, research, management, leadership, and consultation into clinical roles, and they function in collegial relationships with nursing peers and other professionals and individuals who influence the health environment" (ANA, 1996b).

Finally, the American Nurses Association defines the *nurse practitioner* (NP), an APN, as follows:

*The NP is a skilled healthcare provider who utilizes critical judgment in the performance of comprehensive health assessments, differential diagnosis, and the prescribing of pharmacologic and nonpharmacologic treatments in the direct management of acute and chronic illness and disease. Nurse practitioner practice promotes wellness and prevents illness and injury. Nurse practitioners function in various settings for individuals, families, and communities. This includes working autonomously and in interdisciplinary teams as resources and consultants. The role of this provider may include conducting research, providing education, and impacting public policy (ANA, 1996b).*

These elements of basic and advanced nursing practice are intermingled throughout the specific clinical guidelines to improve the quality of life for those patients with a life-limited diagnosis (English & Yocum, 1998). While many APNs practice independently, many state regulations require a collaborative practice arrangement, written or verbally agreed upon between an APN and a physician. End-of-life care often presents clinicians with challenges outside of the scope of practice and expertise of many nurses. We urge you to identify possible interdisciplinary resources, including a physician versed in end-of-life care who can act as a consultant. In addition, we urge you to identify other resources available for assistance with intervening in complicated family and grief situations.

These definitions encourage the APN to define and develop specific guidelines with a collaborative physician. A carefully developed practice agreement that includes practice guidelines between the APN and collaborating physician allows the APN to practice independently within the scope of nursing practice and without the need to adhere to a rigid, preset course of action. Rather, the APN can use his or her own level of expertise and defined scope of advanced practice, nursing expertise, and continued relationship with the patient and family to provide individualized and compassionate care.

## ■ DEFINITION OF PROTOCOLS

*Protocol,* typically used in diplomatic circles, is defined as prescribed rules of etiquette but has come to mean the proper way of doing things (Yarnell, 1974). Scientists have long used the term to define their experiment or research designs. The dictionary defines protocol as a rigid, long-established code prescribing complete deference to superior rank and strict adherence to due order of precedence and precisely correct procedure (Merriam-Webster OnLine, 1997).

By definition, the autonomous APN is precluded from performing independent clinical decision-making. Yarnell (1974) and colleagues define protocol as a specific strategy for handling patient care problems, defining both what data should be collected and what therapeutic approaches should be considered.

## ■ HOW GUIDELINES AND PROTOCOLS GUIDE CLINICAL DECISION MAKING

Guidelines and protocols provide a systematic approach for specific patient care situations, for example, disease-specific management or management of symptoms. They allow individual practitioners to establish mutual communication and agreement about treatment for specific situations with the collaborating physician (Yarnell, 1974). For the purposes of this publication, each specific guideline will include the following information; definition, etiology, history and physical, pertinent diagnosis, interventions, evaluation, follow-up, education, and a case study example. It is important to update clinical guidelines with the use of current research-based interventions to maintain ongoing state-of-the-art interventions (evidenced-based practice). The use of guidelines incorporates proven therapies used to benefit patients in everyday practice instead of relying on personal intuition or anecdotal experiences.

## ■ THE USE OF GUIDELINES AND PROTOCOLS IN A COLLABORATIVE PRACTICE AGREEMENT

Guidelines and protocols should permit the practitioner to incorporate the use of sound clinical judgment, as opposed to a rigid adherence to each step of a process. The "cookbook" approach to symptom management never takes into account the individual situation and the resultant needs and responses. The pharmacological management of frequently occurring symptoms in a patient with end-stage illness and his or her family requires careful assessment, individualized trials of treatment, and ongoing evaluation assessment. The management of any symptom requires patience, experience, and ongoing education of the patient and family. While this is true in all clinical situations, it is especially important in end-of-life care. Applying algorithms specific to an individual symptom such as pain, dyspnea, or restlessness may not necessarily produce the desired outcome. While the use of algorithms and care maps should not be discouraged, careful attention should be given to individual patient and family variations, their responses, and the context of care.

Managing the complex symptoms of a patient with end-stage illness requires knowledge of the pathophysiology associated with advanced diseases; knowledge of disease progression, clinical manifestations, and anticipated symptoms; and a detailed understanding of the pharmaceutical metabolite profile and the application of sound research-based interventions to encourage positive outcomes. The physical effects of the dying process may often mask frequently misdiagnosed and inappropriately treated symptoms. In dehydration, for example, a patient may be experiencing restlessness, which may be aggressively treated with benzodiazepines. Because of dehydration and the increased metabolite profile of the benzodiazepine, the patient's restlessness may be a direct result of the very medication intended to alleviate this symptom. However, if this patient is lightly hydrated (e.g., hypodermoclysis), renal perfusion is increased, the benzodiazepine metabolite is eliminated, and restlessness is reduced. Individual patients metabolize medications uniquely—due largely in part to the different disease processes. The normal effects of the dying experience, compounded with advanced disease and the emotional and existential dimensions that interact within each individual patient, require individual assessment, individual specific interventions, and careful titration to promote a symptom-free dying experience. This benefits both the patient and family.

## ■ COLLABORATIVE PRACTICE ARRANGEMENTS AND AGREEMENTS

Hospice health care providers have long understood the usefulness of a collaborative relationship with all members on the interdisciplinary team. Moreover, establishing a collaborative practice is essential in obtaining Medicare reimbursement and may also be mandated by the state boards of nursing to function within the specific scope of advanced nursing practice of an individual state.

To *collaborate* means to "work together." In 1971, the ANA and the American Medical Association (AMA) worked in partnership to develop the National Joint Practice Commission (NJPC). This commission, after prolonged investigation into the specific roles and relationships between nurses and physicians, defined collaborative practice to be nurses and physicians working as colleagues to provide care (Lysaught, 1986). This commission also called for a shared responsibility in defining roles and relationships in consonance with state laws and professional practice acts (Kedziera & Levy, 1994). However, successful collaborative practice requires a rethinking of the traditional medical hierarchical model of practice. In collaboration, both APN and physician can better focus on holistic interventions that can improve patient and family outcomes (Lysaught, 1986). Certainly the role of the APN and the physician may blur at times, but collaborators are partners and not substitutes for one another. Collaborators agree to ongoing participation in a process to achieve specific goals. These goals can be delineated by specific practice protocols that endorse interdependent practice and act as a mutual contract between the nurse and the physician.

## ■ MEDICARE REIMBURSEMENT FOR THE APN

As part of the Balanced Budget Act of 1997, Congress instructed the Health Care Financing Agency (HCFA) to cover the services performed by NPs and clinical nurse specialists (CNSs) within their scope of practice. On June 5, 1998, the HCFA released their Notice of Proposed Rule Making (NPRM), which outlines changes in the Medicare Part B Physician Fee Schedule for 1999 (Buppert, 1999; Sharp, 1998). These proposed changes required Medicare Part B to reimburse NPs and CNSs for services set by HCFA in a *Physician Fee Schedule*. NPs and CNSs now receive 85% of the fee schedule amount set for that of physicians. Fees may vary depending upon the Current Procedural Terminology (CPT) code billed by the APN. Medicare carriers may either pay the clinician directly or the assigned group or employer. The three areas where they cannot bill for direct services include a federally designated rural health clinic, federally qualified health centers, and health maintenance organizations—these settings already have a fee set that includes the combination of physician and APN services (Buppert, 1999; Federal Register, 1998).

In order to be eligible for Medicare reimbursement, regardless of state practice acts, a collaborative practice arrangement must exist (Buppert, 1999; Sharp, 1998). The definition issued in June, 1998 stirred controversy from NPs and CNSs practicing in the eight states that do not require collaboration with a physician—causing reevaluation of the definition (Buppert, 1999). The final proposed ruling states that NPs and CNSs practicing in a state that does not require a collaborative relationship must document the scope of practice and indicate a consulting or supportive physician relationship should their clinical decision making occur outside the scope of their practice (Buppert, 1999). In the individual states requiring an APN to practice within a collaborative arrangement, the HCFA (now the Centers for Medicare and Medicaid Services [CMS]) has amended its definition to include "collaboration" as found in the June 5, 1998 NPRM:

*Collaboration involves systematic formal planning and assessment and a practice arrangement that reflects and demonstrates evidence of consultation, recog-*

*nition of statutory limits, clinical authority, and accountability for patient care, according to a mutual agreement that allows the physician and the nurse practitioner to function independently as appropriate (Buppert, 1999; Federal Register, 1998; Sharp, 1998).*

## ■ STATE NURSE PRACTICE ACTS

The APN must know his or her specific state practice act to practice within the defined scope of practice. The ANA and the national certification examination determining the APN's specific specialty, in most states, identifies the standards of practice for the APN. (The certification examination is set forth by the American Nursing Credentialing Center [ANCC], a subsidiary of the ANA.) Each state's individual practice act determines the scope of individual practice arrangements and licensure specifically. APNs have prescriptive authority in over half of the states in areas including controlled substances, although some states require physician involvement and/or limit schedules from which the APN can prescribe (Pearson, 1999). The appropriate state board of nursing can provide further information about specific state practice requirements. The state board of nursing can also assist with Medicare and Medicaid reimbursement information. Information available from state boards of nursing includes:

■ Definition, scope of practice, licensure, and requirements for certification as a specialist.
■ Prescriptive authority, limitations, and application requirements, including controlled substance registration (if prescriptive privileges include controlled substances) and state laws regarding the need for separate controlled substance registration (a few states require this).
■ The requirements for collaborative practice agreements and arrangements, guidelines, and protocols.
■ Legislative agendas that pertain to APN practice regulations.
■ Medicare and Medicaid information for reimbursement.

The website for the National Council of State Boards of Nursing (NCSBN) has links to most individual boards of nursing, as well as e-mail addresses. For further information on how to obtain a Medicare provider number for Medicare reimbursement, call 1-202-307-7255 or 1-800-882-9539.

## ■ ADDITIONAL INFORMATION

For more information on the collaborative practice arrangement write, call, fax, or e-mail:
American College of Nurse Practitioners (ACNP)
503 Capitol Court, NE, Suite #300
Washington, DC 20002
Phone: (202) 546-4825
Fax: (202) 546-4979

E-mail: ACNP@nurse.org

To review the final rules see the *Federal Register* (63)211, November 2, 1998. This can be found in law libraries and federal depository libraries or by writing:

New Orders
Superintendent of Documents
PO Box 371956
Pittsburgh, PA 5258-7954

A nominal fee is required. These rules can also be located on the internet at: http://www.access.gpo.gov/su_docs/aces/aaces112.html (Buppert, 1999; Sharp, 1998)

Once the NP receives a Medicare Provider Number, Blue Cross and Blue Shield or another insurance company acting as the fiscal intermediary will request further information from the APN to issue a provider number for Medicare billing and secondary coverage for Medicare beneficiaries. In many areas, the intermediary offers education and technical support on how to bill Medicare and the intermediary for reimbursement. The Medicare website provides a current list of each state's intermediary and carrier with contact information by clicking on "Professional/Technical Information": http://www.hcfa.gov/medicare/medicare.htm

*Nurse Practitioner,* each year in its January issue, features a state-by-state update on regulations and legislative issues affecting advanced nursing practice. Regulations and rules related to advanced nursing practice change frequently, and the role and value of the APN in the care of all patients and families becomes apparent. The annual update includes information relating to legal authority (e.g., scope of practice, education and certification requirements), reimbursement, and prescriptive authority.

# References

AMERICAN Nurses Association. (1996a). *A social policy statement.* Washington, DC: American Nurses Publishing.

AMERICAN Nurses Association. (1996b). *Scope and standards of advanced practice registered nursing.* Washington, DC: American Nurses Publishing.

BUPPERT, C. (1999). *Nurse practitioner's business practice and legal guide.* Gaithersburg, MD: Aspen.

EDDY, D. (1990). Designing of practice policy, standards, guidelines, and options. *Journal of the American Medical Association, 263,* 3077-3084.

ENGLISH, N., & Yocum, C. (1998). *Guidelines for curriculum development on end-of-life and palliative care in nursing education.* Arlington, VA: National Hospice and Palliative Care Organization.

FEDERAL Register. (1998, November 2). *Federal Register, 63*(211). Washington, DC: Author.

KEDZIERA, P., & Levy, M. (1994). Collaborative practice in oncology. *Seminars in Oncology, 21,* 705-11.

Lysaught, J. (1986). Retrospect and prospect in joint practice. In: J. Steel, (Eds.). *Issues in Collaborative Practice*, 15-33, Orlando, FL: Grune & Stratton.

Merriam-Webster OnLine: WWWebster Dictionary. (1997). *Protocol.* http://www.mw.com/dictionary.htm. Accessed September 3, 2000.

Pearson, L. (1999). Annual update of how each state stands on legislative issues affecting advanced nursing practice. *The Nurse Practitioner, 24,* 47-83.

Sharp, N. (1998). From incident to telehealth: New federal rules and regulations affect NPs. *The Nurse Practitioner, 23,* 68-69.

Yarnell, S. (1974). *What is a protocol? Design and use of protocols* (monograph). Seattle, WA: Medical Computer Services Association, 11-14.

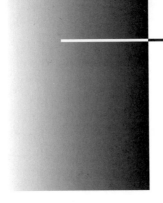

CHAPTER **3**

# *End-of-Life Care*

KIM K. KUEBLER, PATRICIA H. BERRY

*You matter because you are you, and you matter until the last moment of your life. We will do all we can, not only to help you die peacefully, but also to live until you die.*
(DAME CICELY SAUNDERS, FOUNDER OF THE MODERN DAY HOSPICE MOVEMENT)

E nd-of-life care in the United States has evolved into two models of care: (1) "traditional" care under the Medicare Hospice Benefit and (2) palliative care. This dual development continues with some aspects of care coinciding and some diverging. Where some authorities note certain distinctive characteristics of either "hospice" or "palliative" activities, others regard any differences between the two as primarily a matter of semantics.

In the material that follows, we will discuss the evolution of the hospice movement, the development of palliative care models, the status of end-of-life care in the United States, the role of the APN in end-of-life care, important issues associated with advance care planning, and outcome evaluation in end-of-life care.

## ■ HISTORICAL PERSPECTIVES OF HOSPICE CARE

Hospice care traces its philosophic roots to the Middle Ages. The term "hospice" is derived from the Latin root word *hospes,* meaning both host and guest. The interaction of guest and host implies mutual caring for one another (Amenta & Bohnet, 1986).

The concept of caring for weary pilgrims until they were rested or died dates from around 400 A.D. In the Middle Ages, the terms *hospital, hostel,* and *hospice* were used interchangeably. During the Crusades, clerics in facilities called *hospitia* provided shelter and care for sick pilgrims. These were often located adjacent to monasteries, and two of the most famous, the Great St. Bernard and the Little St. Bernard hospices, located in the Swiss Alps, are still in operation today. They trace their beginnings to the tenth century (Amenta & Bohnet, 1986). During that time, the dying were often honored and treated carefully. Seen as travelers on the metaphysical journey, they were viewed as moving on more rapidly than others and were frequently asked to make special prayers on behalf of mankind, as heaven was now directly open to them.

As medical practice advanced over the intervening centuries, medicine focused more intently on curative treatments and acute physical problems. Holistic care, which encompassed values the monks and nuns held dear—care of the soul, nurturing the mind and spirit, and honoring and caring for the dying—was displaced.

The modern hospice movement began in the late 1960s with the work of Dame Cicely Saunders. Dame Saunders, first practicing as a nurse and later as a medical social worker, volunteered at St. Luke's Home for the Dying. Motivated by her tenure at St. Luke's, Saunders entered medical school. After graduating in 1957, Dr. Cicely Saunders studied drug actions in relation to pain in the terminally ill while at St. Joseph's Hospice in London. Here, working with the nuns in caring for the patients, she observed and learned that pain has physical, emotional, social, spiritual, and economic dimensions. In the next few years, Dr. Saunders organized St. Christopher's Hospice, where the modern definition of hospice care evolved. Saunders is credited with founding the modern hospice movement and was honored as Dame Cicely Saunders for her tireless efforts in the care of the terminally ill. She believed that only a skilled interdisciplinary team of professionals could support these multiple needs (Bennahum, 1996). Her vision led to the development of St. Christopher's Hospice in London, England, which evolved a unique focus of patient-centered care and expert pain and symptom management. The precepts of the philosophy of care she integrated into St. Christopher's Hospice include what is traditionally known today as the hospice philosophy (Finn, 1985) (see Box 3-1).

Cicely Saunders introduced this hospice philosophy to the United States through an invited presentation on hospice and pain management at Yale–New Haven Hospital in 1966. Resigning her position as Dean of Yale School of Nursing, Florence Wald then devoted herself full-time to the development of the hospice concept of care in the United States. In 1971, Hospice, Inc. was formed, to be later named The Connecticut Hospice (Bennahum, 1996; Doyle, Hanks, & MacDonald, 1998). While hospice care in the United Kingdom is mainly institutionally based, for a variety of reasons, hospice care in the United States evolved mainly based on a home-care delivery model.

Meanwhile, Dr. Elizabeth Kübler-Ross, a psychiatrist, began her famous work studying death and dying, culminating in her 1969 book *On Death and Dying*. She stressed the importance of open communication and encouraged caregivers to express their feelings about caring for the dying (Kübler-Ross, 1969). Dr. Kübler-Ross' work also gained public attention for the long-ignored problems in the care of dying patients and their families in the United States.

| BOX 3-1 | *The Hospice Philosophy of Care* |
|---------|----------------------------------|

Regardless of the setting of care, hospice care embodies the following characteristics:
- The patient and family are the unit of care (however the patient defines his or her family).
- An interdisciplinary team cares for the needs of the patient and family.
- Emphasis is on control of pain and other symptoms, as well as a relief of suffering.
- The patient and family are recognized as the best judges of their needs, and thus control and choice are afforded them in all decisions regarding their care.

# ■ HISTORICAL PERSPECTIVES OF PALLIATIVE CARE

Canada saw the birth of palliative care when Balfour Mount defined the term and opened the first hospital-based palliative care service at the Royal Victoria Hospital at McGill University in Montreal in 1975 (Doyle, Hanks, & MacDonald, 1998). The McGill model of care was the first to include research and education centered in the area of pain management (Bennahum, 1996; Doyle, Hanks, & MacDonald, 1998).

All of these pioneers believed that professionals educated in the provision of symptom management and psychosocial and spiritual assistance for the dying and their families would support and improve upon a more humane dying process. "To be able to live until one dies at their maximum potential, performing to the limit of their physical activity and mental capacity, with control and independence whenever possible"—these words of Dame Cicely Saunders reverberate the theme for end-of-life care throughout the world (Doyle, Hanks, & MacDonald, 1998).

# ■ HOSPICE CARE TODAY

The care demonstrated by St. Christopher's Hospice and the Connecticut Hospice, along with the attention generated by Elizabeth Kübler-Ross, gained national attention for the hospice philosophy of care (Bennahum, 1996; Doyle, Hanks, & MacDonald, 1998). The National Hospice Organization, now the National Hospice and Palliative Care Organization, was founded in 1978 to promote improved care for the terminally ill in the United States.

The increasing development of hospice programs across the United States and lack of payment for hospice under Medicare prompted the Senate to take up an unprinted amendment during the debate of the budget reconciliation bill of 1982. This amendment provided hospice care as a covered Medicare benefit for persons with a life-limiting illness (Mahoney, 1998). Following widespread endorsement, the Medicare Hospice Benefit was agreed to and passed into law in 1982 (Mahoney, 1998). Since that time, hospice programs have multiplied extensively across the country. Fifteen years after the Senate agreed to endorse the Medicare Hospice Benefit in the United States, there were almost 3000 Medicare hospice programs nationally caring for approximately 450,000 patients annually (Mahoney, 1998).

Would the original pioneers, many still alive at the time of this publication, ever have dreamed that their influence would have led to the exceptional growth of hospice and palliative care worldwide? Western societies' increased awareness of hospice and palliative care services led to much greater availability of acceptable care at life's end.

# ■ THE SUPPORT STUDY—HOW ARE AMERICANS DYING?

The results of the SUPPORT (Study to Understand Prognoses and Preferences for Outcomes and Risks of Treatments), published in the *Journal of the American Medical Association* in 1995, revealed that Americans were dying in pain and often without dignity. This study, conducted at five medical centers across the country over a 10-year period, revealed that 80% of Americans were dying in institutional settings, often with unmanaged pain, in isolation, on mechanical ventilation, or in intensive care units. Furthermore, the use of living wills and health care proxies was often nonexistent and communication efforts between the patients and their physicians often proved futile (SUPPORT Principal Investigators, 1995).

The unexpected results of the SUPPORT study stirred a massive interest to improve the care of dying Americans and prompted a series of reports published by the Hastings Center. Many patients were found to have died after experiencing prolonged hospitalization, intensive care stays, or unrelieved pain. Half of "do not resuscitate" (DNR) orders were written near death and 10% of such patents died after spending 4 weeks in an ICU (Lo, 1995). The investigators noted that the physicians within their study were often uncertain about a patient's prognosis, and that this uncertainty contributed to the overuse of technology. They also identified that physicians did not know about their patient's preferences for life-sustaining interventions and failed to discuss care options with their patients and families, resulting in traditional biomedical interventions. The findings from the SUPPORT study are a powerful reminder of the difficulty associated with discussing death and dying in the context of medical decision-making. On a positive note, however, the SUPPORT team successfully developed specific information related to disease trajectory and prognostic indicators, as well as suggestions to improve communication between patients, their caregivers, and their families (Marshall, 1995).

Today the care of the dying is often termed *end-of-life care* (Kinzbrunner, 1998) and has undergone substantial restructuring since the inception of the Medicare Hospice Benefit in 1982. Despite the tremendous growth of hospice programs across the United States, the average length of stay (LOS) for most patients is estimated at less than 3 weeks. Unpublished data suggests the average LOS for hospice patients across the country is actually decreasing (Kinzbrunner, 1998). Currently only 17% of the terminally ill patients in the country receive hospice services and these are predominately Caucasian, educated, informed, middle-income consumers (Kinzbrunner, 1998).

In 1996, a study published in the *New England Journal of Medicine* suggested hospice care was often "too little, too late," largely because of late referrals and confusion over the Medicare Hospice Benefit admission criteria (Christakis & Escarce, 1996). The financial constraints of hospice and the recognition that the Medicare Hospice Benefit was designed for the care of cancer patients at the end of life further causes perceived limitations. Fallout from the SUPPORT study, current data from the National Hospice and Palliative Care Organization, and the lack of standards and competencies have spurred several initiatives across the country to reevaluate the delivery of care to those with life-limiting illness. We must be open to change. Though hospice has "growing pains," it continues as an endorsed, funded program within which thousands of patients and families receive excellent care and which can be improved by forward-thinking health care providers, legislators, patients, families, and the general public. Perhaps the Medicare Hospice Benefit can be enhanced to improve access and care to all (Lynn, 1998).

## ■ PALLIATIVE CARE

Palliative care is associated with the hospice philosophy and extends the traditional hospice approach of care to include a broader approach of services for the terminally ill (Billings, 1998). Palliative care is often initiated earlier in the course of end-stage disease and is not dependent upon the Medicare Hospice Benefit–defined requirement for a 6-month or less prognosis. Though the prerequisite for admission to a Medicare hospice program is a determination by two physicians that the patient has a prognosis of 6 months or less, provided the disease runs its usual course, palliative care has no such requirement. Persons with advanced illness are often "falling through the cracks" with minimal support before death, largely due to poor prognostication—physician reluctance to discuss care options at the end of life and reluctance to deliver the less than 6-month prognosis, a requirement of the Medicare Hospice Benefit (Christakis & Escarce, 1996; SUPPORT Investigators, 1995). Palliative care encourages skilled interventions sooner in the course of the patient's illness, promoting improved quality of life.

Palliative Care is defined by the World Health Organization (WHO) as:

*The active total care of patients whose disease is not responsive to curative treatment. Control of pain, of other symptoms, and of psychological, social, and spiritual problems is paramount. The goal of palliative care is achievement of the best quality of life for patients and their families. Many aspects of palliative care are also applicable earlier in the course of the illness in conjunction with anticancer treatment. Palliative care affirms life and regards dying as a normal process, neither hastens nor postpones death, provides relief from pain and other distressing symptoms, integrates the psychological and spiritual aspects of care, offers a support system to help patients live as actively as possible until death, and offers a support system to help the family cope during the patient's illness and in their own bereavement (WHO, 1990).*

Palliative care can also be contrasted with traditional or curative care. Palliative care requires a marked shift in the goals of care and the way in which care is delivered. In palliative care, symptom management and comfort are the primary goals; in curative care, prolonging survival and eradication of the disease are the primary goals (see Table 3-1).

## Palliative Care Today

Some experts believe that palliative care is a direct result of hospice care (Kinzbrunner, 1998). Others believe that hospice care in the United States has held back the growth of palliative care (Walsh, 1998). Ira Byock (1998) describes the differences between what he identifies as the *loyalists* and the *progressives* in the hospice field. He defines the loyalists as those who are devotees of the hospice philosophy—particularly those involved with hospice since the grassroots initiatives. He defines the progressives as those who recognize the need to improve the care of the dying and are earnestly trying to do so. The loyalists, as Byock further describes, are threatened by the new players in the field and believe that their presence may actually dilute end-of-life care. The progressives, on the other hand, tend to believe that the rigidity of the hospice benefit does not meet the needs of many dying patients who deserve better care and are pushing for a palliative care specialty in the United States (Byock, 1998).

| TABLE 3-1 | |
|---|---|
| **Curative versus Palliative Care** | |
| **Curative Care** | **Palliative Care** |
| ▪ Cure is the goal | ▪ Symptom control is the goal |
| ▪ Analytical and rationalistic | ▪ Subjective |
| ▪ Based on diagnoses | ▪ Based on symptoms |
| ▪ Scientific and biomedical | ▪ Humanistic and interpersonal |
| ▪ Aimed at disease process | ▪ Aimed at comfort |
| ▪ Views patients as parts | ▪ Views patient as a whole |
| ▪ Based on "hard" sciences | ▪ Based on "soft" social sciences |
| ▪ Impersonal care | ▪ Individualized care |
| ▪ Hierarchical | ▪ Interdisciplinary |
| ▪ Death is seen as failure | ▪ Death accepted as normal |

Lipman, A. (2000). Personal communication.

# ■ THE ROLE OF THE ADVANCED PRACTICE NURSE

Regardless of whether you regard yourself as loyalist or progressive or how you feel the end-of-life care leaders in your community stand, we strongly urge you to identify your local hospice and palliative care resources. Thoroughly acquaint yourself with the services they offer and the state laws and regulations, if any, that further govern the provision of hospice and palliative care services in your state. Use your practice as an advanced practice nurse (APN) to promote the finest end-of-life care beyond the semantics of "hospice" or "palliative" care.

Acquaint yourself with the National Hospice and Palliative Care Organization's *Medical Guidelines for Determining Prognosis in Selected Non-Cancer Diseases, Second Edition*. These guidelines can provide you with information essential in guiding discussions about shifting goals of care and in offering additional resources to your patients and families regarding end-of-life care. The guidelines for heart disease, pulmonary disease, dementia, human immunodeficiency virus (HIV), liver disease, renal disease, stroke and coma, and amyotrophic lateral sclerosis are found in Appendix A.

# ■ ADVANCED PLANNING: EVOLVING CHOICES AND GOALS OF CARE

When patients are well, health care decisions are easier—a patient has an infection, antibiotics are prescribed, and the problem resolves. As a person with a serious illness advances along the disease trajectory, the choices become less clear as their intent may be misunderstood and their consequences less certain. These decisions may have grave implications for continued quality of life.

Most life-threatening illnesses have accepted and documented natural clinical courses. Providing patients and their families with this information can open the discussion about goals of care—including how those goals may change over time—and provide at least a framework from which care planning may begin. However, advance planning discussions are best initiated prior to or early in a potentially life-threatening disease process.

Initiating such discussions is never easy. Recall the model of helping relationships presented in Chapter 1. Asking the following questions with an approach of genuineness, unconditional positive regard, and empathy will go a long way in establishing a trusting and supportive long-term therapeutic relationship critical to successful outcomes in end-of-life care:

- Would you like to talk about the future?
- Do you have any concerns that I can help you address?

If the patient seems more ill, a leading statement may open a much-needed discussion of fears and concerns about impending death. For example: "It seems you are not as active as you were before."

Initiating a discussion in this manner often opens the door for further discussion and decision making about such documents as a Durable Power of

Attorney for Health Care or a Living Will. Another approach to advance care planning is the *Five Wishes* document (Commission on Aging with Dignity, 2000), recognized in 34 states and the District of Columbia as meeting their respective health care decision statutes. Even in states where *Five Wishes* is not recognized, completing it can serve as a way to think about these decisions; converse with family, close other, and the health care team; and serve as the basis for completing the appropriate form. *Five Wishes* includes:

1. The person I want to make care decisions for me when I can't.
2. The kind of medical treatment I want or don't want.
3. How comfortable I want to be.
4. How I want people to treat me.
5. What I want my loved ones to know.

*Five Wishes* assists patients in expressing, in an easy-to-read form without medical or legal jargon, what kind of care is desired when death is expected because of a serious illness. *Five Wishes* also addresses the personal, emotional, and spiritual wishes of a seriously ill person.

While end-of-life discussion should, with rare exceptions, include a close family member, because their involvement assures support when decisions are actually implemented, the competent patient is always the decision maker. When patients lack decision-making ability, decisions are best made by a consensus approach using a family conference format with an interdisciplinary team, if possible. If documents such as the *Five Wishes, Durable Power of Attorney for Health Care,* or *Living Will* are available, they are, of course, the guides in considering the patient's wishes for care. In this case, the surrogate decision maker, usually the person named as the Health Care Power of Attorney (HCPOA) or the close family members, should be known to all staff caring for the patient and be actively involved in the care of the patient (Karlawish, Quill, & Meier, 1999). Thoroughly acquaint yourself with your state's health decision laws so you can provide accurate information and effectively advocate for your patients and families.

Decisions by patients and families, of course, cross the spectrum of care and are often changing, especially as the disease progresses and death nears. They range from continuing treatment for the actual disease (e.g., undergoing chemotherapy or renal dialysis, use of medications) to the act of cardiopulmonary resuscitation (CPR). Ideally, the health care provider facilitates decision making for specific treatments and the timing of their discontinuance within a clear and logical framework—the patient's personal framework and goals of care. For example, patients and families may want to consider the following options for themselves for what their personal goals are or what unfinished business they may have, among other individual factors:

- Treatment and enrollment in any clinical studies for which the patient is eligible
- Treatment as long as there is statistically a greater than 50% chance of response

- Full treatment as long as the patient is ambulatory and able to come to the clinic/office
- Treatment only of "fixable" conditions (e.g., infections, blood glucose levels)
- Treatment only for controlling symptomatic aspects of disease

For example, a patient may want to be well enough to attend a special event, such as a wedding. Given that, the framework of care may be to maximize strength and treat conditions that can be treated (e.g., anemia, an infection). That framework of care may not be appropriate for everybody. The important considerations here, however, are twofold: (1) Discuss the possible frameworks of care and (2) assist the patient and family in identifying what is important—their own goals based on their own lives and context (Berry & Griffie, 2000).

Once a goal framework has been established with the patient, the appropriateness of interventions such as CPR, renal dialysis, or intravenous (IV) antibiotics is clear. For instance, if the patient states he/she desires renal dialysis as long as transportation to the clinic is possible without the use of an ambulance, the end point of dialysis treatment is quite clear. At this point, the futility of CPR would also be apparent. Conversation with patients and families about the pros and cons of certain treatments (e.g., CPR, renal dialysis) is essential to good decision making. In CPR, for instance, generally a poor outcome is predicted in patients with advanced terminal illnesses, dementia, or poor functional status. In renal dialysis, a life-sustaining treatment, it is important to recognize and agree upon the limitations of treatment as death approaches. Inviting patients and families to consider their own goals and value systems when deciding if the treatment is an unjustified burden in the context of disease and quality of life is the most central point in the clarity of goals and the management of care (Berry & Griffie, 2000).

## ■ DISEASE TRAJECTORY AND CLINICAL DECISION MAKING

It is important to note where the patient falls along the disease trajectory (or continuum) of the disease process. The disease trajectory reflects the patient's course of disease experience—from the initial diagnosis of a life-threatening illness until death. Most of all, understanding where the patient is on the disease trajectory provides a valuable context in which decisions to offer certain treatments are made.

When considering the patient's progress along the continuum of the disease trajectory and evaluating specific diagnostics and interventions, the health care provider should review pertinent factors that include underlying disease; patient and family goals; and level of comfort, realistic expectations, functional status, and cost effectiveness. Specific diagnostics and interventions may or may not always be appropriate.

Consider the example of a newly diagnosed, 45-year-old ambulatory and active patient with metastatic lung disease who suddenly develops symptoms of spinal cord compression. Based upon this patient's place on the disease trajectory, the health care provider decides on active treatment to reverse the underlying cause and arranges for diagnostic studies and a subsequent referral to radiation therapy. For a dying patient with spinal cord compression, given the patient's place on the disease trajectory, symptomatic treatment in the form of analgesics and corticosteroids is the more appropriate choice. Bruera and Lawlor (1998) have outlined a four-step approach for clinical decision making when considering palliative interventions that also help the clinician in communicating with patients and families regarding the benefits of palliative care:

1. Define the nature of the patient's clinical findings and/or symptoms. This will require a thorough history and physical examination, a review of current and attempted medications, and a minimal set of diagnostics, which can often differentiate underlying pathophysiology from reversible symptoms.
2. Consider the problem within the context of the patient's situation and priorities. For example, compare urinary infection in a dehydrated and bedridden, cognitively impaired patient to urinary infection in a cognitively intact patient with good symptom control—how the clinician and the family prioritize these problems may be quite different.
3. Define the cost of diagnostic and therapeutic interventions highlighting potential differences between patients. What may be considered appropriate therapy for one patient may be different for another; for example, compare the appropriateness of a 1-week course of oral antibiotics with a 1-week hospital admission for intravenous antibiotics.
4. Discuss the different options with the patient and family, encouraging informed decision making. There is a "middle-of-the-road" approach specific to each individual patient and family situation that falls somewhere between aggressive and palliative. Keep in mind that what may be considered aggressive may result in significant symptom relief, whereas a "passive" approach may result in unnecessary symptoms (Bruera & Lawlor, 1998).

Joanne Lynn (1997a) identifies a good end-of-life care clinician as one who acts as a companion and guide through the unfamiliar and threatening territory of the dying process and who is also an excellent diagnostician. She identifies four critical elements that lend excellence to end-of-life care:

1. Understanding the patient's story, including the role of the family and how they perceive life.
2. Understand the body, including the limitations and effects from chronic disease over time.
3. Understand the current health care system and what can be done routinely and in exceptional situations. It is important to know regional legislation, resources, and ethics.

4. Understanding oneself; this allows for listening and the opportunity to understand the patient and family.

Despite the use of individualized interventions for each patient care situation, patients and families are frequently reassured by the overall approach to their care. Patient confidence and trust comes from establishing a well-crafted care plan created together with the clinician, patient, and family (Lynn, 1997a). Consider this in your own practice; consider your overall approach to care. Are your actions reassuring to the patient and family? These are important considerations in the quality of care and its outcomes. We urge you to consider them in the context of your own practice and how, perhaps, you can improve.

## ■ OUTCOMES OF CARE AND THEIR MEASUREMENT

Intuitively, we know that quality end-of-life care provides positive outcomes, including decreased costs, increased quality of life for the patient and family, and thus a comfortable death for the patient. We in health care are called upon to measure outcomes and prove the effectiveness of our care and interventions. Regulatory agencies, reimbursement systems, and patients and families are demanding outcome measurements, and they all, for differing reasons, deserve information with which they can make decisions (Sanoshy, 1999). Finally, outcome measures often drive the focus of care. For example, if one of the outcome measures important to your setting is advance care planning, including discussion of preference for CPR, you may expect the clinicians will follow through on this aspect of care more consistently.

How exactly should end-of-life care outcomes be determined? Who should be included? What should be measured? How should the data be gathered? Given not all patients are unable to answer questions during the last week of life, is a family member proxy the next best thing? Given also that end-of-life care includes the patient and also the family, how should the family members' perspectives be included in the evaluation?

First, and most importantly, it is critical to define who should be counted in the category of "dying" (Teno & Coppola, 1999). While it may be easy to identify such patients in a hospice or palliative care setting, it may not be as elementary within a general practice setting. Teno and Coppola (1999) suggest consensus should be reached on which patients should be the basis of the measurement of quality, or as they state, the denominator in the quality equation. Indeed, the needs, perspectives, and thus outcomes of care will be radically different for patients who are dying rapidly and their families versus patients experiencing a gradual decline over several years.

Another challenge is determining what should be measured. As with much of the palliative care literature, the study of outcomes has been centered mainly in Canada and England. Be mindful of this if you consider using an already established tool or measure. Many contend that the differences in how end-of-life care is delivered in the UK—through a family physician who accesses other services as needed from a variety of resources—and the US, where the care is largely provided from one central location and access to palliative care services is largely determined by prognosis, make the measures not applicable and therefore not valid (Hearn & Higginson, 1998).

One guide for measuring outcomes in end-of-life care is to refer to consensus statements regarding what outcomes to include. In 1997, led by Joanne Lynn, the American Geriatrics Society released a consensus statement, endorsed by 41 organizations, including the Hospice and Palliative Nurses Association, Oncology Nursing Society, and the National Hospice and Palliative Care Organization, outlining ten domains important to consider in measuring the quality of end-of-life care (Lynn, 1997b). The domains, if measured, would produce a comprehensive assessment of the quality of the end-of-life care provided. They are (Lynn, 1997b):

1. Physical and emotional symptoms
2. Support of function and autonomy
3. Advance care planning
4. Aggressive care near death—site of death, CPR, and hospitalization
5. Patient and family satisfaction with care, including satisfaction with the outcomes achieved and the extent to which opportunities were provided to complete life in a meaningful way
6. Global quality of life
7. Family burden, including financial and emotional effects
8. Survival time
9. Provider continuity and skill
10. Bereavement

Others have turned to focus group methodology to ascertain the most important areas for the evaluation of palliative care outcomes. A focus group of dialysis patients, persons with HIV, and nursing residents identified the following domains: receiving adequate pain and symptom management, avoiding artificial prolongation of dying, achieving a sense of control, relieving burden, and strengthening relationships (Singer, Martin, & Kelner, 1999). Similar areas were identified by patients, family members, and health care professionals (Steinhauser et al., 2000). Finally, Teno and colleagues used the results of focus groups of bereaved family members to create a survey instrument based on a conceptual model of patient-focused, family-centered medical care. The focus group participants defined high-quality end-of-life care as having the following five characteristics, one of which, the burden of advocating for the care of a loved one, was different from what others had identified. The five characteristics are (Teno, Casey, Welch, & Edgman-Levitan, in press):

1. Providing dying persons with the desired physical comfort.
2. Facilitating the dying person in taking control of decisions about their medical care and daily routine.
3. Relieving the family of the burden that they must be present at all times to advocate for the care of their loved one.

4. Educating the family so they feel confident in caring for their loved one at home.

5. Providing the family with emotional support both before and after the patient's death.

The challenge in the evaluation of end-of-life care, however, remains surmounting the lack of measures comprehensive and sensitive enough to capture both the patient and family perspective. Teno and colleagues, of particular note, have worked with a group of experts from all disciplines to develop outcome measures based on retrospective bereaved family interviews and prospective patient interviews (Teno et al., in press). Their project, which is still in progress and is entitled "Toolkit of Instruments to Measure End-of-Life Care" promises sensitive and meaningful measures for the important outcomes of end-of-life care.

Some challenges remain in outcome measurement in end-of-life care (Higginson, 1999):

- How do we differentiate what we know, as palliative care clinicians, versus what we actually do in clinical practice?
- What do quality of life and quality of death mean?
- How can we get better at using and interpreting proxy reports and views?
- Can outcome and process assessment become a part of day-to-day practice?

Consider the domains of quality end-of-life care and the characteristics of high-quality end-of-life care discussed above in the context of your own practice. We urge you to choose a few domains or characteristics and systematically evaluate the outcomes of the care you deliver. We also urge you to track utilization data, which are helpful in determining cost. Finally, we urge you to review the literature in the area of outcome evaluation in end-of-life care, as progress is continuous.

Whether end-of-life care is ultimately known as "hospice" or "palliative," a growing public sophistication and increased demand for quality in the delivery of this care will enter into the process. The emergence of palliative care physicians ensures the presence of the newer movement as an alternative, or perhaps an ally, of traditional hospice. The APN should participate freely and constructively as this unfolds, with the ultimate goal of improved care of dying patients and their families.

## References

AMENTA, M. O., & Bohnet, N. L. (1986). *Nursing care of the terminally ill.* Boston: Little, Brown & Co.

BENNAHUM, D. (1996). The historical development of hospice and palliative care. In D. Sheehan, W. Forman (Eds.). *Hospice and Palliative Care* (pp. 1-10). Sudbury, MA: Jones & Bartlett.

BERRY, P. H., & Griffie, J. (2000). Planning for the actual death. In B. R. Ferrell & N. Coyle (Eds.). *Textbook of palliative nursing* (pp. 382-394). New York: Oxford University Press.

BILLINGS, J. (1998). The hospice Medicare benefit: An appraisal at 15 years. *Journal of Palliative Medicine, 1,* 123-127.

BRUERA, E., & Lawlor, P. (1998). Defining palliative care interventions. *Journal of Palliative Care, 14*(2), 23-24.

BYOCK, I. (1998) Hospice and palliative care: A parting of ways or a path to the future? *Journal of Palliative Medicine, 1*(2), 165-175.

CHRISTAKIS, N., & Escarce, J. (1996). Survival of Medicare patients after enrollment in hospice programs. *The New England Journal of Medicine, 335*(3), 172-202.

COMMISSION on Aging with Dignity. (2000). *Five Wishes.* Tallahassee, FL: Author. (Forms are available online: www.agingwithdignity.org)

DOYLE, D., Hanks, G., & MacDonald, N. (1998). Introduction. In D. Doyle, G. Hanks, & N. MacDonald. (Eds.). *Oxford textbook of palliative medicine* (2$^{nd}$ ed.) (pp. 3-8). New York: Oxford University Press.

FINN, P. L. (1985). The development of hospice in America. *The Hospice Handbook.* Rockland, MD: Aspen Publications.

HEARN, J., & Higginson, I. J. (1998). Do specialist palliative care teams improve outcomes for cancer patients? A systematic literature review. *Palliative Medicine, 12,* 317-332.

HIGGINSON, I. (1999, June). *Going to sea in a sieve—Evidence-based policy making in palliative care* (Paper presented at the Eleventh Annual Assembly of the American Academy of Hospice and Palliative Medicine). Snowbird, UT: Author.

KARLAWISH, H. T., Quill, T., & Meier, D. (1999). A consensus-based approach to providing palliative care to patients who lack decision-making capacity. *Annals of Internal Medicine, 130,* 835-840.

KINZBRUNNER, B. (1998). Hospice: 15 years and beyond in the care of the dying. *Journal of Palliative Medicine, 1*(2), 127-137.

KÜBLER-ROSS, E. (1969). *On Death and Dying.* New York: Macmillan.

LO, B. (1995). End-of-life care after termination of SUPPORT. *Hastings Center Report* (special supplement), *25*(6), S6-8.

LYNN, J. (1997a). An 88-year-old woman facing the end of life. *Journal of the American Medical Association, 227,* 1633-1640.

LYNN, J. (1997b). Measuring quality of care at the end of life: A statement of principles. *Journal of the American Geriatrics Society, 45,* 526-527.

LYNN, J. (1998). Complaints about hospice: growing up or going wrong? *ABCD Exchange, 1*(9), 2-7.

MAHONEY, J. (1998). The Medicare hospice benefit—15 years of success. *Journal of Palliative Medicine, 1*(2), 139-146.

MARSHALL, P. (1995). The SUPPORT study: Who's talking? *Hastings Center Report* (special supplement), *25*(6), S9-S11.

SANOSHY, J. (1999). Outcomes benefit patients by helping nurses to incorporate proven therapies. *ONS News, 14*(2), 1-5.

SINGER, P. A., Martin, D. K., & Kelner, M. (1999). Quality end-of-life care: Patients' perspectives. *Journal of the American Medical Association, 281,* 163-168.

STEINHAUSER, K. E., Clipp, E. C., McNeilly, M., Christakis, N. A., McIntyre, L. M., & Tulsky, J. A. (2000). In search of a good death: Observation of patients, families, and providers. *Annals of Internal Medicine, 132,* 825-832.

SUPPORT Principal Investigators. (1995). A controlled trial to improve care for seriously ill hospitalized patients: The study to understand prognoses and preferences for outcomes and risks of treatments (SUPPORT). *Journal of the American Medical Association, 274,* 1591-1598.

Teno, J. M., Casey, V. A., Welch, L., & Edgman-Levitan, S. (in press). Patient-focused, family-centered end-of-life medical care: View of guidelines and bereaved family members. Unpublished manuscript. *Journal of Pain and Symptom Management.*

Teno, J. M., & Coppola, K. M. (1999). For every numerator, you need a denominator: A simple statement but key to measuring quality in care of the dying. *Journal of Pain and Symptom Management, 17,* 109-113.

Walsh, D. (1998). The Medicare hospice benefit: a critique from palliative medicine. *Journal of Palliative Medicine, 1*(2), 147-149.

World Health Organization. (1990). *Cancer pain relief and palliative care* (Technical Report Series 804). Geneva: Author.

# *The Dying Process*

PATRICIA H. BERRY, JULIE GRIFFIE
DEBRA E. HEIDRICH

*How people die remains in the memories of those who live on.*
(DAME CICELY SAUNDERS, FOUNDER OF THE MODERN DAY HOSPICE MOVEMENT)

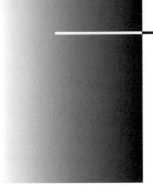 **A**s the disease progresses and death nears, the focus, goals, and rhythm of care change. Patients are often too ill for an office visit. Family may be assisting with care more and more as the patient becomes increasingly unable to care for himself or herself. A home care hospice program may be responsible for the patient and family in their own home or in a hospice, assisted living, or nursing home facility.

Your role as an APN, depending on your setting and scope of practice, also undergoes a shift in rhythm, focus, and goals. At the very time patients and families need consistency, follow-through, and a feeling of connection, they may—and rightly so—feel more and more distant from the relationship with you and the expert care you provide. We strongly urge you to explore the possibility of making visits to the patient's home or care facility. Offer to assist the facility staff hospice interdisciplinary team to care for the patient and family.

Symptom management needs often change as well. Symptoms may intensify, subside, or even appear anew. The research on the incidence of symptoms appearing in the last few days to weeks before death is disheartening. In one multisite U.S. hospital study, the majority of participants did not have a death where symptoms were well managed (SUPPORT Study Principle Investigators, 1995). Studies from New Zealand, Italy, Canada, and the United Kingdom reveal up to 52% of persons have refractory symptoms at the very end of life that require aggressive interventions and, at rare times, terminal sedation (Fainsinger, Miller, Brurera, Hanson, & Maceachern, 1991; Lichter & Hunt, 1990; Twycross & Lichter, 1998; Ventifridda, Ripamonti, De Conno, Tamburini, & Cassileth, 1990). Dyspnea may worsen as death approaches; the final "crescendo" of pain is supported in some studies and not in others. Noisy and moist breathing, urinary incontinence and retention, restlessness, agitation, delirium, and nausea and vomiting appear in many patients as death nears (Lichter & Hunt, 1990; Ventifridda et al.,

1990). Sweating, myoclonus, and confusion also appear, but with less frequency (Ventifridda et al., 1990). In one study, most patients (91.5%) died peacefully, but the remainder (8.5%) experienced symptoms requiring additional intervention on the final day of life, including hemorrhage or hemoptysis (2%), respiratory distress (2%), restlessness (1.5%), pain (1%), myocardial infarction (1%), and regurgitation (1%) (Ventifridda et al., 1990). Pain, dyspnea, restlessness, and agitation are the physical symptoms requiring maximum diligence in assessment, prevention, and aggressive treatment during the final day or two before death.

Psychosocial symptoms may appear as well, including most commonly anxiety, as well as fear, profound loss and grief, and spiritual distress (Working Party on Clinical Guidelines in Palliative Care, 1997). Likewise, symptoms such as agitation, restlessness, and moaning may be signs of physical, emotional, or spiritual discomfort. A thorough assessment is required. Persons with these symptoms who do not have apparent physical causes or who do not improve with usual interventions may require different interventions such as heavy (terminal) sedation (Twycross & Lichter, 1998).

Regardless of their apparent or suspected cause, careful evaluation of all symptoms is required. Ideally, intervention addresses and relieves the underlying cause rather than just treating the outward symptom. For example, restlessness related to the discomfort from urinary retention is best relieved with catheterization, not benzodiazepines. However, frequently the underlying cause is not identifiable or treatable. In those circumstances, interventions are used to lessen the uncomfortable symptom. Refer to the specific clinical practice guidelines for further information.

The presence of the APN is critical in anticipating and monitoring for physical and psychosocial symptoms, educating the patient and family and other caregivers, and thus assuring a good quality of death. Remember, each situation is unique because the patient and family, based on their own perspectives, ascribe meaning to their experiences. For each patient and family, psychologic, spiritual, cultural, and family issues converge and contribute to the end-of-life experience—no two of which are alike.

While the psychosocial issues are varied, the physiology of dying is, in essence, the same for most expected deaths. As the death nears, in addition to anticipating and controlling symptoms and providing support, the APN has the opportunity to normalize the dying process for the patient and family.

In the material that follows, we will discuss the care issues associated with the changing rhythm of care as death nears, common signs and symptoms of death and their management, and care of the patient and family at time of death. With few exceptions, we have only one chance to "get it right" when we care for patients and families as death nears; there are no dress rehearsals. Anticipating and monitoring for treatable symptoms, normalizing the physiologic process of dying, and thoughtful planning are all essential in ensuring the best possible outcome for all involved. Always be mindful of the words of Dame Cicely Saunders: "How people die remains in the memories of those who live on."

## ■ THE CHANGING RHYTHM OF CARE AS DEATH APPROACHES

Persons in the final stages of illness tolerate symptoms very poorly, largely because of weakness and general debility. Uncontrolled symptoms, especially at this stage of the disease process, can escalate rapidly into a crisis (Working Party on Clinical Guidelines in Palliative Care, 1997). Thus the aim of care is prevention and control of distressing symptoms; the use of medications, treatments, and assessments contribute to this end. We discuss some of the ways the rhythm of care changes for the patient near death, including discontinuation of unnecessary medications, concern about dehydration, and vital sign assessment.

### Medications

Considerable tact and kindness, as well as knowledge of the patient and family, are necessary in assisting them to make decisions about discontinuing medications. Every situation is unique. Antihypertensives, replacement hormones, vitamin supplements, iron preparations, hypoglycemics, long-term antibiotics, antiarrhythmics, laxatives, chemotherapy, hormones, and diuretics, **unless they are essential to patient comfort,** should be discontinued (Working Party on Clinical Guidelines in Palliative Care, 1997). As oral medications essential to patient comfort become impossible to administer, the medication may be offered in a liquid or other dosage form if available. The Working Party on Clinical Guidelines in Palliative Care (1997) suggests that the only drugs necessary in the final days of life are analgesics, anticonvulsants, antiemetics, antipyretics, anticholinergics, and sedatives. It is important to note that some patients may require very few medications to be comfortable while others may require a combination of many different medications. Additional medications that may be helpful in managing symptoms in the final days of life include corticosteroids and psychotropics. It is essential that the APN review every medication the patient is taking and critically evaluate the importance of each for managing current symptoms.

The discontinuation of corticosteroids in intracranial malignancy deserves special consideration, as these drugs control the symptoms of headache and seizure secondary to intracranial swelling. However, when the patient is nearing death and no longer able to swallow, the corticosteroids may be discontinued with minimal or no tapering (Working Party on Clinical Guidelines in Palliative Care, 1997), with the understanding that this action may lead to increased cerebral edema and, consequently, headache and progressive neurological dysfunction (Weissman, 1988). Needless to say, addition or adjustment of analgesics and anticonvulsant medications may be necessary for continued comfort.

Because corticosteroids decrease intracranial swelling, they are also viewed by some health care providers as medications that prolong life. As a result, a patient may request to stop treatment with corticosteroids because of continued deterioration and poor quality of life. The corticosteroid should be tapered while an anticonvulsant medication, usually oral, is gradually added, along with careful assessment of the patient's comfort (Twycross & Lichter, 1998). This demonstrates the importance of critically evaluating the effect of each medication on the individual's comfort. While corticosteroids may be helpful for some patients, they may not contribute to comfort in others.

## Dehydration

The provision of fluids and food is fundamental to traditions of care and nurturance, and therefore a change in the ability of the patient to drink raises all sorts of issues, but most importantly symbolizes progression towards death—most patients and families are aware that without fluids, death will occur in a short period of time. Current literature suggests fluids should not be routinely administered to dying patients, nor automatically withheld from them, but rather be given based on the goals of care and a careful assessment of the patient's comfort. The following questions, to clarify the goals of care, are suggested (Zerwekh, 1997):

- Will the patient's well-being be enhanced by artificial hydration?
- Are there symptoms that could be relieved?
- Are there symptoms that could be aggravated?
- Could hydration enhance the patient's mental status or level of consciousness?
- Will it temporarily prolong the patient's life?
- Is that desired by the patient and family?

Some dying patients benefit from dehydration; others may manifest symptoms such as confusion or opioid toxicity that may be corrected or prevented by parenteral hydration (Fainsinger & Bruera, 1997).

In any case, the decision to provide artificial hydration should be considered carefully. Initiating artificial hydration is easily done; discontinuing it is much more difficult. Artificial hydration has the potential to cause fluid accumulation, resulting in distressful symptoms such as edema, ascites, nausea and vomiting, and pulmonary congestion. There is no correlation between reported thirst and dehydration (Ellershaw, Sutcliffe, & Saunders, 1995). Consideration of the goals of care, the patient's overall condition and underlying disease process, along with careful assessment and discussion of the risks and benefits of artificial hydration are essential elements of this decision.

Dry mouth is a consistently reported and sometimes troublesome symptom of dehydration, which can effectively be relieved with sips of beverages, ice chips, or hard candies (Smith, 1995). The mouth may also be kept moist by spraying normal saline in it with the use of an atomizer. (Normal saline can be made by mixing one teaspoon of table salt in a quart of water.) Careful and frequent oral care is essential in end-of-life care and especially for dehydration.

## Vital Signs

With the exception of temperature, the routine measurement of vital signs is usually unnecessary as death approaches. Oftentimes, however, vital signs (pulse and blood pressure) are helpful in assessing symptom distress in an unresponsive patient.

Measuring temperature using the axillary or another noninvasive route should continue until death. The actions taken for an increased temperature are guided by the degree of distress and patient discomfort, not the level of the temperature (Cleary, 1998). An elevated temperature may suggest infection or dehydration, but interventions must be guided solely by the patient's level of discomfort.

## ■ SIGNS AND SYMPTOMS OF THE IMMINENT DYING PROCESS

With few exceptions, there are predictable signs and symptoms that signal death is nearing, due to an interaction of gradual hypoxia, respiratory acidosis, renal failure, and hypoxia of the central nervous system (Kelly & Yetman, 1987; Smith, 1999; Twycross & Lichter, 1998). The APN can use these symptoms as a guide to help the patient and family plan for the death and to clarify with family members their desires and needs at the time of death. Do they wish to be present? Do they know of others who wish to now say a final goodbye? Have they said everything they wish to say to the person who is dying? Do they have any regrets? Are they concerned about anything? Do they wish something could be different? Every person in a family has different and unique needs that unless explored, can go unmet. Family members recall the time before the death and immediately afterwards with great acuity and detail. There usually is no chance for dress rehearsal—rather, there is one chance to get it right and make the experience individualized and memorable (Berry & Griffie, 2000).

Attempting to pinpoint a time of death is problematic, at best; any anticipations should be limited to time periods such as "within a number of hours." In their own way, patients often appear to "choose" such a time—influenced by the presence or absence of a family member or the passing of a significant date or time. This mandates that the APN include in family discussions the likelihood a loved one may be absent at death and their reactions to such an event, given the unpredictability inherent in the situation (Berry & Griffie, 2000).

The signs and symptoms that emerge days before death include (Twycross & Lichter, 1998; Working Party on Clinical Guidelines in Palliative Care, 1997):
- Profound weakness
- Usually bedbound

- Requires assistance with all or most of care
- Gaunt and pale physical appearance (most common in persons with cancer when corticosteroids have not been used as treatment)
- Drowsiness or a reduction in awareness, insight, and perception
- Extended periods of drowsiness
- Extreme difficulty in concentrating; severely limited attention span
- Limited ability, if at all, to cooperate with caregivers
- Disoriented to time and place
- Increasing disinterest in food and fluid with diminished intake
- Increasing difficulty in swallowing oral medications

During the final days and hours, the signs and symptoms described above become more pronounced and, as oxygen concentrations begin to drop, new ones appear. We are not suggesting measurement of oxygen concentration, rather an awareness that the resultant signs and symptoms can help guide the family in their care decisions, normalizing the dying process for the family. Table 4-1 summarizes this physiologic process of dying and suggests interventions for both patients and families.

As the dying person takes less and less food and fluids, third-spaced fluids such as peripheral edema, ascites, or pleural effusions may be reabsorbed. Breathing and pain may be eased, and the patient may be temporarily more alert. This "improvement" must be gently explained to the family. This is often a good time for families to gather, express their feelings, and say their final goodbyes.

Death often occurs when no health care professionals are present. Preparing the patient and family for the time before death and at death is essential—families are known to panic and call for an ambulance. Many hospice home care programs provide educational materials. Figure 4-1 is an example that, with an empathetic tone, reassures families that dying is a natural process and that each person dies in their own way and on their own time. Acquaint yourself with your local laws regarding death, especially when occurring outside of a health care institution, and inform the family so they can prepare.

## ■ CARE AT THE TIME OF DEATH

If present at the time of death, you have a unique opportunity to support the family and care for the body, thus facilitating the early process of grieving. The rhythm of care changes with the death of the patient and focuses more on the family.

Postmortem care is an important nursing function and by caring for the body gently, the care and concern for the person who has died is communicated to the family. In addition, the nurse can continue to communicate his or her care and concern for the patient and family members and model helpful behaviors as the family members begin this phase of their grief work.

## TABLE 4-1

### The Physiologic Process of Dying and Suggested Interventions

| Early Stage Symptoms in the Normal Progression of Dying | Suggested Interventions |
| --- | --- |
| **SENSATION/PERCEPTION** | |
| Impairment in the ability to grasp ideas and reason; periods of alertness along with periods of disorientation and restlessness are also noted | Interpret the signs and symptoms to the patient (when appropriate) and family as part of the normal dying process, for example, assure them the patient's "seeing" and even talking to persons who have died is normal and often expected. Urge family members to look for metaphors for death in speech and conversation; for example, describing a place, choosing a time of death, requesting reconciliation, symbolic dreams, talking of a long journey, needing maps or tickets, or preparing for a trip in other ways (Callahan & Kelley, 1993). Encourage the use of these metaphors as a departure point for conversation with the patient. Urge family to take advantage of the patient's periods of lucidity to talk with him or her and ensure nothing is left unsaid. Encourage family members to touch and speak slowly and gently to the patient without being patronizing. Maximize safety (e.g., use bed rails, schedule people to sit with the patient). |
| Some loss of visual acuity; increased sensitivity to bright lights while other senses, except hearing, are dulled | Keep sensory stimulation to a minimum, including sounds, light, and other visual stimulation; reading to a patient who has enjoyed reading in the past may provide comfort. Urge the family to be mindful of what they say "over" the patient while the patient can still hear; also continue to urge family members to say what they wish not to be left unsaid. |
| **CARDIORESPIRATORY** | |
| Increased pulse and respiratory rate Agonal respirations or sounds of gasping for air without apparent discomfort | Normalize the observed changes by interpreting the signs and symptoms as part of the normal dying process and assuring the patient's comfort. |

*Continued*

## TABLE 4-1

### The Physiologic Process of Dying and Suggested Interventions—cont'd

| Early Stage Symptoms in the Normal Progression of Dying | Suggested Interventions |
| --- | --- |
| **CARDIORESPIRATORY—cont'd** | |
| Apnea, periodic, or Cheyne-Stokes respirations | Assess and treat respiratory distress as appropriate. |
| Inability to cough or clear secretions efficiently, resulting in gurgling or congested breathing (sometimes referred to as the "death rattle") | Assess use and need for parenteral fluids, tube feedings, or hydration. (It is generally appropriate to either discontinue or greatly decrease them.) |
| | Reposition the patient in a side-lying position with the head of the bed elevated. |
| | Suctioning is rarely needed, but when appropriate, suction should be gentle and only at the level of the mouth, throat, and nasal pharynx. |
| | Administer anticholinergic drugs (transdermal scopolamine, hyoscyamine) as appropriate, recognizing and discussing with the family that they will not decrease already existing secretions. |
| **RENAL/URINARY** | |
| Decreasing urinary output, sometimes urinary incontinence or retention | Insert catheter and/or use absorbent padding. |
| | Assess carefully for urinary retention; restlessness can be a related symptom. |
| **MUSCULOSKELETAL** | |
| Gradual loss of the ability to move, beginning with the legs, then progressing to the arms | Reposition every few hours as appropriate. |
| | Anticipate needs, such as sips of fluids, oral care, and changing of bed pads and linens. |

| Late Stage Symptoms in the Normal Progression of Dying | Suggested Interventions |
| --- | --- |
| **SENSATION/PERCEPTION** | |
| Unconsciousness | Interpret the patient's unconsciousness to the family as part of the normal dying process. |
| Eyes remain half open, blink reflex is absent; sense of hearing remains intact and may slowly decrease | Provide total care, including incontinence of urine and stool. |

## TABLE 4-1

### The Physiologic Process of Dying and Suggested Interventions—cont'd

| Late Stage Symptoms in the Normal Progression of Dying | Suggested Interventions |
| --- | --- |
| **SENSATION/PERCEPTION—cont'd** | |
| | Encourage family members to speak slowly and gently to the patient with the assurance that hearing remains intact. |
| **CARDIORESPIRATORY** | |
| Heart rate may double, the strength of contractions may decrease, and rhythm may become irregular | Interpret these changes to family members as part of the normal dying process. |
| Patient feels cool to the touch and becomes diaphoretic | Frequent linen changes and sponge baths may enhance comfort. |
| Cyanosis is noted in the tip of the nose, nail beds, and knees; extremities may become mottled—when progressive, indicates death within a few days; absence of a palpable radial pulse may indicate death within hours | |
| **RENAL/URINARY** | |
| A precipitous drop in urinary output | Interpret to the family that the drop in urinary output is a normal sign that death is near. |
| | Assess carefully for urinary retention; restlessness can be a related symptom. |

From Berry, P. H., & Griffie, J. (2000). Planning for the actual death. In B. R. Ferrell & N. Coyle (Eds.), *Textbook of palliative nursing* (pp. 382-394). New York: Oxford University Press.

During this time, rituals are a sound, desirable aspect of the grieving process, and any pertinent ones should be explored fully. Rituals are social practices that facilitate understanding and coping with the contradictory and complex nature of human existence. They provide a release for emotions, a reinforcement of the psyche, where needed, and a framework for behavior during emotional trauma (Romanoff & Terenzio, 1998). Rituals include unique methods of body preparation (e.g., in Orthodox Judaism) and various kinds of gathering (e.g., wakes). The social interaction of these rituals eases the pain of loss (O'Gorman, 1998). Importantly, remember that family members alone must provide the basis for these rituals as their cultural background determines what activities are useful and expected. There are wide differences among the needs of persons, even within one

## SYMPTOMS AND WHAT TO DO

This list may appear frightening, but knowing what to expect may reduce some of your anxiety about the approaching death.

Each person approaches death in their own way, bringing to this last experience their own uniqueness. Our list is a map to the goal of a peaceful death. Like all maps, there are many different routes to the same destination.

You may see all of these symptoms or none. Death will come in its own time and its own way to each of us. It is important to remember that **dying is a natural process**.

| | |
|---|---|
| 1. Withdrawal—physical and emotional; increased sleep | There is a natural process of withdrawing from everything outside of one's self, looking inward, and reviewing one's self and one's life. Your loved one may turn inward, withdraw physically and emotionally. This occurs in an attempt to cope with the many changes that are occurring. |
| 2. Reduced food and fluid intake | There is decreased **need** because the body will naturally begin to conserve energy that is expended on these tasks. Dehydration is a **natural comfort measure** requiring the body to handle less fluids in all the systems. At no time should food or fluids be **forced**. |
| 3. Confusion or agitation can vary—from mild confusion to end-stage agitation, which may include trying to get out of bed, picking at covers, and seeing things that are not apparent to us. | Talk calmly and assuredly. Keep lights on and use times when patient is alert for meaningful conversation. Music can be very calming. Medication is often used to control this symptom. |
| 4. Changes in breathing patterns | This is common. You may see irregular breathing: very rapid, very slow, or 10 to 30 seconds of no breathing at all (this is called apnea). These symptoms are very common and indicative of a decrease in circulation. It does not mean that your loved one is uncomfortable or struggling. |
| 5. Collection of oral secretions in the back of the throat, causing noisy respiration | The swallowing reflex may be absent. The patient may be breathing through secretions, which can be more uncomfortable for us as observers than the patient experiencing it. Elevate the head of bed or turn the patient on his or her side. |
| 6. Incontinence of urine and stool | Reduced intake results in reduced output with darker color. Bed pads and diapers can be used to protect bed linens. Cleanse the patient and change linens frequently to maintain comfort and protect skin. |
| 7. Changes in skin temperature and color | Decreased circulation can cause coolness and discoloration of skin. Use light covers, turn side to side frequently to maintain comfort and prevent skin breakdown (bedsores). Heating pads and electric blankets are **not recommended.** |

Hearing is the last sense to be lost, so the patient can hear all that is being said. This is a good time to say goodbye and reassure them that you will be all right even though you will miss them greatly. (You may tell them it's okay to "let go.") This permission is often helpful for a peaceful death.

How would you know death has occurred?
- No breathing
- No heartbeat or pulse

If you believe that death has occurred, call Hospice. Do not call 911 or the physician. We will come to your home to help you. (You may want to use the time until we arrive to say your last goodbyes.)

**FIG. 4-1** Educational material for families. *(Courtesy Hospice of Boulder County, Colorado.)*

cultural or religious group. This is an important part of the APN's ongoing assessment.

The APN can do much at this point by taking the initiative to create opportunities for family to spend time with the body, if they wish. The degree of involvement will vary with cultural or religious backgrounds, but any activities, even as basic as combing hair, should be encouraged. Children may often be included, depending on circumstances and their maturity. Conversation—a valuable ritual in itself—during these times allows memories to surface and begins to move loved ones through the healing process (Passagno, 1997). Offer family contact with the patient's body, including helping to dress him or her in other clothes, if desired. When turning a body, air may escape from the lungs causing a "sighing" sound—this should be mentioned to family ahead of time. These respectful, gentle, and attentive guiding activities by the APN will go far to ensure positive memories for the family and a rewarding professional experience for the practitioner.

The care of patients and their families near death and afterward is an important nursing function—arguably one of the most important. Be mindful of Dame Cicely Saunders' words, "How people die remains in the memories of those who live on." As you provide and facilitate care, let this theme guide you. Your principal goal is a positive experience for the family, ensuring helpful memories to carry into the bereavement period and beyond.

## References

BERRY, P. H., & Griffie, J. (2000). Planning for the actual death. In B. R. Ferrell & N. Coyle (Eds.). *Textbook of palliative nursing* (pp. 382-394). New York: Oxford University Press.

CALLAHAN, M., & Kelley, P. (1993). *Final gifts: Understanding the special awareness, needs, and communications of the dying.* New York: Bantam Books.

CLEARY, J. (1998). Fever and sweats: Including the immunocompromised hosts. In A. Berger, R. Portenoy, & D. Weissman (Eds.). *Principles and practice of supportive oncology* (pp. 119-31). New York: Lippincott-Raven.

ELLERSHAW, J. E., Sutcliffe, J. M., & Saunders, C. M. (1995). Dehydration and the dying patient. *Journal of Pain Symptom Management, 10,* 192-7.

FAINSINGER, R. L., & Bruera, E. (1997). When to treat dehydration in a terminally ill patient? *Supportive Care in Cancer, 5*(3), 205-11.

FAINSINGER, R., Miller, M. J., Brurera, E., Hanson, J., & Maceachern, T. (1991). Symptom control during the last week of life on a palliative care unit, *Journal of Palliative Care, 7*(1), 5-11.

KELLY, C., & Yetman, L. (1987). At the end of life. *Canadian Nurse, 83*(4), 33-34.

LICHTER, I, & Hunt E. (1990). The last 48 hours of life. *Journal of Palliative Care,* 6(4), 7-15.

O'GORMAN, S. M. (1998). Death and dying in contemporary society: An evaluation of current attitudes and the rituals associated with death and dying and their relevance to recent understanding of health and healing. *Journal of Advanced Nursing, 27,* 1127-35.

PASSAGNO, R. A. (1997). Postmortem care: Healing's first step. *Nursing 97, 24*(4), 32a-32b.

ROMANOFF, B. D., & Terenzio, M. (1998). Rituals and the grieving process. *Death Studies, 22,* 697-711.

SMITH, S. A. (1995). Patient-induced dehydration: Can it ever be therapeutic? *Oncology Nursing Forum, 22,* 1487-91.

SMITH, J. L. (1999). The process of dying and managing the death event. In: R. S. Schoenwetter, W. Hawke, & C. F. Knight (Eds.). *Hospice and palliative medicine core curriculum and review syllabus.* Dubuque, IA: Kendall/Hunt.

SUPPORT Study Principal Investigators. (1995). A controlled trial to improve care for seriously ill hospitalized patients: The study to understand prognoses and preferences for outcomes and risks of treatments (SUPPORT). *Journal of the American Medical Association, 274,* 1591-98.

TWYCROSS, R., & Lichter, I. (1997). The terminal phase. In: D. Doyle, G. Hanks, & N. MacDonald (Eds.). *Oxford textbook of palliative medicine* (2nd ed.) (pp. 977-92). New York: Oxford University Press.

VENTIFRIDDA, V., Ripamonti, C., De Conno, F., Tamburini, M., & Cassileth, B. R. (1990). Symptom prevalence and control during cancer patients' last days of life. *Journal of Palliative Care, 6*(3), 7-11.

WEISSMAN, D. (1988). Glucocorticoid treatment for brain metastases and epidural spinal cord compression: A review. *Journal of Clinical Oncology, 6,* 543-551.

WORKING Party on Clinical Guidelines in Palliative Care. (1997). *Changing gear: Guidelines for managing the last days of life.* London: National Council for Hospice and Specialist Palliative Care Services.

ZERWEKH, J. (1997). Do dying patients really need IV fluids? *American Journal of Nursing, 97*(3), 26-31.

# PART TWO

## Holistic Care
## at the End of Life

# CHAPTER 5

# Grief and Bereavement

KATE FORD ROBERTS, PATRICIA H. BERRY

*When asked what the death of her husband means to her,* Mrs. A replied:
*"The biggest part of my life is gone—there is a big empty space where he once was..."*
*When asked the same question,* Mrs. B replied:
*"Relief, not grief—a release, freedom, a new chance at happiness."*

T o be alive and human is to face the inevitability of loss. The nature of the losses associated with death leads to a complex and intensely emotional experience that should not be oversimplified. Consider Mrs. A and Mrs. B. While Mrs. A relates the usual, and in many cases, culturally acceptable reaction to the death of her husband, Mrs. B relates a perspective that is quite the opposite. Which woman is grieving in the "right" way? Which may be at risk for abnormal or complicated grief? How comfortable or uncomfortable are you with these reactions? As uncomfortable as it may make us, the experience of losing a close person to death is as individual and unique as the persons involved. Persons individually ascribe meaning to their relationships and, accordingly, individualize their grief reactions.

Our culture denies and defies death. Death is often seen as a defeat, a failure, and an outcome to be resisted at all costs. As a result, the bereaved often feel profoundly isolated. Consider, even perhaps in your own practice setting, how the patient serves as the link to many of the health care services you provide. Family support services are often linked to the administrative and financial connections provided by the patient (Shapiro, 1994). Once the patient dies, family members are often not entitled to these services—further contributing to their sense of disconnection and isolation.

Finally, while our culture generally fears death, many persons experiencing the loss of a close other observe that most people can act or discuss grief as if they have taken "Grief 101"—or are experts on the stages of grief—yet find it impossible to tolerate the depth of pain of the bereaved or acknowledge the effect of the death on everyday life (Shapiro, 1994). We must acknowledge that when a close other dies, survivors are forced to rebuild their lives, recreate their close relationships, and examine and reconstruct their assumptions about themselves and the control they have (or do not have) over their everyday lives. Grief, as anyone who has experienced it will tell you, is hard work.

The purpose of this chapter is to examine the reaction to the loss of a close other, including key term definitions, uncomplicated and complicated grief, and guidance on how best to provide support to a bereaved person. The special needs of children are also discussed. It is important, especially in the area of grief and loss work, for the APN to recognize the scope and therefore the limitations of his or her practice. As you read this chapter and consider how best to provide grief support in your practice setting, think about the resources available to you for providing grief support, as well as referral sources to assist you with complicated grief reactions. Regardless of the resources in your area, it is important to realize that most APNs, unless specifically prepared in mental health, should not manage complicated grief without expert assistance. Consider meeting the staff from the hospice serving your area and acquainting yourself with the resources they provide. Do they offer support groups to community members? Do they present special programs for children or programs about the special challenges surrounding holidays? Having a working knowledge of the grief resources in your area—and even a brief listing of them for your clients—can be helpful and supportive.

## ■ DEFINITION OF TERMS

The following terms, used often in the grief and loss literature, as well as in professional and lay conversation, are important to understand. In addition, the terms *loss, bereavement, grief,* and *mourning* are often used interchangeably, creating confusion.

*Anticipatory grief:* Anticipatory grief refers to the process of mourning an impending loss. This includes, in the context of a death loss, an acknowledgment and working through of myriad losses associated with the death itself—hopes, dreams, expectations, and unfinished business (Rando, 1986). It serves as a kind of rehearsal for all the changes and losses the death represents. Implied in anticipatory grief is the individual nature of grief and the reaction to anticipated loss. An APN can suggest someone consider the many losses associated with the death by gently asking a question such as: "Have you thought about what ____'s death may mean to you?" It is important to listen intently and without judgment to the reply.

*Primary loss:* A physical loss of something tangible or a psychosocial loss of something intangible (Rando, 1993).

*Secondary loss:* Physical or psychosocial loss that coincides with or develops as a consequence of the initial, primary loss (Rando, 1993). Each of these secondary losses carries with it a special grief of its own and often goes unacknowledged and unrecognized (Koeppl, 1996).

*Bereavement:* The state of having suffered a loss—in these examples, a death loss (Rando, 1993).

*Grief:* The emotions and feelings—for example, anger, frustration, loneliness, sadness, guilt, regret—related to the perception of the loss (Rando, 1993). Grief is a natural and expected reaction and continues to develop and change over time. The key is the notion of perception, and the need to accept this perception—without question—as real to the bereaved person. Truly the perception and emotion of grief belongs to the grieving person.

*Mourning:* The process one undergoes to resolve the grief, which involves processes related to the deceased, the self, and the external world. The nature of mourning and the public display of grief is strongly determined by culture and tradition (Rando, 1993).

*Complicated grief:* Simply put, a failure to grieve (Berry, Zeri, & Egan, 1997). The many factors that contribute to the development of complicated grief are discussed later in the chapter.

*Grief counseling:* Facilitation and assistance for persons experiencing uncomplicated or normal grief (Worden, 1991). Grief counseling, as defined here, is in the scope of most APNs, provided he or she is prepared in the basics of grief, loss, and normal grief reactions.

*Grief therapy:* The specialized treatment techniques necessary to help persons with complicated grief reactions (Worden, 1991). Grief therapy, as defined here, is out of the scope of the APN, unless he or she is prepared to provide mental health counseling, psychotherapy, or other psychiatric services. Again, it is crucial for the APN to identify resources for assistance with complicated grief reactions, and promptly consult the resources, and if necessary refer the patient for grief therapy.

## ■ THEORIES OF GRIEF AND LOSS

A brief discussion of some of the significant theories of grief is important in putting the topic of grief and loss in a historical context. It seems most appropriate to begin with Sigmund Freud. In 1917, he published his classic paper "Mourning and Melancholia," in which he defined aspects of normal grief. He wrote that mourning is "the reaction to loss of a loved person, or to the loss of some abstraction which has taken place, of such as one's country, liberty, and ideal, and so on" (Freud, 1957). This quotation implies that grief is a response to loss, and that the loss may not always be due to death. According to Freud, the work of mourning takes time. He indicates that the end of mourning is "when the work of mourning is completed and the ego becomes free and uninhibited again" (Freud, 1957). However, grief affects our past, our present, and our future, and being open to an individual's perception and process of grief is essential to being helpful.

Erich Lindemann was the first person to address grief and bereavement in a systematic way, thereby providing impetus for further research and writings in this area. He interviewed survivors of persons who perished in a nightclub fire and discovered that people experienced somatic symptoms, feelings of guilt and hostility, and a preoccupation with the deceased. The emphasis of Lindemann's work is on acute traumatic grief and thus does not apply to all grief situations. While Parkes (1972) and others, however, describe many limitations to Lindemann's work, it is considered a classic in the field of loss.

Lindemann (1944) described three stages of grief: shock and disbelief, acute mourning, and resolution of the grief process. He concluded that grief is not only natural but is a necessary reaction for the survivor's mental health. In identifying the many factors affecting the progress of mourning, he suggested that the duration of a grief reaction depended upon the success with which a person does the grief work. He describes three tasks of grief: emancipation from the bondage of the deceased, readjustment to the environment in which the deceased is missing, and the formation of new relationships (Lindemann, 1944).

Attachment theory provides a way for us to understand the tendency in humans to make strong affectional bonds with others and what happens when those bonds are threatened or broken (Bowlby, 1980). Attachment behavior is characteristic of many species because it contributes to their survival. It also comes from a need for security and safety. It is the similarity in responses to attachment and separation by humans and higher order primates that convinced Bowlby that grief responses are adaptational and valuable for survival. However, it is important to keep in mind that there are features of grieving that are specific only to human beings.

Based on attachment theory, Bowlby (1980) and Parkes (1972) described four phases of mourning:

- *Phase of Numbness.* People generally feel numb and are in varying degrees of denial. In some ways this is a protective mechanism that allows people to get through the first weeks of bereavement. Sometimes people say that they do not remember if certain people were at the funeral because they felt as if they were in a daze.
- *Yearning and Searching.* In this phase people are trying to find their loved one. They may actually sense his or her presence, hear his or her foot steps, smell his or her scent, and mistake a person in the street for their lost loved one. The bereaved often feel angry when unable to find their loved one and fear they might forget what he or she looks like. This phase is where reality of the death begins to register, and the bereaved may experience disbelief, tension, sobbing, and irritability.
- *Disorganization and Despair.* This phase is characterized by giving up the search to recover the deceased. Bereaved people often feel there is no hope or purpose in life at this point. It would be understandable for the bereaved to feel apathetic and perhaps depressed. The idea of a future without their loved one is a reason for despair.
- *Reorganization.* In this phase the bereaved seeks ways to remake his or her life. It is important for the bereaved to break down attachments to the

lost love one and establish new ties. This can be a phase of growth and a beginning of a new definition of their life without that person they love.

Finally, Kübler-Ross' stages of death and dying (Kübler-Ross, 1969)—denial, anger, bargaining, depression, and acceptance—are often used by health care professionals to define and intervene in the grief process. It is nearly impossible to find a basic nursing textbook that does not feature these stages when discussing the care of dying patients and families or grief and bereavement. While Kübler-Ross later explained she had not meant to imply that her stages were sequential "steps" to accepting death or loss, the use and application of her work continues. Kübler-Ross' work is credited with increased interest in grief, loss, and end-of-life care in the United States. Regardless of the clinical relevance of her work, we must not underestimate its effect on how Americans view death, dying, and loss.

What is the best conceptual framework for helping someone who has lost a close other? How helpful are the theories that describe stages, phases, and thus a correct or preferred way to resolve a loss? Clinical experience teaches us that most bereaved persons do not move through stages or phases in a set manner. There is also the risk that an inexperienced, albeit well-meaning counselor will take the stages too "literally," and perhaps attempt to push people along a premature or inappropriate path. For example, consider the women quoted at the beginning of the chapter. Would it be helpful to approach Mrs. A as if she had the same feelings and relationship with her husband, as did Mrs. B? We feel it is essential to view grief and loss from the perspective of tasks, rather than phases or stages.

Mourning does not involve clear-cut stages but rather certain tasks that need to be accomplished (Worden, 1991). Grief is work and thus demands time, effort, and concentration. Furthermore, viewing grief and loss from a task perspective implies that everyone's grief experience is different and unique, based on the multitude of factors each individual brings to the experience. Worden (1991) proposed four tasks of mourning as essential to the mourning process. They represent a guide for the APN to follow in assisting those who have lost someone close. They are:

1. To accept the reality of the loss
2. To work through the pain of grief
3. To adjust to the environment in which the deceased is missing
4. To relocate the deceased emotionally and move on with life

These tasks will be discussed in more depth in the section entitled "Providing Grief Support." Just as there is a great deal written on theories of grief, much is written concerning normal and abnormal grief. The following section presents discussion of some of the similarities and differences.

# ■ NORMAL GRIEF

Given the experience of losing a close other is individual and widely variable, the definition of *normal grief* is also widely variable. Much of the theory, "clinical lore," and public perceptions surrounding grief and loss has led to unrealistically limited views regarding what actually constitutes a normal grief reaction (Wortman & Silver, 1989). Recognizing the wide variability of "normal" grieving is essential in treating those who have experienced a loss with the respect, sensitivity, and compassion they deserve at this difficult time (Hyrkas, Kaunonen, & Paunonen, 1997; Pilkington, 1993; Wortman & Silver, 1989). In considering normal grief, we will discuss several factors to be considered when helping a person who has lost a close other. These include determinants of grief, manifestations of normal grief, and finally—using the tasks of grief as a guide—specific ways to be helpful. Determinants of grief (Worden, 1991):

1. *Who the person was:* All losses are different, just as all relationships are different. The loss of a spouse will be grieved differently than the loss of a child.
2. *The nature of the relationship:* Was the relationship strong? Secure? Ambivalent? Conflicted?
3. *The mode of death:* How did the person die? Was the death considered natural, accidental, a suicide, or a homicide? These deaths are grieved differently. Did the death happen nearby or far away? Was it sudden or was there some advance warning? Does the survivor feel responsible?
4. *Past loss and life crisis history:* Are there past losses? How did the survivor grieve? Is there a history of depression? Has the survivor experienced many losses and crises in his or her lifetime? Is there a history of alcohol or other drug use?
5. *Personality variables:* Age and sex of the survivor, how they handle feelings and anxiety, need for dependency, and personality disorders are factors to consider here.
6. *Social variables:* What is the survivor's cultural tradition or background? How much social support is available to the survivor? Does the survivor feel supported? Does the survivor have a confidant—someone close who has agreed to provide support and listening? Keep in mind that the presence of a confidant is a predictor of successful grieving.
7. *Concurrent stresses:* Were there marked changes or crises before or after the death? Are there ongoing crises or stresses aside from what was caused by the death?

## Manifestations of Normal Grief

In supporting someone who has lost a close other, it is crucial for the APN to be familiar with the wide range of behaviors that are manifestations of normal grief. They will be discussed in the following four categories: feelings, physical sensations, cognitions, and behaviors. (Refer to Worden [1991] for a more extensive discussion of this topic. This is also a helpful and easy-to-use reference on grief and loss.)

**Feelings.**   There are wide ranges of feelings that accompany grief. While keeping in mind that these represent normal grief, feelings that exist for long periods of time and/or at heightened intensity may herald the development of a complicated grief reaction. Again, it is essential that the APN has someone available to consult regarding complicated grief reactions. Feelings accompanying normal grief include sadness, anger, guilt or self-reproach, anxiety, loneliness, fatigue, helplessness, yearning, emancipation, relief, and numbness.

**Physical sensations.**    Physical sensations are especially important to note because they are very common, often overlooked, and may also be a reason why a grieving person seeks health care. Certainly, assessing a client's loss history is important, but on the other hand it should never preclude a complete investigation into physical symptoms. Physical sensations include hollowness in the stomach, chest and throat tightness, over-sensitivity to noise, a sense of unreality, feeling short of breath, muscle weakness, lack of energy, and dry mouth.

**Cognitions.**    As with feelings and physical sensation, certain thought patterns are characteristic of the normal grief response. While some may disappear after a short time, others persist and can activate feelings leading to depression and anxiety. Common cognitions include disbelief, confusion, preoccupation/obsessiveness, a sense the deceased person is close by, and visual and auditory hallucinations.

**Behaviors.**    Many behaviors are reported after a loss and often correct themselves over time. Normal behaviors include sleep disturbances, appetite disturbances, absentminded behavior, social withdrawal, dreams of the deceased, avoiding reminders of the deceased, searching and calling out, sighing, restless overactivity, crying, treasuring or carrying objects as reminders, and visiting places as reminders of the deceased.

## Ways to Be Helpful

Worden's (1991) tasks of grief provide a helpful framework for interventions to assist those who are mourning the loss of a close other. Interventions relevant to each of the four tasks will be discussed in turn, followed by a list of general suggestions.

Task 1—To accept the reality of the loss:
- Listen actively and without judgment.
- Encourage gentle exploration of what the future may look like without the person who has died.
- Assess and encourage the development of a social support system; remember, the availability of a confidant is very important.
- Encourage time with the body of the deceased at the time of the death, if possible.
- Offer ample opportunity to repeat the story of the death; listen patiently and attentively.
- Normalize feelings through personal contacts and written materials regarding grief and loss.
- Avoid the use of platitudes.
- Attend the funeral and/or visitation if at all possible. Send a personal letter or card to the family.

- Respect the survivor's feelings without judgment; remember, grief has no rules.

Task 2—To work through the pain of grief:

- Assist in identifying feelings or behaviors and normalize them. For example, you might say: "Sometimes persons feel anger; some people have told me they see or hear the voice of the person who died."
- Assist the survivor in placing a meaning on the death. For example, you might ask: "What does the loss of your spouse mean to you? What will you miss? What won't you miss?"

Task 3—To adjust to the environment in which the deceased is missing:

- Assist the survivor in further identifying the meaning of the loss in practical terms (e.g., what roles and functions will be vacant after the death, how their life will be different, how they may have to, in essence, redefine themselves).
- Provide practical assistance with developing needed skills.
- Advise the survivors to minimize change and to grieve where things are familiar; discourage moving or any similar large life change.

Task 4—To relocate the deceased emotionally and move on with life:

- Provide a nonjudgmental and supportive ear as the survivor explores this task.
- Validate and normalize feelings associated with moving the thoughts and memories of the deceased to an effective place that allows for a reinvestment in life.
- Encourage attendance at grief and loss support or educational groups.

Some general suggestions (Worden, 1991):

- Help the survivor to identify and express feelings
- Provide time to grieve
- Interpret "normal" grief behavior
- Allow for individual differences
- Provide continuing support—long after others in the survivor's close personal circle have stopped
- Identify pathology and refer as appropriate

## ■ NORMAL GRIEF VERSUS DEPRESSION

Normal grief and depression share several "classic" symptoms, including sleep and appetite disturbances and profound sadness. What they don't share is a profound and morbid preoccupation with worthlessness, prolonged and marked functional impairment, and marked psychomotor retardation common in depression (Worden, 1991). An APN should never make such a determination alone; consult with persons who are more familiar with the diagnosis and treatment of depression and refer for additional treatment. Table 5-1 summarizes the key differences between normal grief and depression.

## TABLE 5-1

### Key Differences Between Grieving and Depression

| | Grieving | Depression |
|---|---|---|
| Loss | Recognizable and current | May not be recognizable or the loss is seen as punishment |
| Mood states and reactions | Labile, but acute, not prolonged; heightened when thinking of loss | Sadness mixed with anger; mood consistently low, prolonged, and pervasive |
| Behavior | Variable; may shift from sharing one's pain to wanting to be alone; accepts some invitations | Either completely withdrawn or afraid of being alone; no enthusiasm for activity; consistent restriction of pleasure |
| Expression of anger | Open anger and hostility | Turned inward; not expressed |
| Expression of sadness | Periodic weeping and/or crying | Little variability—either inhibited or uncontrolled |
| Cognitions | Preoccupied with loss, confusion, or feelings of helplessness | Preoccupied with self, worthlessness, negative sense of self and future, self-blame, hopelessness |
| History | Little or no history of depression or other mental health issues | Probable history of depression or other mental health issues |
| Dreams, fantasies, and imagery | Vivid, clear dreams; fantasy and capacity for imagery, particularly involving the loss | Relatively little access to dreams; low capacity for fantasy or imagery (except self-punitive) |
| Sleep disturbance | Disturbing dreams; episodic difficulties in getting to sleep | Severe insomnia, regular early morning awakening |
| Self-concept | Sees self as to blame; for example, for not providing adequately for person who has died | Sees self as bad because of being depressed; tendency to experience self as worthless; preoccupation with self; suicidal ideas and feelings |
| Responsiveness | Responds to warmth and reassurance | Responds to pressure and urging or is unresponsive |

Adapted from Berry, P. H., Egan, K., Eighmy, J. B., Kalina, K., Gallagher-Allred, C. R., Murphy, P. L., Nahman, E. J., Rooney, E. J., Smith, S. A., Volker, B. A., & Zeri, K. (1999). *Hospice and palliative nurses' practice review* (3rd ed.). Dubuque, IA: Kendall/Hunt.

## ■ COMPLICATED GRIEF

Complicated grief, also commonly termed abnormal grief, pathologic grief, unresolved grief, chronic grief, delayed grief, or exaggerated grief, can appear in multiple forms. *Complicated grief* is commonly defined as an intensification of grief to the level where the person is overwhelmed, resorts to maladaptive behavior, or remains interminably in the state of grief without progression through the mourning process to completion (Worden, 1991). However, characteristics of complicated grief reactions are also found in normal grief and there may be more of a continuous relationship between complicated and uncomplicated grief reactions. Several authorities on this topic agree that pathology is more related to the intensity or duration of the grief reaction rather than the presence or absence of a specific suspect behavior (Worden, 1991).

In determining a complicated grief reaction, consider the following clues. While the appearance of one may not alone represent a complicated grief reaction, this possibility should be nonetheless considered:

1. The survivor cannot speak of the deceased without experiencing intense and fresh grief.
2. A relatively minor event triggers an intense and fresh grief reaction.
3. Loss is often a theme in interview and discussion.
4. The survivor is unwilling to move items belonging to the deceased and wishes to maintain the environment just the way it was when the person died.
5. The survivor develops physical symptoms like those the deceased experienced before death.
6. Radical changes in lifestyle, friends, and activities after a death.
7. A history of subclinical depression with guilt and low self-esteem and/or a false sense of euphoria after the death.
8. A compulsive need to imitate the deceased person.
9. Self-destructive impulses or behaviors.
10. Unaccountable sadness at certain times of the year.
11. A fear of the illness or circumstance that caused the death of the deceased.
12. Avoidance of the grave site or funeral or other rituals around the time of the death.

If an APN suspects a complicated grief reaction, referral to a grief therapist is imperative. As discussed previously, it is essential to have access to a colleague who can provide the needed consultation and specialized follow-up care.

## ■ CONCLUSION

Grief has no timetable and has been likened to a raw, open wound. With great care it will eventually heal but will always leave a scar. The experiences of grief have also been compared to enduring a fierce storm at sea, where the waves are peaked and close together. Eventually the sea becomes calmer, but occasionally the storm hits without any warning.

> *Grief is a tidal wave that overtakes you, smashes down upon you with unimaginable force, sweeps you up into its darkness, where you tumble and crash against unidentifiable surfaces, only to be thrown out on an unknown beach, bruised, reshaped (Ericsson, 1993).*

APNs play an important role in anticipating grief reactions and providing the needed support to client's families and close others after the death. However, APNs must also be aware of the signs and symptoms of depression and complicated grief and, by recognizing the limits of their practice, arrange for the necessary referrals and follow-up care and support.

## References

BERRY, P. H., Egan, K., Eighmy, J. B., Kalina, K., Gallagher-Allred, C. R., Murphy, P. L., Nahman, E. J., Rooney, E. J., Smith, S. A., Volker, B. A., & Zeri, K. (1999). *Hospice and palliative nurses' practice review* (3rd ed.). Dubuque, IA: Kendall/Hunt.

BERRY, P., Zeri, K., & Egan, K. (1997). *The hospice nurse's study guide: A preparation for the CRNH candidate.* Pittsburgh: Hospice Nurses Association.

BOWLBY, J. (1980). *Attachment and loss: Loss, sadness, and depression* (Vol. 3). New York: Basic Books.

ERICSSON, S. (1993). *Companion through the darkness.* New York: Harper Collins Publishers.

FREUD, S. (1957). Mourning and melancholia. In J. Strachey (Ed.), *Standard Edition of the Complete Psychological Works of Sigmund Freud* (Vol. 14). London: Hogarth Press. (Original work published 1917.)

HYRKAS, K., Kaunonen, M., & Paunonen, M. (1997). Recovering from the death of a spouse, *Journal of Advanced Nursing, 25*(4), 775-779.

KOEPPL, J. (1996). Beyond the emptiness: Helping young widows to name the depth of their loss. *Thanatos, 21*(3), 22-23.

KÜBLER-ROSS, E. (1969). *On death and dying.* New York: Macmillan.

LINDEMANN, E. (1944). Symptomatology and management of acute grief. *American Journal of Psychiatry, 101,* 141-149.

PARKES, C. M. (1972). *Bereavement: Studies of grief in adult life.* New York: International University Press.

PILKINGTON, F. B. (1993). The lived experience of grieving the loss of an important other. *Nursing Science Quarterly, 6*(3), 130-139.

RANDO, T. (1986). *Loss and anticipatory grief.* Lexington, MA: Lexington Books.

RANDO, T. (1993). *Treatment of complicated mourning.* Champaign, IL: Research Press.

SHAPIRO, E. R. (1994). *Grief as a family process: A developmental approach to clinical practice.* New York: The Guiliford Press.

WORDEN, J. W. (1991). *Grief counseling and grief therapy: A handbook for the mental health practitioner* (2nd ed.). New York: Springer Publishing Co.

WORTMAN, C. B., & Silver, R. C. (1989). The myths of coping with loss. *Journal of Consulting & Clinical Psychology, 57*(3), 349-57.

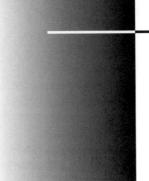

CHAPTER **6**

# Complementary Therapies in End-of-Life Care

NANCY K. ENGLISH

C omplementary therapies are considered nonpharmacologic interventions that are used to enhance and support the patient's palliative plan of care. The art and aesthetics of nursing care is reflected in the therapeutic use of touch, sound, and aroma. An APN who integrates complementary interventions into his or her practice is able to provide a therapeutic environment for the patients as they face the end of life.

## ■ OVERVIEW

A *Journal of the American Medical Association (JAMA)* editorial (Jones, 1998) identified that consumers are spending nearly $100 billion annually for herbal medicines, massage, and various other therapies outside of standard medical care. Jones further suggested that the medical community should acknowledge these trends and create a new paradigm of health care, offering consumers more options to ease their pain and suffering.

The establishment of the Federal Commission on Complementary and Alternative Medicine (CAM) in March of 2000 was in response to numerous professional and consumer groups advocating for alternative approaches to traditional medical care. This commission was charged to:

1. Coordinate research on complementary and alternative medicine (CAM) practices and products
2. Identify appropriate education and training for CAM practitioners
3. Disseminate and review reliable information on CAM for both health care providers and the general public

The commission is currently requesting information from various professional organizations on educational standards, practitioner and instructor qualifications, and a variety of other related topics.

The National Hospice and Palliative Care Organization (NHPCO) (2001) published an educational and informational compendium on complementary

**65**

therapies used in end-of-life care. This resource is intended to help palliative care settings integrate complementary therapy interventions into existing practices. The following outlines the use of art, healing touch, hypnosis, massage, and music therapies.

## ■ COMPLEMENTARY INTERVENTIONS IN THE PALLIATIVE CARE SETTING

Introducing complementary therapies into a palliative plan of care may be best understood in the framework of the now well-documented body/mind interaction. The landmark studies of Wallace and Benson (1972) outlined the physiologic benefits of a "calm mind" as a result of repeated practice of conscious breathing and silently repeating the phrase "I am at peace." The collection of phenomena that results from this exercise is known as the "relaxation response," which can be observed and measured. It is described as an alert predominate parasympathetic nervous system response with decreased sympathetic nervous system activity (Benson, 1984)— in other words, the body resting while the mind remains engaged.

The patient's perception of pain, fear of the unknown, further decline, and death initiates a threat to the body/mind integrity. In response to this threat, an instantaneous chain reaction of biochemical events within the neurologic structures of the brain is activated. This results in an increase in autonomic nervous system (ANS) activity (Ganong, 1987; Pert, 1997). This psycho-neuro-physiologic response can result in fatigue, insomnia, appetite changes, and constipation, all of which influence the patient's sense of well-being. The introduction of complementary therapies (e.g., touch, aromatherapy, guided relaxation, music) can interfere with this chain of events in the body/mind.

In their early discussion of noninvasive pain relief measures, McCaffery and Beebe (1989) outline the following benefits of relaxation with regard to pain management. They concluded that relaxation would benefit the pain experience by:
- Decreasing the anxiety associated with painful situations, such as wound care and dressing changes
- Easing the muscle tension pain of skeletal muscle spasms
- Decreasing fatigue by interrupting the "fight or flight response"
- Providing a period of rest
- Helping the client fall asleep quickly
- Increasing the effect of pain medications
- Helping the client disassociate from pain

The palliative care of plan can evolve around the patient's and family's preferences for specific interventions. Often, discussing complementary interventions reveals unfamiliar options that may be very beneficial and meaningful to both the patient and his or her family.

The APN utilizing complementary interventions can assess patient preferences with the use of the Complementary Therapies Assessment: Inventory (Box 6-1). Understanding and implementing what is most appropriate for individual patients thus prompts improved outcomes.

| BOX 6-1 | *Complementary Therapies Assessment: Inventory* |
|---|---|

1. In the past year, how many times have you received:
   Massage:                    0-5 ____6-15 ____16 or more ____
   Therapeutic Touch:          0-5 ____6-15 ____16 or more ____
   Other Touch Therapies:      0-5 ____6-15 ____16 or more ____

   How would you describe your response to these therapies?
   Pleasurable  1 – 2 – 3 – 4 – 5 – 6 – 7 – 8 – 9 – 10  Not enjoyable
   Relaxing    1 – 2 – 3 – 4 – 5 – 6 – 7 – 8 – 9 – 10  Increased tension
2. Do you practice any relaxation, meditation, or visualization/imagery method?
   Yes ____ No ____
   If "yes," specify method and estimate how frequently you practice it:
   0-5 ____6-15 ____16 or more ____ (times per week)
   Your response from the practice of meditation or visualization could best be described as:
   Relaxing 1 – 2 – 3 – 4 – 5 – 6 – 7 – 8 – 9 – 10 Anxious or unable to maintain a quiet space
3. What is your favorite type of music?
   Select music for a specific mood (give examples):
   Relaxing_____
   Energizing _____
   Easy Listening _____
4. Do you have a favorite...
   Scent or smell?
   Flowers/plant/tree?
   Perfume?
   After shave?
   Other?
Are there any specific memories that are associated with a particular odor?
Are there any odors that increase feelings of nausea or anxiety? If so, specify:

_____
_____
_____
_____
_____
_____
_____
_____
_____
_____
_____
_____

# ■ AROMATHERAPY

Aromatherapy is the therapeutic use of specially prepared essential or aromatic oils (Gattefosse, 1995). Scent conveys the recognition of the familiar, evoking memories of joy and possibly also of sorrow. Essential oils contain the fragrant intensity of plants, trees, and flowers and have been used since ancient times for sacred as well as medicinal purposes. In the clinical setting, aromatherapy is used in massage as an inhalant and in skin care.

## Background

Pedacius Dioscorides, a Greek healer in the 1st century AD recorded a treatise on the use of plants in healing and devoted a great deal of information to aroma therapeutics (Tisserand, 1988). The King James version of the Bible often cites the sacred use of oils, as in the 23rd Psalm: "Anoint thy head with oil." In many religions and indigenous cultures, shaman, priests, and priestesses burn incense or special plants to impart heightened awareness of an omnipotent presence. They believe that certain aromas act as spiritual conduits. Throughout the ages, in a variety of ways, essential oils have been used to connote, express, and invoke the sacred.

Marguerite Konig Maury, an Austrian nurse, revived the therapeutic use of oils in the United Kingdom and in Europe. While working in France in the early years of World War I, Maury was given Dr. Chabenes' 1838 text, *Les Grandes Possibilities par les Matrieres Odoriferantes (The Great Possibilities of Aromatic Substances)* (Maury, 1995). This sparked her passion, and she began her life's work devoted to understanding the physiologic effects of essential oils in health and healing. Maury is credited with creating formulas and protocols for the topical application of oils through massage. With the guidance of Professor Gattefosse, a French chemist, Maury refined and deepened her study of essential oils by investigating their biochemistry. They began the arduous task of analyzing essential oils from various botanicals and documenting their indications and potential therapeutic effectiveness (Gattefosse, 1995; Maury, 1995).

## Biochemistry of Essential Oils

An essential oil is the distilled "essence" of a flower, plant, or tree resin. It is the volatile (easily evaporated), aromatic chemical that gives the plant a distinct, unique scent (Mojay, 1996). These oils are lipid soluble, have an acidic pH, and are easily absorbed through the epidermis and dermis. Since an oil's specific biochemistry determines its therapeutic properties, the distillation process is crucial to preserving the biochemical makeup and therefore the exactness and integrity of the oil's therapeutic properties (Gattefosse, 1995; Mailhebiau, 1995). For example, lavender oil extracted and diluted for cosmetic use does not conform to the standards for distilling a therapeutic essence. The effect of a commercial preparation may indeed be pleasant, but not necessarily therapeutic. It becomes imperative that the practitioner of aromatherapy uses the highest quality of essential oils.

The criteria for a quality essential oil established in the United Kingdom is done through the Scientific Institute of Aromatology and registered under the seal of botanically- and biochemically-defined essential oil (Mailhebiau, 1995; Schnaubelt, 1998). The three criteria used to judge essential oils are:

1. Botanical species information—this includes the Latin classification or the genus name, followed by the epithet, and the variety. For example, Lavender is of the genus *Lavandula,* its epithet is *angustifolia,* and its fragrance variety is Lamiaceae (Mailhebiau, 1995; Rose, 1999).
2. Plant part—Each specific part of a plant has a distinct biochemistry. The leaf, root, or flower may have different biochemical properties even though all are of the same variety (Rose, 1999).
3. Biochemical specificity (i.e., chemotype)—this refers to the exact biochemical properties of the distilled leaf, root, or flower. For example, *Lavendula angustiflora* (flower) produces the effect of relaxation (Mailhebiau, 1995). Prime consideration in the analysis of biochemical specificity is where the plant is grown and where and what time of day the plant is harvested.

## Clinical Research

Selected clinical studies focusing on the use of aromatherapy massage indicate a positive effect of reducing anxiety in patients from a variety of clinical settings (Buckle, 1993; Corner, Cawley, & Hildebrand, 1995: Dunn, Sleep, & Collett, 1995; Stevenson, 1994; Wilkinson, 1995).

Lavender oil is known for its sedative effect (Mailhebiau, 1995). Three clinical studies of older adults attest to the effectiveness of lavender oil as an inhalant for improving sleep (Cannard, 1995; Hardy, Kirk-Smith, & Stretch, 1995; Hudson, 1996).

The use of aromatherapy in the palliative care setting may indeed have a more subjective, aesthetic quality for patients and the environment. Aromatherapy as a complementary modality offers a natural method of symptom management and psychologic support.

## Summary

- Essential oils:
  - Are the "essence" of a flower, plant, or tree resin
  - Are diluted with carrier oil when applied to the skin surface
  - Are absorbed through the fatty (lipid) tissues
  - Must be of a high quality and obtained from a reputable source
  - Must be clearly labeled and stored in a cool, dark place to prevent oxidation and prolong shelf life
  - Have therapeutic value as an inhalant through the use of a diffuser, as an additive to massage oil, and as a spray
- Aromatherapy—the skilled use of essential oils

**Therapeutic massage.**   A gentle, slow rhythm of long stroking movements (see "Effleurage") in a continuous motion to areas of tension in the body. A massage should include the use of absorbent carrier oil. The massage session has a clear start and finish with specific guidelines for the therapist (Maxwell-Hudson, 1988).

**Effleurage.**   This is also referred to as a smoothing stroke; it is a smooth sliding movement that soothes the skin while distributing the lotion or oil. It is not a deep movement but rather a firm and confident movement always toward the direction of the heart of the recipient.

**Carrier oils.**   Effective carrier oils are usually of fruit or vegetable origin. Grape seed oil is recommended because it is highly absorbent, odorless, and economical.

**Therapeutic massage with essential oil (aromatherapy massage).**   Massage with the addition of specific essential plant oil to the carrier lotion. In the United Kingdom and Central Europe, massage with an essential oil added to carrier oil is referred to as aromatherapy (Maury, 1988).

## ■ ESSENTIAL OILS AND THEIR USES

### Lavender *(Lavendula angustiflora)*

Parts of plant used: Flowers (deep blue in color).

Method of extraction: Steam distillation.

Contraindications: Do not use if patient is receiving anticoagulant therapy (Schnaubelt, 1998).

Side effects: None listed (Kerr, 1998; Valnet, 1990).

History: Throughout the ages, lavender has been known for its cleansing qualities. The word "lavender" is derived from the Latin *lavare,* meaning "to wash." The infamous Roman baths often used it as the scent to induce relaxation. Dioscorides, the early Greek healer and physician, recommended lavender oil for "ye griefs of the thorax" (Mojay, 1996). Because of its antifungal and antibacterial qualities, lavender was recognized as an excellent wound-cleansing agent during World War I (Valnet, 1990).

Laboratory research: In one experiment, essential oil of lavender was diluted with peanut oil (2% solution) and massaged for 10 minutes over the stomach area of one subject. Peak serum levels of lavender oil were obtained in 20 minutes. In a 90-minute time period, serum testing indicated only minimal traces of lavender oil (Jager, Buchbauer, Jirovetz, & Fritzer, 1992). Under standardized experimental conditions, the effect of inhaling lavender oil was observed on the activity of mice that had been injected with caffeine. There was a significant decrease in mobility and activity (Buchbauer, Jirovetz, Jager, Dietrich, & Plank, 1991). Another study conducted on mice showed that lavender oil (diluted 1:60) potentiated the effects of barbiturate (pentobarbital) sedation (Guillemain, Rousseau, & Delaveau, 1989).

**Action:** Primarily on the central nervous system, resulting in a sedative effect and antiinflammatory effect on wounds.

**Indications:**

- Sleep-pattern disturbances (especially in the elderly)
- Anxiety, with pacing
- Acute confusion (delirium), with agitation
- Terminal restlessness
- Alterations in skin integrity (e.g., inflammation, wounds)
- Spiritual distress
- Hopelessness

**Applications:**

- Topical massage:
  - Use 10 to 20 gtts in 30 cc of grape seed oil.
  - Add 9 gtts to 15 cc skin protection cream (i.e., aloe preparations); apply to irritated or inflamed skin.
- Wound care:
  - Cleanse or irrigate wound with sterile normal saline.
  - Apply essential oil (2 to 3 gtts) to gauze sponge dressing with ointment or other prescribed salve or ointment. Lanolin base or zinc oxide is preferred; it prevents oxidation of oil.
  - Apply to wound.
  - Cover wound as per protocol.
- Inhalant:
  - Bath—Add 5 drops to 15 cc shampoo; add to warm bath.
  - Diffuser—Add oil to designated port and place in patient's room for 20 to 30 minutes. Note: molecules of oil are diffused in the air via electric pump and usually a glass dispenser.
  - Compress—8 to 10 moist washcloths with 5 drops of oil added can be placed in an electric "hot pot" on low for 10 minutes. These may be offered to patients as a refreshing face cloth at bedtime (Kyle, 2000).

### Eucalyptus *(Eucalyptus globulus)*

Parts of plant (tree) used: Leaves of pale blue-green color.

Method of extraction: Steam distillation (Mailhebiau, 1995; Schnaubelt, 1998).

Safety data: Not for use with small children; avoid contact with eyes.

**History:** The name "eucalyptus" is derived from Greek *eucalyptos,* meaning "well covered." Just prior to blooming, the eucalyptus flower is covered by a membrane to protect the fragile bloom. The Aboriginal people of Australia first used the essential oil for medicinal purposes, primarily to treat infections and fevers. It became known as "the fever tree" because the eucalyptus roots absorbed a great deal of moisture, drying up the marshy soil (Mojay, 1996; Tisserand, 1988).

**Action:** Primary action is on the respiratory system, increasing the depth of respiration (Gattefosse, 1995; Mailhebiau, 1995; Schnaubelt, 1998;

Valnet, 1990). This action may in turn assist the patient in productive coughing.

**Indications:**

- Dyspnea (breathlessness) related to end-stage pulmonary disease
- Dyspnea with congestion
- Moist, noisy breathing when death is impending

**Application:**

- Topical massage:
  - 2 gtts in 15 cc of grape seed oil, applied to chest and gently massaged into the skin; may also be massaged in same manner to the back at the midthoracic area.
  - Inhalant:
  - Place 5 gtts in 60 cc of distilled water and use as spritzer.
  - Diffuser—Use 2 to 3 gtts in designated port and place in patient's room for 30 minutes.

## Frankincense (Boswellia carteri)

Parts of plant (tree) used: Resin (an orange-brown gum).
Method of extraction: Steam distillation of the gum.
Safety data: Nontoxic; nonirritant.

**History:** This small tree, with its narrow leaves and pale-pink flowers, creates a resin (gum) in its trunk. The oil is distilled from the hardened resin. Throughout the ages, frankincense, or olibanum, has played a role in religious and tribal ceremonies. One of the most expensive oils of the ancient world, its name is derived from the Medieval French word *franc,* meaning "pure" or "free," and from the Latin *incensium,* meaning "to smoke." In Western culture, frankincense is familiar as one of the gifts given to the baby Jesus, and is mentioned in the Bible 22 times (Frankincense and Myrrh—History, 1997; Mojay, 1996).

**Action:** It is thought to act on the nervous system by calming, yet energizing (Tisserand, 1988).

**Indications:**

- Spiritual distress
- Hopelessness, with agitation
- Fatigue
- Impending death

**Application:**

- Topical Massage:
  - 10 gtts in 30 cc of grape seed oil for hands, feet, or back massage; also may be added to cream or lotion for massage.
- Inhalant:
  - Place 5 gtts in 60 cc of distilled water and use as spritzer.
  - Diffuser—Add 3 gtts to designated port and place in patient's room for 30 minutes.
  - Bath—Use 2 to 3 gtts in 15 cc of milk or shampoo; add to warm bath.

## Geranium *(Pelargonium odorantissimum)*

Parts of plant used: Leaves.

Method of extraction: Steam distillation.

Safety data: Nontoxic; nonirritant; avoid use close to eyes (Mojay, 1996; Raymen, 1991; Rose, 1999).

**History:** The name "pelargonium" derives from the Greek *palargos,* referring to the pelican's (i.e., stork's) bill, similar in shape to the fruit of this small perennial shrub. The plant originated in South Africa and was brought to France in the 19th century where the oil was first distilled and utilized by an Italian physician in the treatment of anxiety states (Mojay, 1996; Tisserand, 1988).

**Laboratory research:** Pelargonium has not yet been investigated according to the Aromatherapy Database (1998), a computer search of professional journals worldwide. Tisserand (1988) quotes a Japanese study (without reference) attesting to the use of geranium oil for individual needs. For example, some subjects in the study experienced a sedative effect, while others found the geranium oil to be energizing. Because of its adaptable, individualistic nature, Tisserand suggested that geranium oil could be used in combination with other oils in massage.

**Action:** May act to stimulate the function of the liver and pancreas (Mojay, 1996).

**Indications:**
- Constipation
- Anxiety

**Application:**
- Topical Massage:
  - Add 3 gtts of essential oil to 15 cc of grape seed oil; massage in counterclockwise movement on abdomen above umbilicus and a clockwise movement on colon area.
- Inhalant:
  - Diffuser—Add 3 gtts to designated port and place in patient's room for 30 minutes.

## Tea Tree *(Melaleuca alternifolia)*

Part of plant (tree) used: Leaves.

Method of extraction: Steam distillation (Carson, 1998; Mojay, 1996).

Safety data: Always use in a diluted form to avoid allergic contact dermatitis; do not use near eyes or as an inhalant (Mojay, 1996).

**History:** The ingenious Aboriginal people have found that every part of this small tree can be used in a purposeful way, including soaking the leaves in hot water to treat respiratory problems. When Captain Cook explored the coast of Australia, the English settlers enjoyed a spicy beverage brewed from the leaves, which led to Cook's coining the name, "tea tree." More recently, the oil of the tree has been called "the Australian wonder," due to its many uses (Mojay, 1996; Rose, 1992).

**Laboratory research:** Tea tree oil is one of the most highly researched oils, primarily in the science laboratories of Australia and New Zealand. A 5% solution of tree tea oil was compared with 5% benzoyl peroxide for the treatment of acne. Both solutions were effective, yet the subjects treated with tea tree oil had fewer side effects (Bassett, Pannowitz, & Barnetson, 1990). The effectiveness of the oil as an anti-fungal agent was indicated in the treatment of 28 patients for vaginitis *(Candida albicans).* After 30 days of treatment, 75% of the patients were asymptomatic and indicated a negative culture for *C. albicans* (Belaiche, 1985).

Tea tree oil has been the subject of the research laboratories at the University of Western Australia. Here, microbiologist Christine Carson has studied antimicrobial activity of tea tree oil for the past 6 years. Her recent work attests to the effectiveness of 0.25% solution of tea tree oil against the highly resistant MRSA (Carson, 1998).

**Indications:**
- Alteration in skin integrity
- Wounds: Stages II, III, IV
- Infected and odorous wounds: highly sensitive to MRSA
- *C. albicans*

**Application:**
- Topical:
  - Wound irrigation: Use a 0.25% solution with sterile normal saline (0.9%). Moisten sponges with 2 to 3 gtts of tea tree oil; apply to wound and cover as per protocol. (Tea tree oil can be used in a similar manner to lavender for wound care.)

### Summary

Little has been said in the professional literature regarding how use of a subtle scent can change the ambiance of a palliative care setting or relieve the stress of a caregiver in the home. Although the gathering of qualitative and quantitative data is still formative, anecdotal evidence and a long history of use across cultures supports the effectiveness of essential oils. The introduction of these tiny molecules of fragrance can offer strength to a caregiver and solace to a patient. An environment filled with carefully chosen oil can communicate comfort, wisdom, awareness, and compassion. The gentle power of scent may serve to ease suffering and pain in end-of-life care in ways that we are only beginning to acknowledge.

## ■ ENERGY BALANCING THERAPIES
### Overview

In Chinese and Ayurvedic medicine, all living things in the universe are seen as being multidimensional energy fields. These fields of light energy (*chi,* or *prana*) in the human include the physical body and extend to subtle or invisible energy fields surrounding the physical body (Kaptchuk, 1983; Lad, 1984). Health in the body-mind are viewed as a balanced energy system, and thus disease or symptoms such as pain, nausea, or dyspnea represent an energy field disturbance or an imbalance in energy, referred to as blocked or stagnant energy. Diagnoses of blocked or stagnant energy in the Eastern healing systems are identified through the quality of the patient's pulses, color of the tongue, and color and quality of the skin. In energy balancing interventions, the practitioner's hands assess the energy field imbalances by either scanning the entire body or by the tension at a designated acupressure point. For example, when a Therapeutic Touch (TT), Healing Touch, or Reiki practitioner scans the energy field of a patient who is experiencing dyspnea (i.e., breathlessness), the field may be warm in the chest compared with other areas of the body. A practitioner of Jin Shin Jyutsu acupressure would assess the tension or tightness surrounding Lung 1 (acupoint). Once an assessment is made, the practitioner plans an intervention to restore balance in the recipient's energy field. The practitioner's hands, as transmitters of energy, repattern the energy field and often relieve the patient's experience of dyspnea or other symptoms.

## Acupressure

Origin: A spiritual practice, called Jin Shin Jyutsu (The Art of the Creator through the Person of Compassion), brought to the United States in the late 1940s from Japan by Mary Iino Burmeister (Burmeister & Monte, 1997). In 1978, Iona and Ron Teegarten, students of Mary Burmeister, included concepts from Traditional Chinese Medicine and Transpersonal Psychology and refer to this as Jin Shin Do (The Way of the Compassionate Spirit) (Teegarten, 1978).

Description: A gentle finger pressure is applied to acupuncture points found on the "extraordinary meridians" as outlined in Traditional Chinese Medicine (Matsumoto & Birch, 1986). The acupoints are held until the tension at the acupoint is relaxed. Specific patterns of acupoints, referred to as *energy flows,* address a variety of problems affecting the body and mind of the recipient.

Requirements for entry-level practice: From 15 to 20 hours of didactic and supervised practice from a certified instructor of Jin Shin Jyutsu or Jin Shin Do.

## Healing Touch

Origin: Healing Touch is a combination of energy-based therapeutic approaches to healing. Janet Mentgen, a nurse and student of Dolores Krieger, developed the practice in 1989 (Healing Touch Notebook Level I, 2001).

Description: The core practice of Therapeutic Touch, described in the following section, forms the foundation for planning a Healing Touch intervention. A wide variety of energy balancing modalities are used in approaching the recipient's problem.

Requirements for entry-level practice: 15 hours of didactic and supervised practice from a certified instructor of Healing Touch. Advanced courses are offered through Healing Touch International (see internet resources).

## Reiki

Origin: Reiki is a laying-on-of-hands technique thought to have originated as a Tibetan Buddhist meditative healing practice. In the late 1800s, Mikao Usui began the practice known today as the Usui Method of Reiki healing (Stein, 1995).

Description: The practitioner places their hands in a specified pattern with the intention of balancing the recipient's energy field. The hand placements of the practitioner on the recipient's body are sequential, with minimal variation from the ancient practice as taught by Master Usui (personal communication, T. Vargus, April, 2001).

Requirements for entry-level practice: 12 hours of didactic and supervised practice from a Master Level Reiki Instructor.

## Therapeutic Touch

Origin: Therapeutic Touch (TT) is derived from the ancient and traditional method of "laying on of hands." TT was introduced to the nursing profession in the 1970s by Dolores Krieger, a professor of nursing at New York University. A specific method outlined by Krieger and her mentor, Dora Kunz, is a standardized approach known as the Krieger-Kunz method of Therapeutic Touch (Krieger, 1997; Macrae, 1994). Numerous investigations testify to the effectiveness of TT as nursing intervention (see "Clinical Research").

Description: TT is a contemporary interpretation of ancient healing practices in which the practitioner's hands facilitate balance in the recipient's energy field. The practitioner's intention to help another is the core of the practice of TT (Nurse Healers Professional Associates International, 1992) (see "Method").

Requirements for entry-level practice: 15 hours of didactic and supervised practice from a certified Therapeutic Touch instructor.

## ■ THERAPEUTIC TOUCH

TT is a contemporary interpretation of several ancient healing practices and is a consciously directed process of energy exchange, during which the practitioner uses the hands as a focus to facilitate healing (Nurse Healers Professional Associates International, 1992).

### Clinical Research

TT has been the subject of numerous clinical studies. The following discussion highlights selected TT studies.

The relaxation response is the most reliable response of recipients of a TT intervention (Krieger, 1997). Participants in numerous investigations of TT report warmth in the extremities, slower and deeper respirations, decrease in pain perception, and decrease in anxiety (Gagne & Toye, 1994; Heidt, 1990; Quinn, 1989; Simington & Laing, 1993).

A clinical trial of the elderly in long-term care settings reported pain relief after receiving TT interventions over 3 consecutive days for 20 minutes. The control group, receiving a mimic touch intervention for the same period of time, reported little or no effect on their pain (Mast, 1998). In a second trial, tension headaches of 60 college students who also received a TT intervention reported a significant reduction in pain (Keller & Bzdek, 1986).

Qualitative studies provide promising avenues for documenting the effects of TT. A study by Samarel (1992) of the experience of patients' receiving TT indicates that recipients report an increase in personal awareness. Sameral describes this increase in personal awareness as having three aspects—physiological, mental/emotional, and spiritual. The twenty patients who participated in this investigation experienced the phenomena as a linear-cognitive process. This process follows a course of "the perceived need," "the decision to seek treatment," "receiving treatment," and "following treatment" (Samarel, 1992). The following excerpt of one subject's description of this process illustrates the phenomena (Samarel, 1992):

> *It seems as if the pain was the most important reason I sought TT, but now it's not the pain that's important. I mean, I have less pain but what really is important is how I feel as a whole person.*

As Samarel concludes, additional qualitative data is needed to make the depth of this unique nursing practice of TT clear to practitioners and patients.

Fanslow-Brunjes, a nursing pioneer in the practice and teaching of TT in hospice settings throughout the United States, created an intervention, referred to as the *Hand-to-Heart Connection™*, for patients approaching death. She observed that her patients became calm and relaxed after receiving this simple yet profound intervention (Fanslow-Brunjes, as cited in Versagi, 1999).

## Methods

- *Intention* is a prerequisite for the nurse or practitioner of TT. *Intentionality* is defined as the centered, focused intent of the practitioner to be a conduit of universal life energy and to direct this energy to the recipient (i.e., the patient) (Complementary Therapies Workgroup, 1997). *Centered, focused intent* is defined as a silent, inward focus where the intent is to help the patient in whatever way possible.
- Explanation of TT, which includes its role in relaxation, is provided to the patient and/or family.
- Evaluation of the recipient's response to the intervention consists of observing their nonverbal response and also their verbal response. Indicators of change, such as visual analogue scales are of value. This can quantify the degree of change as a result of the TT intervention.

Step 1—Centering: The practitioner relates to the inner self, finding an inner stable center. A silent intention to help the recipient is repeated.

Step 2—Assessment (scanning): The hands of the practitioner are held 2 to 3 inches from the recipient's body, starting at the top of the head and slowly moving down to the feet. Imbalances in the energy field of the recipient may be sensed as (Healing Touch, Level 1, Notebook, 2000; Macrae, 1994):

- Dense
- Congested
- Tingling
- Vibrating
- Electric
- Hot
- Cold

Step 3—Unruffling the Energy Field: The hands of the practitioner return to an area of the body where any of the above sensations are sensed. Slowly the practitioner's hands brush down and away from the body with the palms of the hand facing the recipient.

Step 4—Repatterning or Modulating: After unruffling the recipient's energy field, the practitioner gently lays his or her hands on the area that was assessed.

Step 5—Closure: The TT intervention is complete when the practitioner perceives that the recipient's energy field is balanced.

Step 6—Evaluation: The recipient may want to talk and relate their experience of TT. If the recipient is asleep, note the relaxation of the breath, eyes, and facial muscles.

Step 7—Documentation: Document the encounter on the recipient's medical record.

## Precautions

- Children, older adults, and the severely debilitated—May be more sensitive to TT; therefore, the length of treatment should be of a shorter duration—generally 10 minutes or less.
- Impending death—The treatment duration should be five minutes or less.

## Intervention: Hand-to-Heart Connection™

Indications:
- Anxiety
- Terminal agitation
- Impending death

Methods:
- Centering: The practitioner relates to the inner self, finding an inner stable center. A silent intention to help the recipient is repeated.
- Sitting at patient's left side: Take the patient's left hand in your left (palm-to-palm) and place your right hand over the left.

- Slowly move the right hand to the patient's left shoulder remaining there for 2 to 3 seconds.
- Quietly move your right hand down from the shoulder and place the right hand lightly over the patient's heart area.
- Remain in this position in silent prayer or meditation.
- Return the right hand to the patient's left shoulder and slowly move your right hand down the patient's left arm, placing it again over the left hand. Let go of the patient's left hand slowly.
- Teach to significant caregivers as appropriate (Fanslow-Brunjes, as cited in Versagi, 1999).

### Summary

Energy-balancing therapies such as TT, Reiki, Healing Touch, and acupressure offer the APN therapeutic venues for providing the patient relaxation and symptom relief. These interventions can easily be taught to family members who may want to participate in comfort care during the last days of life.

## ■ RELAXATION, IMAGERY, AND MUSIC

Relaxation exercises and imagery sessions center on words scripted to quiet the body and mind. Basic to all practices of relaxation and imagery is the patient's concentrated awareness of his or her own breath. This is accomplished by focusing on the rhythm of the breath for a specified period of time. Boerstler, who has developed a method referred to as "comeditation" in his work with dying patients, relates: "The breath is the pulse of the mind and there is a direct correlation between breathing and thinking" (Miller, 1991, p. 65). The soft voice of the guide helps focus the patient on the rhythm of the breath, while suggesting letting go of all tension.

When specific music is added to a relaxation or imagery session it can potentiate the relaxation response. Few question that music and rhythm affect mood. The sounds of the National Anthem can create a sense of unity that one shares with a larger group. These unifying sounds speak to those ancient voices heard within each individual, whether it is the steady beat of a drum or an old familiar rhythm. Music has the effect of intensifying the underlying emotion (Guzzetta, 1991).

Writing in *Music Therapy: Nursing the Music of the Soul*, Guzzetta (1991) states that the goal of adding music and rhythm to a patient's therapeutic regimen is to achieve a deep state of relaxation and decreased pain and anxiety. She adds that appropriate music serves as a vehicle for achieving the relaxation response and quieting ceaseless thinking. Choosing the appropriate music to achieve the desired outcome in the clinical setting is important, as individuals differ in their responses to the multitude of beats and rhythms. Music without words is preferred because listening to words forces the patient to listen to the message of the lyrics rather than attending to the voice of the guide. Musical sounds of nature, such as the sound of the ocean, can help achieve a deeper state of relaxation. Using music may facilitate the images deep within the patient's mind during a guided imagery session.

## Clinical Research

In the mid-70s, Carl and Stephanie Simonton published groundbreaking work outlining the use of relaxation and imagery interventions with patients who had cancer. The Simontons reported that those patients who participated in the relaxation and imagery sessions had double the survival time when compared with those who received standard protocols for chemotherapy and radiation treatments (Simonton, Simonton, & Creighton, 1978).

The health care community reluctantly became aware of the power of the mind-body connection and the meaningful part that patients can play in their own health and well-being. As a result, relaxation methods and guided imagery sessions are an integral part of cancer treatment in many oncology settings. The National Institute of Health (NIH), in 1995 after reviewing a series of studies, recommended that relaxation methods be included in the treatment of chronic pain and insomnia (Taylor, 1999).

A series of studies reviewed by Good (1996) on the effects of relaxation exercises and music on patients' response to postoperative pain showed that these interventions were most effective on the emotional nature of the pain experience. Patients reportedly were better able to cope with the pain (Good, 1996).

Sims (1987) reviewed the literature on how consistent relaxation practice is used to help people cope with cancer. Her findings suggest that patients with cancer who receive a relaxation intervention with a guide indicate an improvement in their quality of life and increased sense of well-being. She concluded, from her review, that studies involving a person-guided relaxation practice had positive results, while those in which an audiotaped relaxation instruction was given did not show as positive results. She also suggested that attention must be given to the environment in which the instruction is given. Her advice is to offer the relaxation intervention in a setting away from where the patient receives painful or other invasive treatments such as their chemotherapy or radiation (Sims, 1987).

In summary, the literature reviewed indicates positive results from offering relaxation and music as an interventions in palliative care. Variables that can influence outcomes of a relaxation and music or imagery session include:

- The presence of a guide, giving instruction to the patient
- Repeated sessions over time (the exact number has not been determined)
- Environment where the instruction is given
- The presence of a guide, facilitating the learning process for patients
- Selected music, facilitating relaxation or evoking images

## Methods

- Providing privacy: Be aware of distractions in the environment and minimize.

- Patient identifies problem or goal for imagery session.
- Positioning: Assist the patient to a comfortable position, either in bed or in a comfortable chair. Instruct the patient to scan their body to note areas of tension that may need special attention.
- Explain the intervention according to the selected method (explanation may be to family, partner, or other caregiver):
  - Time involved
  - Purpose
  - Body-mind connection
- Relaxation response is a process that is learned over time; practice on a daily basis is recommended.
- Complementary music or rhythm: Consider patient and family preference. Suggest music without words.
- Documentation: Document session according to the symptom or behavior assessed.
- Family and caregiver teaching: Can be given to family or partners with instructions on how and when to offer intervention.

### Precautions

Avoid in the following:
- Confused or psychotic patients

## ■ INTERVENTIONS
### Relaxation: Focusing on the Breath

Time: 2 to 3 minutes
Indications:
- Anticipatory anxiety
- Invasive and potentially painful procedures
- Wound care
- Preceding a massage or therapeutic touch intervention
Suggested Music: *White Rose* (harp music)

The practitioner (guide) coaches the patient, pausing after each statement allowing the patient to silently follow the voice of the guide:

> *"Close your eyes... Focus on the rhythm of the breath. Inhale to a count of 3; exhale to a count of 5. Repeat 5 times; complete the exercise by taking a full deep breath... Open your eyes."*

### Relaxation Method: Affirmations

Time: 5 to 7 minutes—for 10 days, practicing twice daily
Indications:
- Nausea
- Acute or chronic pain after medication

- Breathlessness (dyspnea)
- Fatigue

The practitioner or guide reads the script, pausing after each statement allowing the patient to repeat the statement silently (personal communication, Reagan, 1984):

*"I close my eyes and take a calming breath.*
*I empty my mind of all concern and worry.*
*As these leave my mind, I notice and let them go.*
*I let all thoughts flow like a river through my mind.*
*My mind empties and the cool river calms my body.*
*I allow my mind and body to rest.*
*I appreciate the rest and peace.*
*I take a slow and calming breath."*

## Progressive Muscle Relaxation (General Relaxation)

Time: 10 minutes. This can precede any of the exercises outlined; it is recommended to precede comeditation (see below) and guided imagery sessions.
Indications:
- Sleep disturbance
- Pain/muscular tension

Suggested music: *White Rose* (harp music)

The practitioner (guide) reads the script slowly, allowing the patient to sense the relaxation:

*"Focus your awareness on your feet, toes...*
*Letting the tension flow out the soles of your feet.*
*Slowly move your awareness to any tension in your calves... knees...*
*Letting go... and relaxing your calves and knees.*
*Now bring your awareness to your lower back, hip, and pelvis, relaxing...*
*And letting go of all tension, tightness... Now take two deep breaths...*
*Breathing slowly in and out... saying silently... 'I am relaxed...'*
*Moving your awareness to any tension in your stomach... middle of your back...*
*Repeating... 'I am relaxed...'*
*Focusing again on your breathing and notice how the breath moves through*
*your chest, your throat, your upper back and shoulders. Taking a deep, slow*
*breath and as you exhale, repeating: 'I am relaxed.'*
*Become aware of your jaw, mouth, eyes, ears, and the top of your head.*
*Noting tightness, soreness, and again silently repeating as you exhale.*
*'I am relaxed.'*
*Now scanning your entire body for any remaining tension or tightness.*
*And with a deep breath, exhaling with an audible 'Ahhhh.'"*

Sit silently with the patient noting their response to the exercise or proceed to Comeditation or Imagery.

## Comeditation or Shared Breathing (Boerstler & Kornfeld, 1995)

Time: Undetermined.

Indications:

- Anxiety
- Fear
- Hopelessness
- Preparing for death
- Impending death

Suggested music: Chants (Gregorian or Tibetan) or *Harp Realm*

The practitioner (guide) communicates to the patient:

> *"There is nothing you have to do except listen carefully to my voice and follow your own breathing.*
> *Begin by taking a deep breath, and as you exhale say 'A-ha.'"* (Make sure the words follow the rhythm of the patient's exhalation.)
> *"This is the great sound of letting go, of clearing and calming the mind."* (Count from 10 to 1, each number synchronized to the exhalation of the patient.)
> *"As we count, visualize the numbers—clear and white—going out over your feet into the horizon.*
> *Thinking is not necessary, just focus on each number."*
> *(Occasionally interject phrases such as "breathing and counting," "clear mind," and "peaceful heart.")*
> *If the patient falls asleep, the guide continues with the pace of the exhalations, repeating on the exhalation: "Sleep is O.K."; "You are safe and loved."*
> *Observing the patient's deeper state of relaxation, continue:*
> *"Imagine you are moving toward a vast, boundless ocean of light.*
> *Picture yourself in the center of light.*
> *As you exhale merge with the light.*
> *There is the light and only the light."*

Close the exercise with words, prayers, or mantras that the patient/family has chosen. If the patient and family have not selected personal words, the guide silently releases the experience to the spiritual light of the soul always residing within the patient (Boestler, as cited in Miller, 1991).

## Moving into the Light

Time: Undetermined (Levine, as cited in Achterberg, Dossey, & Kolkmeier, 1994).

Indications:

- Preparation for death
- Impending death

Suggested music: Therese Shroeder-Sheker's *Chalice of Repose Rosa Mystica* or a selection of the patient or family

The practitioner (guide) communicates to the patient:

*"Fill yourself with an awareness of the brilliance of a clear blue white light.*
*This light is pure and it surrounds you and helps you move forward.*
*As you move forward, release anything that you may see as holding you—*
*keeping you from moving into the vastness of the light.*
*Letting go of all fears, releasing those you love, knowing they will be comforted*
*and cared for.*
*What is called death has arrived and you are not alone—many have gone*
*before you.*
*Letting yourself go—moving into the clear blue white light."* (Levine, as cited
in Achterberg et al., 1994, p. 308)

Close by sitting quietly with the patient, observing changes in patient's
demeanor.

## ■ GUIDED IMAGERY

Guided imagery sessions may be offered by any APN, social worker, or chaplain who offers evidence of advanced instruction and practice in guided imagery and altered states of awareness. The patient, prior to the session, must
agree upon the purpose of the imagery session. Symbolic imagery, as described in the next section, is a collection of self-images or beliefs that are
stored deep within the unconscious and influence the behavior, emotions,
and attitude of the individual. The goal of the session is to facilitate the patient's conscious awareness of how unconscious beliefs, symbols, and fears
can influence the problem he or she has identified to address in the imagery
session.

### Critical Elements
- Mental images (symbols) are stored in the mind and can affect the body,
  mind, and spirit.
- Mental images (symbols) can be changed through active imagination
  and a relaxed altered state of awareness.
- The active imagination is an internal experience and is connected
  through our senses (e.g., sight, smell, touch, taste, hearing).
- The active imagination can be accessed to change symbols of increased
  anxiety and fear into symbols of empowerment, hope, and peace.
Time: 30 to 45 minutes.
### Indications:
- Preparation for invasive treatments, radiation therapy, or chemotherapy
- Spiritual distress
- Unresolved psychologic issues
- Anxiety
- Chronic pain
- Hopelessness
- Powerlessness

Suggested music: *Echoes of Angels*

The following is an example of symbolic imagery and should be preceded by a general relaxation session as outlined previously.

> *"Give yourself permission to become relaxed, going deeper into the innermost part of your imagination. Observe yourself walking down a long hallway in a familiar place.*
>
> *There are many doors. All the doors are closed. Give yourself permission to open one of the doors, knowing that you are safe and you are not alone."*

(Observe the patient's forehead—eyelids remaining closed and relaxed.)

> *"As you enter this room, you notice the familiar furnishings, lighting, and comfortable chairs. Observe yourself finding the most inviting spot in the room and making yourself comfortable. You remember that part of you that has experienced _____ ." (Supply the word that describes the patient's prominent symptom).*

The following is an example of imagery for a patient experiencing pain:

> *"Observe yourself when the pain is most severe. Describe the intensity. What emotion are you sensing when experiencing this pain ... fear? Loneliness? Anger? Is there an image that comes into your awareness?*
>
> *Can you remember a time when you experienced a similar emotion? Where were you? Who was there with you?"*

At this point the patient may remember painful past experiences where resentment and fear reside. Explores these issues and their meaning further at a deeper level and continue as follows:

> *"If you were to name a color that represents your pain what would that color be? What about the shape of the pain . . . round? Jagged? What about size . . . Large? Medium? Small? What about texture . . . hard? Rough? Soft? What about . . . smell? Taste? Sound?*
>
> *Observe this pain that you describe as separate from you, _____ (supply patient's name). What is the pain saying to you? Do you recognize the voice of the pain? Is it someone or something you know?*
>
> *Say whatever you want to the pain, remembering what the pain feels, smells, looks like."*

Help the patient create a metaphor, such as "a stone stuck in mud" or "a snake in a cage."

For example, the patient states: "My pain is like a snake in a cage." You may ask: "Who has the key?" "How can you get the key?" and so on.

Continuing:

> *"Remembering the part of you that is powerful, wise, and creative, know that you are in charge of the pain. Does it change your description of the pain? The size, smell, shape, or color?"*

(This helps the patient create a positive image of being in control and in charge of the pain experience.)

*"As you see yourself in charge of the pain, remember that you may access this image at any time during the day or night."* (Validate the image by reviewing the metaphors the patient has described.)

Closing the session:

*"Observe yourself leaving this room, walking slowly and relaxed toward the door and walking down the hallway. Become aware of your breathing—inhaling, exhaling—become totally aware of your body: where you are sitting, the sounds in this room, being present to this time and place"* (personal experience, Lane, 1987).

The practitioner can sit silently for a moment before discussing this experience with the patient. The imagery session is the patient's way of communicating unfulfilled wishes or irrational fears. The practitioner seizes the opportunity to explore, in depth, the meaning of the symbols through metaphors. The cage, as described in the preceding section, may mean that the patient is feeling powerless and helpless. The practitioner may suggest to the patient that he or she possesses the key to unlock the door to the cage. The "key" becomes the metaphor for a deeper exploration into the unconscious realms of the patient's psyche. In this altered state of awareness, a patient's innate strength and courage may be revealed. The role of the practitioner is to guide the patient to change the symbols of powerlessness to symbols of control—of pain and or any related symptoms that the patient has identified.

Guided imagery sessions are of maximum benefit to the patient early in the course of an illness or treatment. Images and symbols of hope and empowerment can be retained in the mind although the patient's journey through treatment of advancing disease may result in increased stress.

## ■ SUMMARY

The APN can initiate interest among colleagues, review literature, and design practice protocols for offering complementary therapies as options for care. It is through this process that questions regarding the efficacy and benefits of complementary therapies can be explored and evaluated. As outlined in this chapter, many complementary therapies are being investigated and have demonstrated effectiveness as interventions in pain and symptom management. The APN can be an advocate for establishing evidence-based protocols and evaluating complementary therapies in promoting relaxation and a decrease in symptoms in palliative care. Including qualitative methods and quantifiable data, the APN can illustrate how complementary therapies help patients cope with continual change and suffering. Healing—becoming whole in body, mind, and spirit—may eventually be the experience of patients in the journey with a life-limiting disease.

## ■ RESOURCES

### Journals

*Alternative/Complementary Therapies in Health and Medicine*—A bimonthly publication for health care professionals which reviews a wide range of alternative therapies.
(800) M-LIEBERT
infor@liebertpub.com

*Aromatherapy Today Journal*—A quarterly international professional journal from Australia. Health care professionals offer advice and outlines for use of essential oils in health care services in Australia and New Zealand.
http://www.hawknet.com.au/-jkerr
jkerr@haawknet.com.au

*International Journal of Aromatherapy*—A bimonthly journal with a focus on research in aromatherapy in Europe.
http://www.harcourt-international.com/journals/ijar

*Massage*—A monthly journal offering a comprehensive overview of massage as a therapy as well as other touch healing modalities.
(800) 533-4263
http://www.massagemag.com

### Videotape Resources

Stratos Institute for Healthcare Performance (1999). *Complementary therapy: Options for your patients.* Oncology Nursing Today—Educational Video Series. Laguna Niguel, CA: Author.
(949) 249-2885
Institute@home.com

### Professional Organizations

American Holistic Nurses Association (AHNO)
Flagstaff, AZ 86003-2130
http://www.AHNA.org
National organization that emphasizes the concepts of holism in the caring practice of nursing.

National Hospice and Palliative Care Organization (NHPCO)
Alexandria, VA 22314
http://www.nhpco.org
National organization that addresses the education, practice, and political needs of all interdisciplinary professionals in hospice and palliative care settings.

Nurse Healers–Professional Associates International, Inc. (NHPA)
3760 S Highland Dr. #429
Salt Lake City, UT 84106
http://www.therapeutic-touch.org
nh-pai@therapuetic-touch.org
Official organization of therapeutic touch practitioners. Membership offers a variety of benefits, including an extensive database of references on therapeutic touch. An informative newsletter, as well as beginning, intermediate, and advanced classes and intensives are offered throughout the United States and Canada.

Therapeutic Touch Networks of Canada
http://www.therapeutictouchnetwk.com
Professional organization of therapeutic touch in Canada, which offers the outstanding newsletter *In Touch,* conferences, and classes.

National Association for Holistic Aromatherapy
Seattle, WA
http://www.naha.org
Membership includes a newsletter and professional directory. Excellent conferences and trade shows, biannually.

The Canadian Federation of Aromatherapists
Toronto, Ontario, Canada
(888) 578-7815
cica@aromachoppe.com
Excellent international conferences and trade shows.

## Internet

Center for Mind-Body Medicine
http://www.cmbm.org/

International Center for Reiki Training
http://www.reiki.org

American Holistic Nurses Association (AHNA)
http://www.ahna.org

Academy of Guided Imagery
http://www.healthy.net/agi/

Guided Imagery Resource Center
http://www.healthjourneys.com/

International Association of Interactive Imagery
http://www.iaii.org/

## Suggested Music (Compact Discs)

White Rose; harp music. Christina Touring with Kim Robertson and William Jackson. Emerald Harp Productions.

Echoes of Angels; harp and chorus. Christina Tourin. Dedicated to the Memory of Princess Diana of Wales: Emerald Harp Productions. Contains Canon in D, Pachelbel.

Prelude in C. Bach. Available from: Int'l Society of Folk Harpers and Craftsmen, Inc., 14641 Gladebrook Dr. #10, Houston, TX 77068, (281) 469-7885, melody@neosoft.com. Catalogue available.

Rosa Mystica; harp music. Therese Schroeder-Sheker, Celestial Harmonies. Used in palliative/hospice care settings. Available from: Celestial Harmonies, PO Box 30122, Tucson, AZ 85751.

**Chants:**

Shri Ram, On Wings of Song and Robert Gass. Spring Hill Music; a Sanskrit chant which is a synthesis of Eastern and Western influences. Available from: Spring Hill Music, PO Box 800 Boulder, CO 80306. Free catalogue of inspirational music.

Chant. Benedictine Monks of Santo Domingo De Silos. Angel Records; authentic Gregorian chants from the monastery at Santo Domingo de Silos, Spain. Available from major record stores in the USA and Canada.

Gregorian Chants for all Seasons. Choir of the Vienna Hofburgkapele, Josef Schabasser. Vox Box. Classic Gregorian chants. Available from major record stores in the USA and Canada.

An English Ladymass, medieval chant and polyphony. Anonymous 4. Harmonia mundi 13th and 14th Century chant and polyphony in honor of the Virgin Mary. Available from major record stores in the USA and Canada.

Hildegard of Bingen, The Harmony of Heaven. Ellen Oak. Bison Tales Production. Hildegard of Bingen (1098-1179 AD). Poetress, herbalist, and medieval saint composer of inspiration musical sonnets, expressed in the melodious voice of Ellen Oak. Available from major record stores in the USA and Canada.

Hildegard Von Bingen, Symphoniae Geistliche Gesange/Spiritual Song. Sequentia. Harmonia Mundi. Melodious chants from the songs and sonnets of Hildegard of Bingen. Available from major record stores in the USA and Canada.

The Sacred Chorde. Steven Halpern and Fabien Maman; a variety of extraordinary instruments along with piano, blendings sounds of different cultures. Steven Halpern has many arrangements suitable for palliative care settings. Available from: White Swan, 4730 Table Mesa Drive, Ste. E., Boulder, CO 80303, www.stevenhalpern.com. Free catalogue.

Way of the Ocean. Medwyn Goddall. Dolphins and Orca whales sing among the waves along with sounds of the guitar, flute, and keyboard. Available from: White Swan, 4730 Table Mesa Drive, Ste. E., Boulder, CO 80303, www.stevenhalpern.com. Free catalogue.

Medicine Wheel. On wings of Song and Robert Gass; with Native American musicians. Available from: Spring Hill Music, PO Box 800, Boulder, CO 80306.

## Resources for Essential Oils and Diffusers

Amrita Aromatherapy
Fairfield, Iowa
(800) 410-9651

Over 140 therapeutic quality essential oils, personally tested by Christoph Streicher, PhD (physiology and biochemistry); OSHA guidelines, MSDS and catalogue available.

Aromatic Arts
Colorado
(888) 282-2002
http://www.aroma-rn.com
larainek@qwest.net

Laraine Kyle, MSN, RN, CMT has formulated quality oils for use in hospital and long-term care settings; MSDS available.

AromaTherapy International
Michigan
(800) 722-4377
eurolink@umich.edu

Awarded "quality of certification" by the Scientific Institute of Aromatherapy, France; wide range of products including diffusers, books, and journals. Free catalogue.

AromaTherapy Market
New York
http://www.aromatherapy.net

Free catalogue. Offers classes for using essential oils with massage. Sponsor of seminars by Gabriel Mojay, well known in the United Kingdom and Europe for his innovative use of essential oils with principles and practices of traditional Chinese medicine.

Essential Air Diffusers
Available from Leyden House
www.leydenhouse.com
(800) 754-0668

Diffusers that meet safety standards for inpatient settings.

Fragrant Earth Essential Oils
http://www.fragrant-earth.com
all-enquiries@fragrant-earth.com
United States Distributor: Jade Shutes, located in Washington
jades@accessone.com

Quality oils formulated and tested by Jan Kusmirek, a well-known chemist in the United Kingdom. Excellent correspondence course on Aromatherapy and Essential Oils.

Florial

www.florial.com

United States Distributor: Geraldine Zelinsky, located in Shreveport, LA

zelin19@idt.net

Mostly quality organic oils created specifically for herbal medicine and aromatherapy. MSDS available.

Vié Arome

www.viearome.com

Formulas available at Cheryl's Herbs

(800) 231-5971

infor@cherylsherbs.com

Formulated by Nelly Grosjean, French Doctor of Naturopathy.

## References

BENSON, H. (1984). *Beyond the relaxation response.* New York: Berkeley Books.

GANONG, W. (1987). *Review of medical physiology* (13th ed.). Norwalk, CT: Appleton & Lange.

JONES, W. (1998). Alternative medicine: Learning from the past, examining the present, advancing to the future (editorial). *Journal of the American Medical Association, 280,* 1617.

McCAFFERY, M., Beebe, A. (1989). *Pain: Clinical manual for nursing management.* St. Louis: C. V. Mosby.

NATIONAL Hospice and Palliative Care Organization (NHPCO) (2001). *Complementary therapies in end-of-life care.* Alexandria, VA: Author.

PERT, C. (1997). *Molecules of emotion.* New York: Scribner.

WALLACE, K., & Benson, H. (1972). The physiology of meditation. *Scientific American, 226,* 84-90.

## Aromatherapy

Bassett, I., Pannowitz, D., & Barnetson R. (1990). A comparative study of tea tree oil versus benzoyl peroxide in the treatment of acne. *Medical Journal of Australia, 153,* 455-458.

Belaiche, P. (1985). Treatment of vaginal infections of *Candida albicans* with the essential oil of *Melaleuca alternifolia. Phytotherapy, 15,* 13-15.

Buchbauer, G., Jirovetz, I., Jager, W., Dietrich H., & Plank, C. (1991). Aromatherapy: Evidence for sedative effects of the essential oil of lavender after inhalation. *Z Naturforsch, C-46,* 1067-1072.

Buckle, J. (1993). Aromatherapy: Does it matter which lavender oil is used? *Nursing Times, 89,* 32-35.

Cannard, G. (1995). On the scent of a good night's sleep. *Nursing Standard, 9,* 21.

Carson, C. (1998). Antimicrobial activity of tea tree oil: Essential oil against skin microorganisms. In J. Hoard, & V. Gough (Eds.), *Proceedings of World of Aromatherapy II, International Conference* (September 25-28, 1998), St. Louis: National Association for Holistic Aromatherapy, Inc. Complementary Medicine Series (1994). *Nursing Times, 90,* 3-7.

Corner, J., Cawley, N., & Hildebrand, S. (1995). An evaluation of the use of essential oils on the well-being of cancer patients. *International Journal of Palliative Nursing, 1,* 67-73.

Dunn, C., Sleep, J., & Collett, D. (1995). Sensing an improvement: An experimental study to evaluate the use of aromatherapy, massage, and periods of rest in an intensive care unit. *Journal of Advanced Nursing, 21,* 34-40.

Frankincense and Myrrh—History (1997, December). *International Journal of Alternative and Complementary Medicine, 15* (12); 16-18.

Gattefosse, R. M. (1995). *Gattefosse's aromatherapy* (1st ed. translation). Saffron Walden, Essex, England: C. W. Daniel (Original work published, 1937).

Greer, S. (1994). Psycho-oncology: Its aims, achievements and future tasks. *Psycho-oncology, 1,* 87-101

Guillemain, J., Rousseau, A., & Delaveau, P. (1989). Neurodepressive effects of the essential oil of *Lavandula angustifolia. Annals Pharmaceutical of France, 47,* 337-343.

Hardy, M., Kirk-Smith, M., & Stretch, D. (1995). Replacement of drug treatment for insomnia by ambient odour. *Lancet, 346,* 701.

Hudson, R. (1996). The value of lavender for rest and activity in the elderly patient. *Complementary Therapies in Medicine, 4,* 52-57.

Jager, W., Buchbauer, G., Jirovetz, L., & Fritzer, M. (1992). *Journal of Social Cosmetic Chemistry, 43,* 49-54.

Kerr, J. (1998). Essential oil profile... lavenders. *Aromatherapy Today, 8,* 12-17.

Kyle, L. (November, 2000). End-of-life care with aromatherapy. In K. A. Schnaubelt (Ed.), *Essential oils and cancer,* Pacific Institute of Aromatherapy Conference Proceedings, San Francisco, 181-189.

Mailhebiau, P. (1995). *Portraits in oils.* (Susan Y. Chalkley. Trans.) Saffron Walden, Essex, England: C. W. Daniel Co. (Original work published, 1995).

Maury, M. (1995). *The secret of life and beauty.* (McDonald and Co. Trans.) Saffron Walden, Essex, England: C. W. Daniel Co. (Original work published, 1961).

Maxwell-Hudson, C. (1988). *The complete book of massage.* New York: Random House.

Mojay, G. (1996). *Aromatherapy for healing the spirit.* London: Gaia Books, Ltd.

Psalms 23:5. *The Holy Bible* (King James version). New York: Oxford University Press.

Rayman, D. (1991). *Aromatherapy: The complete guide to plant and flower essences for health and beauty.* London: Bantam Books.

Rose, J. (1992). *The aromatherapy book: Applications and inhalations.* Berkeley, CA: North Atlantic Books.

Rose, J. (1999). *375 essential oils and hydrosols.* Berkeley, CA: Frog, Ltd.

Schnaubelt, K. (1998). *Advanced aromatherapy: The science of essential oil therapy.* (J. Michael Beasley. Trans.) Rochester, Vermont: Healing Arts Press. (Original work published, 1995.)

Stevenson, C. (1994). The psychophysiological effects of aromatherapy massage following cardiac surgery. *Complementary Therapies in Medicine, 2,* 27-37.

Tisserand, R. (1988). *Aromatherapy to heal and tend the body.* Wilmot, WI: Lotus Press.

Valnet, J. (1990). *The practice of aromatherapy.* (C. W. Daniel Co. Ltd. Trans.). Rochester, Vermont: Healing Arts Press. (Original work published, 1982.)

Wilkinson, S. (1995). Aromatherapy and massage in palliative care. *International Journal of Palliative Nursing, 1,* 21-30.

## Energy Balancing Therapies

Burmeister, A. (1997). *The touch of healing.* New York, NY: Bantam Books.

Complementary Therapies Workgroup (1997). *The procedure of performing therapeutic touch: Krieger and Kunz Method.* Massachusetts General Hospital, Department of Nursing, Protocol for the Practice of Therapeutic Touch.

Fanslow-Brunjes, C. (1999). *The hand-heart connection.* Cited in Versagi, C. Hands of peace. *Massage Magazine, 82*(November, December), 73.

Gagne, D., & Toye, R. C. (1994). The effects of therapeutic touch and relaxation therapy in reducing anxiety. *Archives Psychiatric Nursing 8,* 184-189.

Healing Touch, Level 1, Notebook (2000). Colorado Center for Healing Touch, Inc. Lakewood, CA. http://www.healingtouch.net

Heidt, P. (1990). Helping patients to rest: Clinical studies in therapeutic touch. *Holistic Nursing Practice, 5,* 57-66.

Kaptchuk, T. J. (1983). *The web that has no weaver: Understanding Chinese medicine.* New York: Congdon/Weed.

Keller, E., & Bzdek, V. M. (1986). Effects of therapeutic touch on tension headache pain. *Nursing Research, 35,* 101-106.

Krieger, D. (1997). *Therapeutic touch, inner workbook.* Santa Fe, NM: Bear & Company.

Lad, V. (1984). *Ayurveda: The science of self-healing.* Wilmot, WI: Lotus Press.

Macrae, J. (1994). *Therapeutic touch: A practical guide.* New York: Alfred A. Knopf.

Matsumoto, K., & Birch, S. (1986*). Extraordinary vessels.* Brookline, MA: Paradigm.

Mast, M. E. (1998). Office of Alternative Medicine supports research to evaluate effectiveness, safety, and cost of alternative and complementary treatments. *ONS News, 13,* 9.

Nurse Healers-Professional Associates International (1992). Therapeutic touch, teaching guidelines: Beginners' level. Salt Lake City, UT: Author. www.therapeutic-touch.org; nh-pai@therapeutic-touch.org

Quinn, J. F. (1989). Therapeutic touch, an energy exchange: Replication and extension. *Nursing Science Quarterly, 2,* 74-78.

Samarel, N. (1992). The experience of receiving therapeutic touch. *Journal of Advanced Nursing, 17,* 651-657.

Simington, J. A. & Laing, O. P. (1993). Effects of therapeutic touch on anxiety in the institutionalized elderly. *Clinical Nursing Research, 2,* 438-450.

Stein, D. (1995*). Essential Reiki: A complete guide to an ancient healing art.* Freedom, CA: Crossing Press.

Teegarten, I. (1978). *Acupressure: A way of health—Jin Shin Do.* Tokyo, Japan: Japan Publications.

## Relaxation, Breathing, Music, and Guided Imagery

Achterberg, J., Dossey, B., & Kolkmeier, L. (1994). *Rituals of healing: Using imagery for health and wellness.* New York: Bantam Books.

Boerstler, R. W., Kornfeld, H. S. (1995). *Life to death: Harmonizing the transition.* Rochester, VT: Healing Arts Press.

Good, M. (1996). Effects of relaxation and music on postoperative pain: A review. *Journal of Advanced Nursing, 24,* 905-914.

Guzzetta, C. E. ( 1991). Music therapy: Nursing the music of the soul. In
    D. Campbell (Ed.), *Music: Physician for times to come* (pp. 146-166). Wheaton, IL:
    Quest Books.
Kolcaba, K., & Fox, C. (1999). The effects of guided imagery on comfort of women
    with early-stage breast cancer undergoing radiation therapy. *Oncology Nursing
    Forum, 26*(1), 67-72.
Kolkmeier, L. G. (1995). Relaxation: Opening the door to change. In B. Dossey,
    L. Keegan, C. Guzzetta, & L. Kolkmeier (Eds.), *Holistic nursing: A handbook for
    practice* (2nd ed.) (pp. 523-560). Gaithersburg, MD: Aspen.
Krieger, D. (1998). *Therapeutic touch: Inner workbook.* Santa Fe, NM: Bear & Co.
Lane, S. (1994). *Inner visions: A guide to physical and spiritual healing.* Laguna Niguel,
    CA: Author.
Miller, O. (1991). A sharing of breaths: An Eastern approach to illness and dying.
    *QUEST,* Autumn, 65-69.
Simonton, C., Simonton, S., & Creighton, J. (1978). *Getting well again.* Los Angeles:
    Tarcher.
Sims, S. (1987). Relaxation training as a technique for helping patients cope with
    the experience of cancer: A selective review of the literature. *Journal of Advanced
    Nursing, 12,* 583-591.
Taylor, A. G. (1999). Complementary/alternative therapies in the treatment of pain.
    In J. Spencer, & J. Jacobs (Eds.), *Complementary/alternative medicine: Evidence-based
    approach* (Chapter 10). Brookline, MA: Redwing Books.

## Suggested Readings

Achterberg, J. Dossey, B., & Kolkmeier, L. (1994). *Rituals of healing: Using imagery for
    health and wellness.* New York: Bantam Books. (Outlines the use of imagery for
    various medical conditions, including a special section on assisting in the death
    ritual.)
Benson, H. (1984). *Beyond the relaxation response.* New York: Berkley Books. (An
    informative and instructive review of Benson's lifelong research of the
    "relaxation response" and its effect on the well-being of individuals.)
Buckle, J. (1997). *Clinical aromatherapy in nursing practice.* San Diego: Singular Press.
    (English RN who outlines how to use essential oils in a variety of clinical
    settings.)
Campbell, D. (1991). *Music: Physician for times to come.* Wheaton, IL: Quest Books.
    (Excellent reference material that offers the reader an overview of the benefits of
    music on various emotional states of mind.)
Cooksley, V. G. (1996). *Aromatherapy: A lifetime guide to healing with essential oils.*
    Paramus, NJ: Prentice Hall. (Excellent resource for health care personal
    addressing common problems in health care; Written by an RN.)
Dossey, B., Keegan, L., Guzzetta, C., & Kolkmeier, L. G. (1998). *Holistic nursing: A
    handbook for practice* (3rd ed.). Gaithersburg, MD: Aspen. (Four nursing leaders
    articulately describe how to integrate alternative and complementary therapies
    in traditional nursing practice.)
Dossey, B., Keegan, L., & Guzzetta, C. (1995). *The art of caring: Holistic healing with
    relaxation, imagery, music, and touch.* Gaithersburg, MD: Aspen.

Ferrell, B., & Coyle, N. (Eds.) (2001). *Textbook of palliative nursing.* New York: Oxford University Press. (The first published text on palliative care nursing. Chapter 27 outlines select complementary therapies and how they can be used in palliative care settings.)

Hoffman, J. (1995). *Rhythmic medicine: Music with a purpose.* Leawood, KS: Macmillan Press. (A self-help book toward understanding the vast benefits of music therapy.)

Lawless, J. (1995). *The illustrated encyclopedia of essential oils.* Rockport, MA: Element Books. (A beginner's guide to understanding the history and use of essential oils today. Illustrations are remarkable and artistic.)

Matzo-LaPorte, M., Sherman, D. W. (Eds.) (2001). *Palliative care nursing: Quality of life to the end of life.* New York: Springer Publishing. (Outlines the 21 nursing competencies for nursing in end-of-life care and includes a comprehensive chapter on complementary therapies.)

Mojay, G. (1996). *Aromatherapy for healing the spirit: A guide to restoring emotional and mental balance through essential oils.* London: Henry Holt. (A beautifully illustrated guide for the use of essential oils along acupuncture energy channels in the body. The only book which discusses the relationship between these two systems of healing. Available from the Aromatherapy Market, 501 S. Meadow Street, Ithaca, NY 14850, 607-277-0440.)

Rose, J. (1992). *The aromatherapy book: Applications and inhalations.* Berkeley, CA: North Atlantic Books. (Descriptive and illustrative ways to apply essential oils. Contains extensive glossary of terms and descriptions of essential oils. Lists resources by state for books, essential oils, and courses on aromatherapy.)

Rose, J. (1999). *375 essential oils and hydrosols.* Berkeley, CA: Frog, Ltd. (A definitive outline of the botanical origins of plants, oils, and their uses.)

Storr, A. (1992). *Music and the mind.* New York: Ballantine Books. (Written by a psychiatrist who takes an in-depth look at why music has such a profound effect on the mind, heart, and soul.)

# CHAPTER 7

# *Psychosocial and Spiritual Care*

DIANE B. LOSETH

C are for the patient at the end of life must extend beyond alleviation of physical symptoms to include emotional or psychologic needs, social needs, and spiritual needs. As nurses, we are taught to care for the whole person, but often we are not given the skills to deal with all of these dimensions. The goal of this chapter is to review the psychologic, social, and spiritual dimensions of care at the end of life.

## ■ PSYCHOLOGIC NEEDS AT THE END OF LIFE

Patients at the end of life may experience a variety of psychologic symptoms such as sadness, grief, depression, or anxiety. These can be normal reactions to a stressful situation, which may become pathologic. For instance, it may be normal for patients to feel sad as they move toward the end of their lives, but if that sadness becomes all consuming, it may require further assessment and intervention. The feelings of sadness may be a result of all the losses for the dying patient. Often the losses are sequential, one loss after another, though sometimes they occur simultaneously. Patients may no longer have the energy to work outside the home or enjoy their hobbies or other interests. They may find it difficult to concentrate due to physical symptoms or to feelings of anxiety or depression. They may feel sad about missing future events. As the disease progresses, adjustments in patients' routines will occur. It is important for the advanced practice nurse (APN) to anticipate these changes and the potential for feelings of sadness and the needs of patients to grieve over the losses.

### Depression

Depression should not be mistaken for sadness. Studies of depression in the terminally ill are few, but the prevalence is as high as 58% in patients dying of cancer (Breitbart, Breura, Chochinov, & Lynch, 1995; Chochinov, Wilson, Enns, & Lander, 1994; Wilson, Chochinov, de Faye, & Breitbart, 2000). The actual prevalence may be higher, due to the failure of physicians and nurses to recognize depression in their patients (Hardman, Maguire, & Crowther, 1989; McDonald et al., 1999; Passik et al., 1998). Knowledge deficits, placing a low priority on psychologic symptoms, time constraints, and fears of polypharmacy and adverse reactions from psychiatric medications are all factors in depression being underdiagnosed and undertreated (Block, 2000; Wilson et al., 2000).

In addition, depression may manifest as uncontrolled or poorly controlled symptoms. Uncontrolled pain may cause patients to feel that life is not worth living and lead them to express suicidal thoughts (Ciaramella & Poli, 2001). With adequate relief of the pain, depression and suicidal thoughts often subside (Roth & Breitbart, 1996). A study of cancer patients with and without breakthrough pain found that those who experience episodes of breakthrough pain during the day or night have higher levels of depression overall (Portenoy, Payne, & Jacobsen, 1999). Knowledge of this fact may encourage earlier assessment and appropriate interventions.

As reviewed, the *Diagnostic and Statistical Manual of Mental Disorders, Fourth Edition (DSM-IV)* criteria for depression may not be useful at the end of life. Dying patients normally experience weight loss, loss of energy, loss of appetite, and changes in sleeping patterns. Further, it is natural to have thoughts about death as death approaches. Therefore, it is often necessary to use other criteria for assessing depression in dying patients. Endicott (1984) identified four symptoms that replace the physical symptoms above. They are:
- Depressed appearance
- Social withdrawal or decreased talkativeness
- Brooding or pessimism
- Lack of reactivity

In place of the vegetative symptoms, Roth & Breitbart (1996) have suggested feelings of helplessness, hopelessness, worthlessness, guilt, and suicidal ideation as better indicators of depression in the terminally ill. Formal tools to screen for depression are reviewed in Chapter 22. However, patients who are debilitated at the end of life may not be able to tolerate long screening questionnaires.

One simple tool that may be more appropriate at the end of life, the "Distress Thermometer," is based on the visual analog scale that is used to assess pain. The thermometer is a vertical scale of 0 to 10 with word anchors of no distress at 0, moderate distress at 5 and extreme distress at 10. Even though this is a global scale, not specific to depression, it is useful. Prostate patients who scored ≥5 on the distress thermometer in a study were then referred to psychiatry for further evaluation (Roth et al., 1998). Chochinov et al. (1997) simply ask "are you depressed?" and found this one question just as effective as the formal screening tools.

## Anxiety

Anxiety is another psychologic symptom that dying patients may experience. Three types of anxiety have been identified. The first type, reactive anxiety, includes adjustment disorders related to having a diagnosis such as cancer or the realization that the disease has reached a terminal stage. The second type of anxiety is seen in those patients with a preexisting anxiety disorder, such as generalized anxiety, panic, phobias, or posttraumatic stress disorder (Massie & Holland, 1992; Payne & Massie, 2000). Patients with preexisting anxiety or panic may worsen as the end of life approaches (Payne & Massie, 2000). With the third type, patients have feelings of anxiety related to a medical illness, which may present as uncontrolled symptoms, such as pain or dyspnea, side effects from medications, and certain medical conditions (Massie & Holland, 1992; Payne & Massie, 2000). For this type of anxiety, the underlying cause should be aggressively treated before anxiolytics are initiated. While anxiety experienced by the patient in pain may resolve with appropriate treatment of the pain, there is evidence that certain types of pain cause higher levels of anxiety. In the study mentioned above on breakthrough pain, the authors also found that those with breakthrough pain had more anxiety overall than those without it (Portenoy et al., 1999). The APN should know that even with adequate pain management, these patients with breakthrough pain may require treatment of their anxiety. Treatment can be initiated earlier if the APN knows that these patients are at a higher risk for anxiety. (See Chapter 16 for detailed discussion of assessment and interventions for anxiety.)

## Concerns and Worries

Terminally ill patients have many concerns, worries, and fears. In fact, worrying was ranked as the second most prevalent symptom in a study of almost 300 cancer patients. Over half of those patients had metastatic disease (Portenoy et al., 1994). By the time curative therapies are no longer effective, the patient or family may have heard, "there's nothing more we can do for you." This statement in and of itself is quite distressing to patients and families. What they usually feel is a sense of abandonment by the health care team. Abandonment or isolation by their family and friends is only one of a number of fears patients express. A study by Heaven and Maguire (1998) elicited the concerns of 87 hospice patients. The average score was 6.5 concerns per patient, and those expressing a higher number of concerns had greater psychologic distress. The five most common concerns were: loss of independence, worries about their family, concerns about physical problems other than pain, pain, and feeling like they are a burden. The patients also completed anxiety and depression scales. Those who scored high on the anxiety scale were found to have concerns about physical symptoms, while those who scored high on the depression scale expressed concerns about losses. Of the 562 concerns disclosed, 385 were rated by the patients for degree of importance, in terms of small, medium, large, and biggest concern. Cancer's impact on daily life, appearance, and pain were rated as being the biggest concerns.

Another study, investigating the defining characteristics of a good death, identified six major components. Most health care providers, patients, and families worried about dying in pain. Adequate pain management in the present and in the future were also concerns. Two other needs identified were participating in decision making and understanding what to expect in the dying process. The final three themes of a good death were related to completion issues, being able to contribute to others, and being affirmed as a whole person (Steinhauser et al., 2000).

Understanding the worries, fears, and concerns patients may experience will give the APN an opportunity to attend to and inquire about these issues. Some patients may fear pain at the end of life, while others may fear the idea of being incontinent or being dependent on others for physical care. Others fear losing the ability to think clearly. Simply asking the patient, "What do you fear most?" or "What worries you the most?" can allow the patient to express his or her fears. In addition, if the patient isn't forthcoming, stating some of the common fears out loud gives credence and a voice to the fear the patient may have but is reluctant to admit. By starting the conversation, the patient is given the opportunity to respond without having to initiate this type of discussion. It is important for the clinician to be able to anticipate these concerns, discuss them, and allay the patient's fears and concerns.

## Physician-Assisted Suicide

It is beyond the scope of this chapter to discuss physician-assisted suicide (PAS) in detail, yet as an APN you most likely will have to confront this at some point in your care of dying patients, because patients and families may want to discuss this difficult issue. *Active euthanasia* means to directly, with intent, cause the death of a patient by administering a lethal dose of a medication; *assisted suicide* refers to patients wishing to end their lives with the assistance of another. This assistance could include simply providing information on committing suicide, being present with the patient during suicide, or even providing the means to end the patient's life (Supanich, Brody, & Ogle, 1998). Euthanasia is not the withholding of nutrition or fluids in dying patients at their request. It is not the administration of enough opioids for pain or dyspnea management in dying patients who are hypotensive. It is not sedating a dying patient for management of other symptoms, such as anxiety, agitation, or delirium (Coyle, 1992).

It is clear that uncontrolled symptoms such as pain or dyspnea can cause a patient to feel depressed and even consider suicide. Uncontrolled symptoms are not the only factors that influence a request for hastened death or PAS. McDonald et al. (2000) identified patients at risk as those with a poor prognosis (advancing illness), uncontrolled symptoms (e.g., pain, depression, delirium), exhaustion, a lack of social support, and feelings of hopelessness/helplessness. In addition, loss of control, perceived loss of dignity, loss of purpose and meaning in life, and preexisting psychopathology were also factors.

In a study of 988 terminally ill patients throughout the United States, 60% would consider PAS in a hypothetical situation, while 10% had personally thought about PAS. Finally, 3% had actually discussed PAS with family, friends, or health care providers. Those who were African-American, older than 65, religious, or felt appreciated were less likely to endorse PAS. Those patients who endorsed PAS had more pain, more caregiver needs, and were more depressed. The underlying disease had no bearing on patients' endorsement. Cancer patients did not endorse PAS significantly more compared with those with other terminal illnesses. Patients in this study were interviewed again 2 to 6 months after the initial interview. For those that could still participate, one half of those who had thought about PAS changed their minds. A slightly smaller number of patients who previously had not considered PAS did so at the follow-up interview (Emanuel E., Fairclough, Slutsman, & Emanuel L., 2000).

Breitbart et al. (2000) also investigated factors related to what they called a desire for hastened death. Of the 92 terminally ill patients, 16% met criteria for a major depressive episode. Based on the tool used to evaluate desire for hastened death, 17% of the 92 patients had a high desire for hastened death. Patients experiencing major depression were four times more likely to wish for hastened death. Further, hopelessness also predicted a desire for hastened death. Hopelessness and depression were independent of each other. Patients who were not depressed or hopeless had a low score on their desire for hastened death. The other factors identified with a higher desire for hastened death were the perception of being a burden to others, physical symptoms and symptom distress, poor quality of life, race (white patients expressed a greater desire), and a lower sense of spiritual well-being. Perceived quality of social support and pain intensity were not factors.

The APN should understand these variables and their influence on a patient's or family's desire for PAS or hastened death. A comprehensive assessment should be undertaken to understand the patient's rationale related to a request for hastened death. All efforts to manage symptoms, address concerns, and allay fears are paramount. This is an issue that is best handled by a team approach, rather than by the individual nurse. It is important to have collegial support when dealing with difficult patient and family situations. Several national organizations (e.g., American Medical Association, Oncology Nursing Society, American Society of Clinical Oncology, American Pain Society, National Hospice and Palliative Care Organization) have issued position statements against PAS. The APN should be familiar with these. Others have developed guidelines related to this issue (Box 7-1).

| BOX 7-1 | *Guidelines for Caring for the Patient Who Expresses Interest in Hastening Death* |
|---------|----------------------------------------------------------------------------------|

I. Policy Statement

Hospice of Boulder County respects the right of dying persons to maintain control and to make choices during the dying process. Nevertheless, patients who express a desire to hasten death must be carefully evaluated for unmet needs. Our goal is to create an environment in which patients will feel permission to discuss their thoughts, plans, and fears. Every effort will be made to palliate physical, emotional and spiritual distress. We recognize that some patients will make this choice in spite of aggressive and supportive interventions. These guidelines do not prescribe specific interventions; rather, they rely upon the judgment of the hospice professional.

II. Patient Assessment

a. When a patient discusses the desire to hasten death, whether that be by ceasing to eat or drink or by a swifter method, more than one team member should explore this motivation. One of the team members should be the social worker. The following questions may be asked:

1. Please tell me what is happening now that makes you consider this action.
2. If we could relieve that problem would you still be interested in dying now?
3. What do you know about the process? What questions do you have? Have you considered the effect of this method on your family?
4. Is this an idea that is yours alone or has someone suggested that you consider this?
5. Have you discussed this with family members, your doctor, or others who are caring for you?

b. The assessment included evaluation of patient's satisfaction with pain and symptom management, depression, anxiety, fears, anger, family pressures, personal philosophy, and spiritual considerations.

c. A safety evaluation should be conducted if there are weapons on the premises.

## ■ SOCIAL NEEDS AT THE END OF LIFE

Social issues at the end of life concern both the patient and the family. Social aspects have to do with one's roles and relationships within and outside of the family, financial issues, and employment. Culture is also part of the social fabric of the patient and family.

As disease progresses and the physical body deteriorates, patients are forced to adjust to those changes. In the early stages of a terminal illness, patients may be able to continue in all of life's activities—though perhaps at a slower pace—fitting health care appointments into their schedules. As disease progresses, symptoms begin to affect those activities. For instance, there will come a time when the patient can no longer work or drive. These can be monumental adjustments. The patient's identity may be wrapped up in his or her work. Furthermore, having to give up work may cause a significant financial burden for

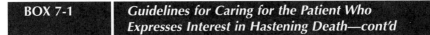

| BOX 7-1 | *Guidelines for Caring for the Patient Who Expresses Interest in Hastening Death—cont'd* |
|---------|------------------------------------------------------------------------------------------|

III. Intervention
  a. The services of the interdisciplinary team should be enlisted and aggressive efforts should be made to alleviate any unmet physical, emotional, or spiritual needs.
  b. It is preferable for patients to initiate the conversation about a hastened death. In some situations it may be appropriate for staff to provide information and counsel about the efficacy of methods that the patient is considering. It may be appropriate to provide information, both verbally and in writing, about the physiologic process of dehydration and starvation, as an alternative.
  c. Persons who are considering a hastened death should be strongly encouraged to discuss this with their family and others who are involved in their care.
  d. The physician and other involved team members will be made aware of the patient's intentions.
  e. If there is reason to believe that clinical depression is present, pharmacological treatment should be considered and offered.
  f. Only staff members who are comfortable with the patient's choice will be assigned to provide care.
  g. An Ethics Committee consultation may be called if there is any conflict surrounding the patient's decision.
  h. If the presence of weapons poses a risk to staff or family members, they should be removed from the home.
IV. Documentation
  a. The patient assessment and all interventions are to be documented in the patient record.
  b. Ethics Committee consult will be noted on the patient record and the usual documentation will be maintained in the Ethics Committee file.
  c. The underlying disease will be listed as the cause of death.

Courtesy Hospice of Boulder County.
Approved by the Hospice of Boulder County Ethics Committee on January 15, 1997.

the patient or family. Is the patient the sole breadwinner? Are there other sources of income? Another role change occurs when the patient has to give up driving. This signifies a loss of independence, one of the greatest concerns mentioned previously. As disease progresses, other roles and relationships are affected, including the amount of interaction with those outside the family or the patient's role within the family. For instance, the patient with metastatic breast cancer with back pain may no longer be able to pick up her 2-year-old child or tolerate the child's jumping up and down on the bed. This is a dramatic change for that mother. As the disease continues to progress and energy levels decrease, patients become less able to participate in usual activities. The person who has been the caregiver now has to become the care receiver. Eventually, there will come a time when the patient is bedridden and needs significant assistance with activities of daily living, eventually moving into the actively dying stage. For the patient, the world around him or her becomes smaller and smaller. During each of these transitions, the patient will feel a loss, whether or not it is expressed. Helping patients through these transitions, acknowledging the losses, and assisting them in the practical needs are important aspects of quality care at the end of life.

## Family and Caregiver Burden

The term *caregiver* refers to anyone who provides assistance to someone else who needs it. Formal caregivers are those who volunteer or are paid to care for a patient. Unpaid individuals are considered to be informal caregivers. Family members and friends fit into this group. It is estimated that there are as many as 54 million informal caregivers in the United States. This data is extrapolated from a survey by the National Family Caregivers Association (NFCA) (NFCA, 2000). This survey showed new trends of more male caregivers and more caregivers living with the patient than several years ago. The burden of caregiving is well documented. In the 1997 survey by NFCA, caregivers reported increased physical symptoms such as headache, backache, stomach problems, sleepless nights, and depression. About 67% of those surveyed felt frustrated and 43% felt isolated from others and perceived a lack of understanding by others. Other feelings experienced by the caregivers were sadness, the stress of making decisions for the patient, loss of personal time, and lack of support from other family members. This survey also explored the positive aspects of caregiving. About 70% reported they found an inner strength unknown to them previously. About 33% developed a closer relationship with the patient and about 33% learned new skills (NFCA, 1997). Most studies have only investigated the burdens associated with caregiving. Carter and Chang (2000) found sleep problems and depression in those caring for terminally ill patients. The authors, not surprisingly, found a strong correlation between poor sleep and depression. Several other studies report higher depression scores in caregivers (Emanuel E. et al., 2000; Given B., Given C., Helms, Strommel, & DeVoss, 1997; Raveis, Karus, & Seigel, 1997). Interestingly, in a comparison of caregivers of patients with a new diagnosis of cancer versus those patients with recurrence, it was not the stage of disease that determined the possibility of depression in the caregiver. It was the patients' symptoms and symptom experience that had a greater impact on caregiver depression (Given et al., 1997). Weitzner et al. (1999) found that higher levels of emotional distress in the caregiver and sickness in the patient correlated with poorer quality of life of the caregiver. Other studies also reported diminished quality of life (Kristjanson, Sloan, Dudgeon, & Adaskin, 1996; Myers & Gray, 2001).

Patients often worry about being a financial burden to their loved ones, which is borne out in the literature. Of 988 terminally ill patients and 893 caregivers across the United States, there was a subjective perception of economic burden. Greater care needs of the patient mean a greater financial burden. The burdens identified in this study were economic hardship; spending ≥10% of household income on health care (exclusive of premiums); and needing to borrow money, sell assets, or obtain an additional job to cover costs (Emanuel E. et al., 2000). From the Study to Understand Prognoses and Preferences for Outcomes and Risks of Treatment (SUPPORT), 20% of the families had to stop working in addition to giving up other activities. Almost a third lost most of their savings (Covinsky et al., 1994; Roth, Lynn, Zhong, Borum, & Dawson, 2000). The concerns of patients are obviously not unfounded.

In developing the FAMCARE instrument, an instrument for determining family satisfaction with care, Kristjanson (1993) identified four domains of care: information giving, physical patient care, psychosocial concerns, and availability. Families have identified such concerns as the physical comfort for the patient, the need for information about the patient and about caregiving, and understanding the dying process.

Families are now expected to provide even more care for the patient with less preparation at the time of discharge. Shortened lengths of stay in the hospital have had the greatest effect. There is often minimal time for family teaching. Technology becomes more advanced and to a great extent moves out of the hospital into the home setting. Many patients and families feel overwhelmed and frightened, wondering how they will manage. Most hospital discharge instructions cover only the basics of the medication name, dosage and frequency, and the doctor's or APN's phone number. This is an opportunity for APNs to develop simple discharge instructions pertinent to their patient population. What are the most common concerns of your patients at the time of discharge? What are the most common symptoms the patients might experience? What are the most common pieces of equipment (e.g., taking care of a Foley catheter, handling a patient-controlled analgesia [PCA] pump)? In addition to the usual instructions, simple fact cards addressing these concerns or symptoms should be provided to the patient and family. Table 7-1 reviews family concerns and the assessment of those concerns or needs.

## Cultural Factors

The face of America has changed over the last century. Caucasians, once in the majority, are becoming the minority. Many people now come from mixed races. Culture encompasses more than just one's ethnicity. Culture refers to learned behaviors, beliefs, and values that frame a person's experience. Ethnicity, on the other hand, refers to one's membership in a group bound by common racial, religious, national, or linguistic backgrounds (Marshall, 1990). For instance, if two of your patients are Hispanic, the one from Mexico may have very different ideas about illness compared with the one from Spain. Further, the culture surrounding the patient and family in their daily lives may or may not be the same as their culture of origin. It is important for the clinician to understand the cultures affecting the patient and family. Culture affects all aspects of our lives, including health, illness, and dying, and life after death.

## TABLE 7-1

### Assessment of Family Concerns

| Family Concern | Family Assessment |
| --- | --- |
| Patient Comfort | Are all symptoms optimally managed?<br>Are there simple comfort measures that the caregiver* can offer?<br>Are the patient's fears being addressed?<br>Are spiritual issues being attended to? |
| Information on Caregiving | Does the caregiver understand how to give the needed care (e.g., administering medications, feeding, turning, bathing)?<br>Does the caregiver understand the operation of the equipment?<br>Does the caregiver know who to call when concerned about physical caregiving issues? |
| General Information about the Patient | Does the caregiver understand the goals of care?<br>Has the caregiver been given information about what to expect as the patient's condition changes?<br>Does the caregiver need help in speaking with others about the patient's condition (e.g., children, grandchildren)? |
| Care of the Dying Patient | Has the caregiver been instructed as to the normal processes of dying (e.g., apnea, cool extremities)?<br>Does the caregiver know who to call for support as the patient's condition deteriorates?<br>Is the caregiver alone?<br>Does the caregiver understand the necessary steps once the patient has died? |
| Family Needs and Resources | How is the caregiver adjusting to being the caregiver?<br>**Acknowledge that the caregiver is doing a good job.**<br>Does the caregiver have a support system?<br>What are the resources available (e.g., home environment, caregiving assistance, financial)?<br>Does the caregiver have a chance to get a break from the caregiving?<br>What are the resources in the patient's community? Is there a hospice? Is there a place for respite care?<br>Is the caregiver coping well physically, emotionally, and spiritually? |
| Emergency Information | Does the caregiver know what to do in the event of an emergency, such as uncontrolled symptoms or the sudden death of the patient?<br>Does the caregiver have access to a health care professional 24 hours per day? **This is essential for the caregiver's well-being.** |

Adapted from Cherny, N. I., Coyle, N., & Foley, K. M. (1996). Guidelines in the care of the dying cancer patient. *Hematology/Oncology Clinics of North America, 10*(1), 261-286.
*Caregiver can be anyone who attends to the care of the patient. **All concerns require an initial assessment and ongoing reassessment.**

There are many ways that culture influences end-of-life care. Latimer (2000) identified the following areas of culture's effect:

- Decision-making
- Truth-telling
- Value and ethics of pain management, as well as the perception of opioids
- Personal values and emotional expression
- Use of physical touch between people
- Care of the dying
- Rituals surrounding the time of death including grieving
- Family systems: authority, tasks, and roles
- Understanding and expectations related to health care providers and institutions

One role of the APN is to be a role model for others. Exhibiting sensitivity to all cultures is paramount. One needs to acknowledge the uniqueness of each patient and family. When there are differing opinions between the health care team and the patient and family, emphasize the common ground rather than the differences. This will be beneficial in the long run. Inquire about the patient's and family's cultural background, asking them to help you have a better understanding of who they are as individuals and as a family. When language is a barrier, it is preferable to use a trained interpreter rather than a family member. It may be burdensome for the family member to be the interpreter, especially when bad news needs to be conveyed.

To help educate others in your practice setting, ask representatives of different cultures to assist you in compiling a notebook or manual that explains their cultures on such topics as health, illness, pain, death, dying, grieving, and rituals. Some institutions have a manual prepared as a resource for staff (Boxes 7-2 and 7-3). The APN should include reference articles whenever possible. This will assist everyone in becoming more sensitive to the specific cultural needs of patients and families.

Interwoven with the cultural effect on the patient and the family is the patient's own personal history. The patient's life story will affect the perceptions of end-of-life issues. What sort of life experiences has the patient gone through? Have there been many trials and tribulations? What is the nature of the family relationships? Have there been other family members who have died? What was that experience about? All these things shape how the patient and family will respond in the uncharted waters at the end of life.

# ■ SPIRITUAL NEEDS AT THE END OF LIFE

Spirituality is an important dimension of humanity. Every person has a spiritual dimension in addition to physical, psychologic, and social dimensions. No dimension can be influenced without affecting the whole person, and the whole includes spiritual aspects. Plato states: "As you ought not to

*Text continued on p. 118*

| BOX 7-2 | *Getting Acquainted with the Chinese Culture* |
|---|---|

This information is meant to help the professional become more sensitive to the nuances of cultures that are unfamiliar. Information should be used as a starting place and guide; this information cannot be generalized to all people of a culture. It is important to ask the patient and family about specific beliefs, practices, and customs that may be relevant and important during medical treatment and hospitalization.

### GENERAL INFORMATION

- People from China tend to be more formal than Americans. Patients may prefer to be "Mr.," "Ms.," or "Mrs.," especially if they are older than the caregiver. Calling an elderly patient "grandmother" or "grandfather" shows respect. Children can be called by their first name, "little sister," or "little brother." Ask your patient how he/she wishes to be addressed.
- The opposite forces of yin and yang are basic to Chinese culture. Yin and yang maintain peace and harmony in society and the body.
- A response to yes/no questions is likely to be "yes," a nod, or "I know." These responses may not indicate understanding; they may simply mean that the patient has heard you. Ask the patient or family to repeat the information.
- To be polite, a patient may decline an offer (e.g., "would you like something to drink?") unless asked twice or more. Do not be afraid to keep asking.
- Assertive and individualistic personalities may be considered crude and poorly socialized. This may mean that patients will not speak up on their own behalf.
- Elderly patients, especially, may be hesitant to ask for help or things if they think they can manage alone.
- Always tell the patient that an interpreter can be provided, even if the only resource available is the AT&T Language Hotline. Patients may feel closer to someone who speaks the same language.

### DECISION MAKING

- Treatment decisions are often made by the family rather than by the individual patient. The patient may want conversations about treatment to take place when the family is present. Ask the patient if this is his/her preference.
- Age plays an important role within the family structure. Children, regardless of their age, commonly defer to their parents, grandparents, and elders.

### EMOTIONS

- Feelings may be divided into two categories, public and private. Public feelings may not be reflective of emotions felt, but personal or private feelings are generally not openly expressed. Some Chinese believe that "excessive" expression of emotion may upset the harmonious functions of the body (yin and yang) and actually cause disease.
- Harmonious relationships are very important and any feeling that might upset these relationships may not be expressed (e.g., disagreement with the family's wishes).

### MEDICAL TREATMENT

- Patients may believe symptom relief should happen quickly, but they may also think the illness is cured when the symptoms go away. Pointing out progress or improvement may make results more obvious and act as as incentive for the patient to continue treatment.

| BOX 7-2 | *Getting Acquainted with the Chinese Culture—cont'd* |

- Blood tests may pose a problem, since they allow the *Chi* (the essence of one's body energy) to leak out of the body.
- Since patients may see both the American physician and a Chinese practitioner, it is important to ask what other medicines or herbs (including teas) the patient is taking. Some can cause an overdose or adverse reaction when combined with medicines prescribed by the physicians in the hospital.
- Illness, especially cancer, may be viewed as a punishment. Patients or their families may believe an elder or grandparent has done something wrong or bad if a young person becomes ill or dies.

### PAIN
- The Chinese vocabulary has specific words that define ranges of emotion. Instead of asking "Do you have pain?" you might ask "How much pain are your having?"
- It is important to emphasize the importance of pain relief; also emphasize that relieving pain is not a bother for the nurse. Asking repeatedly about the level of pain may reinforce our belief in the importance of relieving it. Emphasize that enduring pain does not contribute to recovery. Some patients, however, may view any discussion of pain as a sign of weakness and endurance of it as a sign of character.

### FOOD
- Food, when metabolized, is turned into *Chi* (energy) and becomes either yin, a cold force, or yang, a hot force. When a patient has been diagnosed with an illness, a change in the diet may be indicated. Often hot or cold foods will be used to bring yin and yang into balance. Illnesses caused by yin are treated with hot foods; those caused by yang are treated with cold foods. Cold and hot foods may differ from family to family (cold and hot do not refer to temperature). Cancer is a cold disease and is treated with hot foods. The family may wish to bring these foods to the patient. As long as they do not contradict the patient's medical diet, this should be allowed and encouraged.
- Ice water is considered harmful and most Chinese patients boil water before they drink it. They generally prefer drinking hot water or lukewarm water to cold. If it is not possible to give them hot water, boiled cool water is acceptable. Be sure to tell the patient the water has been boiled.
- Patients may not like western food and may ask family members to bring food from home.

### DEATH
- In the Chinese culture, patients are typically told little of the life-threatening aspects of illness. Explanations are made to the family who will care for the patient.
- The family will usually want to stay at the bedside when the patient dies.
- Age at death may be important. Dying old may be seen as a blessing, while dying young may be seen as a punishment from a higher force.
- If the patient dies, clothing may be left in the hospital for a period of time to allow "evil spirits" to leave. Help the family to make arrangements to pick it up at a later date.
- Families from the Chinese culture may frown on autopsies.
- Patients are often unwilling to permit the donation of body parts.

| BOX 7-3 | *Getting Acquainted with the Orthodox Judaism/Hasidic Judaism* |
|---------|----------------------------------------------------------------|

This information is meant to help the professional become more sensitive to the nuances of cultures that are unfamiliar. Information should be used as a starting place and guide; this information cannot be generalized to all people of a culture. It is important to ask the patient and family about specific beliefs, practices, and customs that may be relevant and important during medical treatment and hospitalization.

### GENERAL INFORMATION

- Casual touching between sexes (e.g., handshakes, placing an arm around shoulder) is strictly forbidden. Staff should not touch patients of the opposite sex without explaining what they are going to do.
- Orthodox Jews are strict in their observance of the Sabbath and many holy days. Sabbath begins at sundown on Friday night and ends at sundown Saturday night. During this time, no work may be performed. Turning on a light switch, signing a document, and pushing a call bell are considered work and therefore these tasks may not be performed. Ask the patient specifically what is and is not allowed. If necessary, consult a rabbi; Jewish law allows the Sabbath to be violated in cases where health is at stake. Holy days, which prohibit work, are Yom Kippur, Rosh Hashana (2 days), Succos (8 days long, 4 prohibit work), Passover (8 days long, 4 prohibit work), and Shavuos (2 days).
- In observance of Sabbath, candles are lit approximately 18 minutes before sundown. Traditionally, two candles represent the commands "Remember" and "Observe," but some people light candles for every member of the family. Symbolically, light represents joy and happiness. Electric candles and grape juice, also used in the celebration of Sabbath, can be obtained from ext. 5982.
- The Bikur Cholim is a service provided by the Jewish community that will arrange housing for family members who wish to remain close to the patient during the Sabbath and Holy days. They can also help with transportation. Their telephone number is (212) 472-3968 or (718) 384-4621.

### INTERPERSONAL RELATIONSHIPS

- Family is very important to Orthodox Jews, but as with all cultures and religions, there is wide diversity. Issues of sterility should be considered extremely important and discussion should take place specifically about side effects of treatments that might result in an inability to have children.

### DECISION MAKING

- Patients and families may want to have discussions with a rabbi before making any serious decision.

### EMOTIONS

- Emotions, especially surrounding a cancer diagnosis, may be complicated by the Orthodox person's belief that God is benevolent, omniscient, and controls the world. Patients and families might feel cancer is a reflection of God's will.
- The religion has a strong emphasis on freewill and the power to influence fate through prayer. Hope is never abandoned.

| BOX 7-3 | *Getting Acquainted with the Orthodox Judaism/Hasidic Judaism—cont'd* |
|---|---|

## MEDICAL TREATMENT

- Members of the Orthodox Jewish community generally actively pursue quality medical care. The basic tenet that God helps those who help themselves will often kindle a desire to be involved in the details of care and in working with the physician.
- Jewish law mandates that one do whatever possible to increase the chance of survival.
- Body parts removed during surgery should be buried. Clarify the patient's and family's wishes before surgery.
- Clarify in advance who will be performing care (e.g., female doctors or nurses for male patients, male doctors or nurses for female patients).

## PAIN

- There are no beliefs or behaviors associated with pain that are particular to the Orthodox Jewish religion. However, traditionally patients are encouraged to verbalize pain and seek relief if possible.

## FOOD

- Dietary laws are extremely strict and patients must be placed on a kosher diet. This diet is available through the dietary department.
- Some patients will require a separate refrigerator for food brought from home that needs refrigeration; others will allow it to be stored, well wrapped, in the patient refrigerator in the pantry.

## DEATH

- Jewish law requires the physician to do everything in his/her power to prolong life but at the same time prohibits the use of measures that prolong the act of dying. General supportive care (e.g., water and nourishment) should always be provided.
- Clarify the family's wishes regarding who should be called as the patient nears death. It may be important for the rabbi and other family members to be present before death occurs.
- Any drains, catheters, or such that have the patient's blood in them should be left attached to the body.
- The family may not want hospital staff to touch the body.
- The family may perform ritual washing after death. Some families will call a special Burial Committee to make sure the body is prepared for burial according to Jewish law. Some branches of the Orthodox religion have particular practices (e.g., the Hasidim place the body on the floor and do not cross the arms or legs). The religion dictates that burial must take place within 24 hours of death. Traditionally, the body is not to be left alone and mourners will gather to pray.
- Often, special arrangements will be made for the body to be wrapped and taken directly to the funeral home rather than the morgue.
- Unless required by law, autopsy is prohibited.

attempt to cure the eyes without the head, or the head without the body, so neither ought you attempt to cure the body without the soul. For the part can never be well unless the whole is well. And therefore, if the head and body are to be well, you must begin by curing the soul."

## Definitions

The word spirit comes from the Latin *spiritus,* meaning breath. This breath of life is what gives us meaning and purpose. Spirituality deals with a person's search for meaning. There are several definitions related to spirituality. One of the earliest definitions in nursing literature comes from Stallwood (1975), who defined spiritual needs as "any factors necessary to establish and maintain a person's dynamic relationship with God (as defined by that individual)." Note that in her definition the concept of "God" is not necessarily absolute or traditional, but rather permeable and unique to each individual.

Colliton (1981), a few years later, defined spiritual need in a more inclusive and expansive way: "Spiritual need is more encompassing than religious need. Spiritual need is that requirement which touches the core of one's being, where the search for personal meaning takes place."

Several sociologists developed the concept of spiritual well-being. Moberg and Brusek (1978) introduced the concept of vertical and horizontal dimensions, in which the vertical dimension describes one's relationship with God and the horizontal dimension describes one's perception of life's purpose and satisfaction. From this framework, Paloutzian and Ellison (1982) developed the Spiritual Well-Being Scale that includes religious well-being (RWB) and existential well-being (EWB).

Highfield and Cason (1983), two nurses, conceptualized spirituality in terms of four needs and then described signs of spiritual health and spiritual problems for each. In the first need, the need for meaning and purpose in life, examples of spiritual problems would be expression of no reason to live, questioning the meaning in suffering and death, or jokes about life after death. Examples of spiritual problems of the second need, the need to receive love, would be expression of feelings of loss of a faith in God, a fear of dependence, or a loss of self-value because of decreasing physical health. In the third need, the need to give love, the patient might express worries about financial status or separation from others in death. In the fourth and last need, the need for hope and creativity, some of the signs of spiritual problems include concerns about loss of control, having overly dependent behaviors, and denial of the reality of his or her condition. The authors identified other signs of spiritual problems for each need, in addition to identifying signs of spiritual health.

Spirituality related to the end of life was addressed by the International Work Group for Death and Dying, who published a document in 1990 on the assumptions and principles of spiritual care. Their definition of spirituality is that which "is concerned with the transcendental, inspirational and existential ways to live one's life, as well as, in a fundamental and profound sense, with the person as a human being. The search for spirituality may be heightened as one confronts death" (International Work Group for Death and Dying, 1990). This is an excellent document, as it addresses spirituality in general, related to the patient, family, and caregivers (i.e., professional). It also speaks of community coordination and education and research.

And finally, spirituality encompasses both religious and nonreligious belief systems. Religion is a formal faith which expresses certain tenets. Religion is an actual practice one may use to express one's spirituality. However, one can be spiritual without being religious.

## Spirituality and Health

The interest and investigation of the relationship between spirituality or religion and health has increased significantly over the past decade. Hundreds of studies have explored a particular faith tradition and its influence on the health of individuals. For instance, a Dutch study showed that Seventh Day Adventists have lower rates of heart disease and cancer than the general population (Berkel & de Waard, 1983). Few studies look at the spiritual dimension of patients as a part of the whole person and barely any studies focus on the end of life. Yates et al. (1981), in one of the earlier investigations, studied patients with advanced cancer whose prognosis was between 3 and 12 months. Patients were visited regularly. Religious activity and connections were associated with higher levels of well-being. Religious variables, such as religious beliefs, activities, and connections, were negatively correlated to pain levels but religious belief or activity was not related to duration of survival.

Peteet (1985), a psychiatrist, also concluded that religious issues were important, in a study in which 32 of 50 hospitalized cancer patients seen in psychiatric consultation identified or were concerned with religious issues. Time since diagnosis ranged from weeks to years for these patients.

One of the first nursing studies examining religious faith and health was conducted by O'Brien (1982). A 3-year longitudinal study of patients with end-stage renal disease receiving hemodialysis was conducted to observe changes in religious faith and the effect of such changes on adjustment to this illness. Initially, 126 patients were interviewed and 63 patients of the original sample were located 3 years later. Her findings showed that those patients who perceived religious faith as associated with acceptance of their condition and its treatment were also the least alienated and the most compliant. When these patients were interviewed again, the content analysis showed that the perception in 27% of the respondents changed from a negative to a positive attitude or had notably increased in the degree of importance of religious faith over the 3 years. Religion was an important variable in the long-term adjustment to end-stage renal disease.

Miller (1985), investigating loneliness and spiritual well-being among healthy and chronically ill adults, found a negative correlation between loneliness and spiritual well-being in both groups. In addition, religion or religious well-being (as a sub-scale of the Spiritual Well-Being Scale) was significantly more important to the chronically ill patients than the healthy adults.

A related study focused on spiritual well-being and anxiety in adult patients with cancer (Kaczorowski, 1989). Spiritual well-being was correlated negatively with anxiety—those patients with a high sense of spiritual well-being had lower levels of anxiety.

Reed (1986, 1987) also investigated spiritual well-being. She conducted two studies, the second being an extension of the first. Reed divided 300 adult patients into three groups: terminally ill hospitalized adults, non–terminally ill hospitalized adults, and healthy nonhospitalized adults. She further matched patients by age, gender, years of education, and religious background. Her results indicated that terminally ill hospitalized adults showed the greatest spiritual perspective, or spirituality, compared with the non–terminally ill hospitalized adults and healthy adults.

More recently, others have found results similar to these initial studies. Patients with a positive spiritual well-being are less depressed (Breitbart et al., 2000; Fehring, Miller, & Shaw, 1997; Koenig et al., 1992) and have a higher quality of life—higher levels of faith meaning acted as a quality of life buffer in patients with pain or fatigue (Brady, Peterman, Fitchett, Mo, & Cella, 1999) and higher levels of meaning also correlated with less of a desire for hastened death (Breitbart et al., 2000).

## The Challenge

We, as APNs, are asked to care for the whole person—for the physical, emotional, and spiritual aspects of each individual patient throughout the course of illness. We pride ourselves on caring for the physical needs by mastering technologic advances. We have become more willing to invest in caring for the psychologic and emotional needs of our patients. However, spiritual needs have not been well addressed. This may be due to nurses' discomfort with this dimension of patient care and lack of knowledge of assessment. Two studies have reported nurses' inability to address spiritual concerns.

In Highfield and Cason's (1983) study, the purpose was to examine oncology nurses' awareness of their patients' spiritual needs and problems. By using a questionnaire, could the nurses recognize spiritual health, identify spiritual problems, and express an awareness that spiritual problems occur in patients? The results showed that the nurses had a limited ability to recognize signs associated with spiritual health, both on individual questions and questions grouped into the four spiritual needs identified by the authors, as discussed previously. The nurses also had a limited awareness of spiritual problems. Of the 31 behaviors and conditions indicating spiritual problems, the nurses were only able to identify five as spiritual in nature. These included four that had direct reference to God and one item concerning questioning the meaning in suffering and death. Often these nurses identified the problems in relation to the psychosocial dimension instead of the spiritual dimension. The authors contend that there are different interventions when a problem is identified as a psychosocial need instead of a spiritual need. For example, if a spiritual problem is identified in the psychosocial domain, a pastoral care referral might be missed when in fact that might be the most appropriate intervention.

Soderstrom and Martinson (1987) conducted a study on patients' spiritual coping strategies, investigating both nurse and patient perspectives. About 88% of the patients used a variety of spiritual activities (e.g., prayer, Bible reading, church attendance, religious objects, music) and resource people (e.g., family, friends, clergy, medical staff) to cope with their cancer. Furthermore, 66% reported increased awareness and practice of spirituality since their diagnoses. From the nursing perspective on spiritual coping, those nurses interviewed had difficulty identifying patients' use of spiritual coping strategies. The results of the nurses' interviews support Highfield and Cason's conclusions that nurses have difficulty identifying patients' spiritual needs.

## Spiritual Assessment

As noted, the literature has looked at spirituality from several perspectives, such as spiritual needs, spiritual health, spiritual well-being, and spiritual distress. There have been a number of assessment models and tools. One of the first to publish a spiritual assessment questionnaire was Ruth Stoll (1979), a nurse. She has four categories of assessment, each of which have four to five specific questions. Her areas of assessment are: concept of deity, a person's source of strength and hope, significance of religious practices and rituals, and a person's perceived relationships between beliefs and state of health.

Another model of assessment comes from the North American Nursing Diagnosis Association (NANDA), which includes a definition, etiology, or related factors and defining characteristics for each nursing diagnosis label. Carpenito (1997), another nurse, takes the nursing diagnosis "spiritual distress" and makes it clinically applicable. She suggests asking about the importance of religion or God and if the patient has a special religious leader. How is the illness affecting spiritual practices? Are there any religious items that are of significance? And finally, how can the nurse help maintain the patient's spiritual strength?

Hay (1989), a chaplain, addressed spiritual assessment in terms of four spiritual problem categories. The first category is religious request—a specified expressed religious need or request. The second category is a problem with the belief system—a lack of conscious awareness of personal or spiritual meaning. The third category is that of an inner resource deficiency. The last category is spiritual suffering, described as intrapersonal or interpersonal anguish of unspecified origin. As in the process of nursing diagnosis, each problem has defining characteristics, assessments, goals, expected outcomes, and interventions. Hay's spiritual assessment was designed so that with minimal training any health care provider could use the tool.

A group of chaplains and nurses developed a model of the spiritual dimension with seven components: beliefs and meaning, vocation and consequences, experience and emotion, courage and growth, ritual and practice, community, and authority and guidance (Emblen, Fitchett, Farran, & Burck, 1992). This model of spiritual assessments is quite cumbersome but can be used for a very thorough and comprehensive assessment.

Highfield (1993, 2000) also developed a model for spiritual care for nurses. She uses the acronym: PLAN. **P**ermission is the first step—the nurse gives the patient permission to talk about spiritual concerns. Next is **L**imited information—giving brief factual information, such as how to contact clergy. The third step is **A**ctivating resources for the patient and family and helping them find resolution to spiritual distress. The last step, **N**onnursing assistance, is for when the scope of the spiritual problem is beyond the nurse either in terms of experience, education, or time. An appropriate referral would be made in this situation.

A final spiritual tool to assess patients is Puchalski's (2000) Spiritual Assessment Tool. She uses the acronym: FICA—**F**aith or beliefs, **I**mportance, **C**ommunity, and **A**ddress. She further suggests some key questions for discussion under each item.

So how is the nurse to assess spiritual issues for the patient at the end of life? A nurse could use any of the assessment tools discussed, though some may not be realistic in today's health care settings, with patients being sicker and having less time for interactions. Spiritual assessment doesn't have to be complicated. It can be as simple as asking:

- What were you raised to believe?
- Where are you now?
- Where would you like to be?
- It takes a lot of strength to go through this period in your life. Where do you get the inner strength to go through this?

Take your cues from the patient/family. Remember, however, that not all cues from patients and families with spiritual concerns are verbal. Notice what is in the patient's room or home. Are there religious objects? Are there cards with a religious theme? Have you noticed any behaviors, such as praying or meditating? Are there undercurrents of hopelessness? Often commenting on these nonverbal cues can be the opening needed to address spiritual issues.

## Interventions

What interventions can the APN provide? Consider the following suggestions:

1. Address the specific concerns that are illuminated by the assessment.
2. Consider offering different types of music. For many, music touches the soul. It is important to identify the particular type of music each patient and family desires. For some, meditative music is soothing; for some, it is a rousing old hymn; and for others, gospel or jazz. Gather a variety of

music and compile a library of tapes and CDs that can be loaned to patients and families.
3. Act as an advocate for the patient. For instance, a Muslim patient may
want to pray towards Mecca five times a day. Determine which direction is east in the patient's room. Help the patient, together with the
nursing staff, to provide time and privacy during prayer times.
4. If you are unsure about the patient's religious practices, ask. Most patients are happy to share this information, as it indicates a sense that
you are caring for all aspects of their being.
5. If you consider praying with the patient, ask their permission first.
6. Make a referral to pastoral care. Sometimes simply inquiring and listening with care is another way to provide spiritual care—the nurse is
touching the spirit of that patient.

It is essential that APNs address this important and often neglected dimension of patient care. It is helpful to understand one's own sense of spirituality to be able to provide support to patients and families. Initially, as
with any new skill, there will be a certain level of discomfort. That discomfort will eventually give way to an ability to discuss these significant issues
with patients and families. The APN who has not yet developed these assessment skills needs to do so. Once the APN is grounded in his or her own
spirituality, has a willingness to be open and present, and has developed the
skills necessary, patients and families will receive quality of care that includes
all dimensions.

## ■ SUFFERING

*To provide cure sometimes*
*To relieve often*
*To comfort always* **16**TH C. ANONYMOUS

### Understanding Suffering

What is suffering? Joyce Travelbee (1971) described it as "a feeling of dis-
pleasure that ranges from simple transitory mental, physical, or spiritual discomfort to extreme anguish and those places beyond anguish." Not every
patient who approaches the end of his or her life suffers. Some think of suffering in the physical domain only. Often pain and suffering are fused, but
pain (or any other symptom at the end of life) may or may not be associated
with suffering. When suffering is related to symptoms, it generally occurs in
the setting of a symptom that is out of control, overwhelming, or ceaseless.
Suffering can also occur when the source of the symptom is unknown
(Cassel, 1991). Any symptom could qualify, though results from the
SUPPORT study (Desbiens, Mueller-Rizner, Connors, & Wenger, 1997;
Levenson, McCarthy, Lynn, Davis, & Phillips, 2000; McCarthy, Phillips,
Zhong, Drews, & Lynn, 2000) found that the four symptoms having the

greatest burden were pain, dyspnea, anxiety, and depression and were associated with the poorest quality of life.

Some think of suffering as only spiritual (i.e., spiritual pain equals suffering). Some see suffering as punishment, a test of moral fiber, or an opportunity to transcend the current situation. Suffering affects all dimensions of the holistic person. Cassel refers to suffering as "a state of severe distress associated with events that threaten the intactness of the person" (Cassell, 1991). Suffering is connected to meaning and finding meaning in life. Viktor Frankl, a psychotherapist who survived the concentration camps of World War II, states that "to live is to suffer, to survive is to find meaning in the suffering" (Frankl, 1962). Despite severe hardship and the atrocities of his years in the concentration camps, he was able to find meaning in his suffering.

Suffering is an intensely personal experience. It is unique to each person, patient, and family member. It is important to remember that the family can be suffering even if the patient is not. Kahn and Steeves (1996) have done extensive research into the phenomenon of suffering. Some of the principles developed from their work are:

- Suffering is a private, personal experience unique to each individual.
- Suffering results when the most important aspects of a person's identity are threatened or lost.
- Suffering cannot be assumed to be absent or present in any given situation.
- Suffering can also be viewed as an experience of lost personal meaning.
- The care environment in which the process of suffering occurs can influence a person's suffering positively and negatively.

What influences suffering? A complete listing is not possible, as the number of influences and aspects of suffering is potentially endless. Box 7-4 lists some of the major influences related to suffering. Even though suffering involves the whole person, suffering can be related to a single domain or all domains of life. Understanding the influences helps the APN focus on the issues for the patient and family as they express their suffering. Cherney et al. (1994) describe a detailed taxonomy of factors contributing to suffering. They discuss suffering of the patient, family, and health care professional. For the suffering of the patient, there are physical symptoms, psychologic symptoms, existential concerns, empathic suffering with the family, and issues related to health care in general. For the family, factors include empathic suffering with the patient, physical illness, family dynamic, impending bereavement, burdens of care, and conflicts. The factors related to suffering for the health care professional are empathic suffering with the patient and family, physical illness, burdens of care, conflict, psychologic symptoms, and existential concerns.

## Managing Suffering

Assessment of symptoms is the first step, followed by aggressive management of physical and psychologic symptoms. Assisting with the existential and spiritual issues is also an expectation. These are detailed elsewhere in the text. Knowing the normal trajectory of the terminal illness is

| BOX 7-4 | *Some Factors Influencing Suffering* |
|---|---|

When listening to patients express their suffering, these are some of the influencing factors to be considered:

- The meaning of the illness
- The meaning of the symptom(s)
- Having the symptom(s) invalidated by family or health care professionals
- The past, including regrets
- Life experiences
- The cultural background of the patient/family
- The religious background of the patient/family
- The present
- Changed roles (e.g., in the family, in the world)
- The perceived future
- Dreams, hopes, fantasies
- Unfinished business
- Fears (e.g., of the unknown, of uncontrollable symptoms, of abandonment, of meaninglessness)
- Exhaustion of the patient/family

imperative. It allows for anticipation of the physical and psychologic symptoms that are associated with a particular illness. Caring for the patient at the end of life with chronic obstructive pulmonary disease may be very different than caring for the patient with metastatic ovarian cancer. A few physical symptoms may be similar and even have identical approaches to treatment, but the psychologic symptoms can be very different from one disease to another. In contrast, spiritual issues often transcend the nature of specific illnesses. To understand your patient's or family's suffering, you must know the disease trajectory and understand these influencing factors.

Finally, understanding the goals of care as expressed by the patient and family is essential. Goals of care that are not clearly understood can lead to suffering of those involved with the patient, including the patient, the family, and the health care provider. As an APN, you will be called on to help the patient and family when there are conflicting goals of care. Clarifying the goals of care may come in the form of a family meeting, with or without the patient, or it may be one on one with a family member or the patient. Who is this person in relation to his or her terminal illness, in relation to the family? Are there cultural or religious factors influencing the suffering? What is underneath the suffering? If you suspect that the patient is suffering but this isn't apparent, then you have to ask directly if suffering is present. As you listen to the person suffering, it is not helpful to say, "I know what you are going through." Remember that suffering is a unique experience to that person. No one can walk in another's shoes. You can walk beside the person. It is interesting that the word patient comes from the Latin *patiens*, which means "to suffer."

Can suffering be relieved? Cassel (1991) believes that if you help the person suffering to find a new meaning, then suffering can be relieved. Frankl (1962) says that "if there is meaning in life at all then there must be meaning in suffering. Suffering is an ineradicable part of life, even as fate and death. Without suffering and death, human life would not be complete" (Frankl, 1962). For some, suffering may even be transforming, offering the opportunity for growth.

# ■ SUMMARY

Quality care at the end of life entails knowing the disease trajectory and being able to anticipate physical symptoms. It also entails addressing the psychologic, social, and spiritual dimensions of each patient and family. All symptoms, issues, and concerns require aggressive management. As we care for these patients we bring ourselves into every encounter, so it is important to understand ourselves emotionally and spiritually. This allows for the nurse to be truly present for the patient and family. This is a very intimate time in their lives. It is a privilege to walk beside them.

## References

BERKEL, J., & de Waard, F. (1983). Mortality patterns and life expectancy of Seventh-Day Adventists in the Netherlands. *International Journal of Epidemiology, 12*(4), 455-459.

BLOCK, S. D. (2000). Assessing and managing depression in the terminally ill patient. ACP-ASIM End-of-Life Care Consensus Panel. American College of Physicians–American Society of Internal Medicine. *Annals of Internal Medicine, 132,* 209-218.

BRADY, M. J., Peterman, A. H., Fitchett, G., Mo, M., & Cella, D., (1999). A case for including spirituality in quality of life measurement in oncology. *Psycho-oncology, 8,* 417-428.

BREITBART, W., Breura, E., Chochinov, H., & Lynch, M. (1995). Neuropsychiatric syndromes and psychological symptoms in patients with advanced cancer. *Journal of Pain and Symptom Management, 10,* 131-141.

BREITBART, W., Rosenfeld, B., Pessin, H., Kaim, M., Funesti-Esch, J., Galietta, M., Nelson, C. J., & Brescia, R. (2000). Depression, hopelessness, and desire for hastened death in terminally ill patients with cancer. *Journal of the American Medical Association, 284*(22), 2907-2911.

CARPENITO, L. J. (1997). *Nursing diagnosis: Application to clinical practice* (7ᵗʰ ed.). Philadelphia: Lippincott.

CARTER, P. A., & Chang, B. L. (2000). Sleep and depression in cancer caregivers. *Cancer Nursing, 23*(6), 410-415.

CASSEL, E. J. (1991). *The nature of suffering and the goals of medicine.* New York: Oxford University Press.

CHERNEY, N. I., Coyle, N., & Foley, K. M. (1994). Suffering in the advanced cancer patient: A definition and taxonomy. *Journal of Palliative Care, 10*(2), 57-70.

CHERNY, N. I., Coyle, N., & Foley, K. M. (1996). Guidelines in the care of the dying cancer patient. *Hematology/Oncology Clinics of North America, 10*(1), 261-286.

CHOCHINOV, H. M., Wilson, K. G., Enns, M., & Lander, S. (1994). Prevalence of depression in the terminally ill: Effects of diagnostic criteria and symptom threshold judgments. *American Journal of Psychiatry, 151,* 537-540.

CHOCHINOV, H. M., Wilson, K. G., Enns, M., & Lander, S. (1997). "Are you depressed?" Screening for depression in the terminally ill. *American Journal of Psychiatry, 154,* 674-676.

CIARAMELLA, A., & Poli, P. (2001). Assessment of depression among cancer patients: The role of pain, cancer type, and treatment. *Psycho-oncology, 10,* 156-165.

COLLITON, M.A. (1981). The spiritual dimension of nursing. In I. L. Beland & J. Y. Passos (Eds.), *Clinical nursing* (4th ed.) (pp. 492-501). New York: Macmillan.

COVINSKY, K. E., Goldman, L., Cook, E. F., Oye, R., Desbeins, N., Reding, D., Fulkerson, W., Connors, A. F. Jr., Lynn, J., & Phillips, R. S. (1994). The impact of serious illness on patients' families. Study to Understand Prognoses and Preferences for Outcomes and Risks of Treatment (SUPPORT) Investigators. *Journal of the American Medical Association, 272*(23), 1839-1844.

COYLE, N. (1992). The euthanasia and physician-assisted debate: Issues for nursing. *Oncology Nursing Forum, 19*(7S), 41-46.

DESBIENS, N. A., Mueller-Rizner, N., Connors, A. F., & Wenger, N. S. (1997). The relationship of nausea and dyspnea to pain in seriously ill patients. *Pain, 71,* 149-156.

EMANUEL, E. J., Fairclough, D. L., Slutsman, J., & Emanuel, L. L. (2000). Understanding economic and other burdens of terminal illness: The experience of patients and their caregivers. *Annals of Internal Medicine, 132,* 451-459.

EMBLEN, J. Q., Fitchett, G., Farran, C. J., & Burck, J. R. (1992). Identifying parameters of spiritual need. *Care Giver Journal, 8*(2), 44-50.

ENDICOTT, J. (1984). Measurement of depression in patients with cancer. *Cancer, 53S,* 2243-2248.

FEHRING, R. J., Miller, J. F., & Shaw, C. (1997). Spiritual well-being, religiosity, hope, depression, and other mood states in elderly people coping with cancer. *Oncology Nursing Forum, 24*(4), 663-671.

FRANKL, V. (1962). *Man's search for meaning.* Boston: Beacon Press.

GIVEN, B. A., Given, C. W., Helms, E., Strommel, M., & DeVoss, D. N. (1997). Determinants of family caregiver reaction: New and recurrent cancer. *Cancer Practice, 5*(1), 17-24.

HARDMAN, A., Maguire, P., & Crowther, D. (1989). The recognition of psychiatric morbidity on a medical oncology ward. *Journal of Psychosomatic Research, 33,* 235-239.

HAY, M. W. (Sept/Oct, 1989). Principles in building spiritual assessment tools. *American Journal of Hospice Care,* 25-31.

HEAVEN, C., & Maguire, P. (1998). The relationship between patients' concerns and psychological distress in a hospice setting. *Psycho-oncology, 7,* 502-507.

HIGHFIELD, M. E. (1993). PLAN: A spiritual care model for every nurse. *Quality of Life—A Nursing Challenge, 2*(3), 80-84.

HIGHFIELD, M. E. (2000). Providing spiritual care to patients with cancer. *Clinical Journal of Oncology Nursing, 4*(3), 115-120.

HIGHFIELD, M. E., & Cason, C. (1983). Spiritual needs of patients: Are they recognized? *Cancer Nursing, 6,* 187-192.

INTERNATIONAL Work Group for Death and Dying. (1990). Assumptions and principles of spiritual care. *Death Studies, 14,* 75-81.

KACZOROWSKI, J. M. (1989). Spiritual well-being and anxiety in adults diagnosed with cancer. *The Hospice Journal, 5*(3/4), 105-116.

KAHN, D. L., & Steeves, R. H. (1996). An understanding of suffering grounded in clinical practice and research. In B. R. Ferrell (Ed.), *Suffering* (pp. 3-27). Boston: Jones & Bartlett Publishing.

KOENIG, H. G., Cohen, H. J., Blazer, D. G., Pieper, C., Meador, K. G., Shelp, S., Goli, V., & DiPasquale, B. (1992). Religious coping and depression among elderly hospitalized medically ill men. *American Journal of Psychiatry, 149*(12), 1693-1700.

KRISTJANSON, L. (1993). Validity and reliability testing of the FAMCARE scale: Measuring family satisfaction with advanced cancer care. *Social Science Medicine, 36*(5), 693-701.

KRISTJANSON, L. J., Sloan, J. A., Dudgeon, D., & Adaskin, E. (1996). Family members' perceptions of palliative cancer care: Predictors of family functioning and family members' health. *Journal of Palliative Care, 12*(4), 10-20.

LATIMER, E. J. (2000, September). *The interplay of ethics, culture and faith.* Presentation at the Thirteenth International Congress on the Care of the Terminally Ill. Montreal, Canada: Author.

LEVENSON, J. W., McCarthy, E. P., Lynn, J., Davis, R. B., & Phillips, R. S. (2000). The last six months of life for patients with congestive heart failure. *Journal of the American Geriatric Society, 48*(5S), 101-109.

MARSHALL, P. A. (1990). Cultural influences on perceived quality of life. *Seminars in Oncology Nursing, 6*(4), 278-284.

MASSIE, M. J., & Holland, J. C. (1992). The cancer patient with pain: Psychiatric complications and their management. *Journal of Pain and Symptom Management, 7*(2), 99-109.

MCCARTHY, E. P., Phillips, R. S., Zhong, Z., Drews, R. E., & Lynn, J. (2000). Dying with cancer: Patients' function, symptoms, and care preferences as death approaches. *Journal of the American Geriatric Society, 48*(5S), 110-121.

MCDONALD, M. V., Passik, S. D., & Coyle, N. (2000). Addressing the needs of the patient who requests physician-assisted suicide or euthanasia. In H. M. Chochinov & W. Breitbart (Eds.), *Handbook of psychiatry in palliative medicine* (pp. 349-356). New York: Oxford University Press.

MCDONALD, M. V., Passik, S. D., Dugan, W., Rosenfeld, B., Theobald, D. E., & Edgerton, S. (1999). Nurses' recognition of depression in their patients with cancer. *Oncology Nursing Forum, 26*(3), 593-599.

MILLER, J. F. (1985). Assessment of loneliness and spiritual well-being in chronically ill and healthy adults. *Journal of Professional Nursing, 1*(2), 79-85.

MOBERG, D. O., & Brusek P. M. (1978). Spiritual well-being: A neglected subject in quality-of-life research. *Social Indicators Research, 5,* 303-323.

MYERS, J. L., & Gray, L. N. (2001). The relationship between family primary caregiver characteristics and satisfaction with hospice care, quality of life, and burden. *Oncology Nursing Forum, 28*(1), 73-82.

NATIONAL Family Caregivers Association (NFCA) (1997). *Caregiver survey.* Kensington, MD: Author.

NATIONAL Family Caregivers Association (NFCA) (2000). *Caregiver survey 2000.* Kensington, MD: Author.

O'BRIEN, M. E. (1982). Religious faith and adjustment to long-term hemodialysis. *Journal of Religion and Health, 21,* 68-80.

PALOUTZIAN, R., & Ellison, C. (1982). Loneliness, spiritual well-being, and the quality of life. In D. Perlman & L. Peplau (Eds.), *Loneliness: A sourcebook of current theory, research and therapy,* (pp. 224-237). New York: J. Wiley & Sons.

PASSIK, S. D., Dugan, W., McDonald, M. V., Rosenfeld, B., Theobald, D., & Edgerton, S. (1998). Oncologists' recognition of depression in their patients with cancer. *Journal of Clinical Oncology, 16,* 1594-1600.

PAYNE, D. K., & Massie, M. J. (2000). Anxiety in Palliative Care. In H. M. Chochinov & W. Breitbart (Eds.), *Handbook of psychiatry in palliative medicine* (pp. 63-74). New York: Oxford University Press.

PETEET, J. R. (1985). Religious issues presented by cancer patients seen in psychiatric consultation. *Journal of Psychosocial Oncology, 3,* 53-66.

PORTENOY, R. K., Payne, D., & Jacobsen P. (1999). Breakthrough pain: Characteristics and impact in patients with cancer pain. *Pain, 81,* 129-134.

PORTENOY, R. K., Thaler, H. T., Kornblith, A. B., McCarthy-Lepore, J., Friedlander-Klar, H., Kiyasu, E., Sobel, K., Coyle, N., Kemeny, N., Norton, L., & Scher, H. (1994). The Memorial Symptom Assessment Scale: An instrument for the evaluation of symptom prevalence, characteristics, and distress. *European Journal of Cancer, 30A*(9), 1326-1336.

PUCHALSKI, C., & Romer A. L. (2000). Taking a spiritual history allows clinicians to understand patients more fully. *Journal of Palliative Medicine, 3*(1), 129-137.

RAVEIS, V. H., Karus, D. G., & Seigel, K. (1997). Correlates of depressive symptomatology among daughter caregivers of a parent with cancer. *Cancer, 83*(8), 1652-1663.

REED, P. (1986). Religiousness among terminally ill and healthy adults. *Research in Nursing and Health, 9,* 35-41.

REED, P. (1987). Spirituality and well-being in terminally ill hospitalized adults. *Research in Nursing and Health, 10,* 335-344.

ROTH, A. J., & Breitbart, W. (1996). Psychiatric emergencies in terminally ill cancer patients. *Hematology/Oncology Clinics of North America, 10,* 235-259.

ROTH, A. J., Kornblith, A. B., Batel-Copel, L., Peabody, E., Scher, H. I., & Holland, J. C. (1998). Rapid screening for psychologic distress in men with prostate carcinoma. *Cancer, 82,* 1904-1908.

ROTH, K., Lynn, J., Zhong, Z., Borum, M., & Dawson, N. V. (2000). Dying with end-stage liver disease with cirrhosis: Insights from Study to Understand Prognoses and Preferences for Outcomes and Risks of Treatment (SUPPORT). *Journal of the American Geriatric Society, 48*(5S), 122-130.

SODERSTROM, K. E., & Martinson, I. M. (1987). Patients' spiritual coping strategies: A study of nurse and patient perspectives. *Oncology Nursing Forum, 14,* 41-46.

STALLWOOD, J. (1975). Spiritual dimensions of nursing practice. In I. L. Beland & J. Y. Passos (Eds.), *Clinical nursing* (3rd ed.) (pp. 1086-1098). New York: Macmillan.

STEINHAUSER, K. E, Clipp, E. C., McNeilly, M., Christakis, N. A., McIntyre, L. K., & Tulsky, J. A. (2000). In search of a good death: Observations of patients, families, and providers. *Annals of Internal Medicine, 132*(10), 825-32.

STOLL, R. I. (1979). Guidelines for spiritual assessment. *American Journal of Nursing, 79,* 1574-1577.

SUPANICH, B. A., Brody, H., & Ogle, K. S. (1998). Palliative care and physician-assisted death. In A. M. Berger, R. K. Portenoy, & D. E. Weissman (Eds.), *Principles and practice of supportive oncology* (pp. 819-829). New York: Lippincott-Raven.

TRAVELBEE, J. (1971). *Interpersonal aspects of nursing* (2nd ed.) (p. 62). Philadelphia: F. A. Davis Co.

WEITZNER, M. A., Jacobsen, P. B., Wagner, H. Jr, Friedland, J., & Cox, C. (1999). The Caregiver Quality of Life Index-Cancer (CQOLC) Scale: Development and validation of an instrument to measure quality of life of the family caregiver of patients with cancer. *Quality of Life Research, 8*(1/2), 55-63.

WILSON, K. G., Chochinov, H. M., de Faye, B. J., & Breitbart, W. (2000). Diagnosis and management of depression in palliative care. In H. M. Chochinov & W. Breitbart (Eds.), *Handbook of psychiatry in palliative medicine* (pp. 25-49). New York: Oxford University Press.

YATES, J. W., Chalmer, B. J., St. James, P., Follansbee, M., & McKegney, F. P. (1981). Religion in patients with advanced cancer. *Medical and Pediatric Oncology, 9*, 121-128.

# PART THREE

## Advanced/End-Stage Disease Process

# Cardiovascular Disease

CAROL L. SCOT

A dvanced cardiovascular disease is virtually synonymous with chronic congestive heart failure (CHF). A badly damaged heart or vascular system cannot fulfill its basic function, which is to circulate blood through the lungs and body at a rate and pressure sufficient to meet tissue needs for oxygen and nutrients (Colucci & Grossman, 1997). Failure presents in two ways. A heart can fail abruptly, as, for instance, from the rhythm disturbance or electromechanical dissociation of an acute infarction—resulting in sudden cardiac death. On the other hand, if the heart fails slowly, the patient lives and dies with CHF.

Clinicians caring for patients with CHF at the beginning of the twenty-first century have far more information about the condition and its care than was available even 20 years earlier, but every advance brings new challenges. Most patients come to palliative care with relief; happy to change to comfort care only. But a patient who had hoped to receive a heart transplant, and who has just been turned down, may seek palliative care in grief and despair.

In addition to the disease process and its management, the clinician must know the trajectory of illness the patient has undergone, the emotional state of the patient and family, and the goals for care. With this scientific and individual knowledge, the clinician can treat the physical symptoms and also support the patient and family in reaching their goals, as well as help them keep those goals realistic.

This chapter provides an overview of CHF and its etiologies, symptoms, physical findings, appropriate diagnostics, and care.

## ■ OVERVIEW

*Congestive heart failure* is defined as the inability of the heart to supply the heart muscle and the rest of the body with adequate arterial pressure and circulatory volume (Berry, Zeri, & Egan, 1997; Packer & Cohn, 1999). Although morbidity and mortality from most cardiovascular diseases have decreased dramatically in recent decades, CHF has dramatically increased. Over the last 30 years the prevalence of CHF has doubled, perhaps because of the increased survival of patients after acute cardiovascular events. As more patients survive these, the number of people living with damaged hearts increases. Approximately 4.8 million persons in the United States have heart failure, and another 400,000 to 700,000 cases are diagnosed each year. CHF causes or contributes to 250,000 deaths per year (Applefeld, Calkins, Creager, O'Gara, & Rubenfire, 1998).

CHF is strongly age associated—it rarely occurs under age 50; increases markedly from ages 50 to 80; and increases greatly after age 80, with an incidence of up to 10% of that population. CHF is the most common hospital discharge diagnosis for persons over 65 (Applefeld et al., 1998). As would be expected, the costs of care for this epidemic are enormous—in 1994, conservatively, estimates were $10 to $15 billion a year (Applefeld et al., 1998). Between 60% and 70% of the cost is for hospitalizations, and it is here that effective palliative care can make not only a significant human contribution but also an economic one (Council on National Cardiac Education for Registered Nurses, 1997).

CHF is known to be a progressive condition, and recent studies have identified the causative mechanisms. Some neuroendocrine events, such as the activation of the sympathetic nervous system and the renin-angiotensin system, which improve function in the short term, have deleterious effects in the long term (Council on National Cardiac Education for Registered Nurses, 1997). Much of the current care of CHF focuses on blocking these neuroendocrine pathways to slow the progression of the disease.

CHF can be differentiated into primarily left ventricular (systolic) failure (LVF), right ventricular (diastolic) failure (RVF), or cardiomyopathy. Approximately 80% to 90% of cases of CHF are due to LVF (Packer & Cohn, 1999); consequently, the many recent large-scale studies of short- and long-term effects of drugs have concentrated on patients with LVF. In spite of the wealth of material now supporting certain drug regimens for these patients with CHF, the challenge remains for the clinician to individualize care for each patient, whether that patient fits the usual profile or not.

## Medications

For patients with LVF, the class of medication that has been shown to slow the progression of the disease are the neurohormonal blockers: the angiotensin-converting enzyme (ACE) inhibitors and beta blockers. Beta blockers are recommended only for patients in class II or III heart failure (Box 8-1) (Packer & Cohn, 1999).

No studies have been done that show the long-term effects of diuretics, but many have shown the positive effect of control of symptoms. The use of diuretics, especially loop diuretics such as furosemide or bumetanide, is necessary for almost every CHF patient. Nonsteroidal antiinflammatory drugs (NSAIDs) can inhibit the action of diuretics and therefore should be avoided in patients taking diuretics (Packer & Cohn, 1999).

> ### New York Heart Association Functional Classification of Patients with Heart Failure
>
> Class I—*No limitation:* Ordinary physical activity does not cause undue fatigue, dyspnea, or palpitation.
> Class II—*Slight limitation of physical activity:* Patient is comfortable at rest. Ordinary physical activity results in fatigue, palpitation, dyspnea, or angina.
> Class III—*Marked limitation of physical activity:* Although patient is comfortable at rest, less than ordinary activity will lead to symptoms.
> Class IV—*Inability to carry on any physical activity without discomfort:* Symptoms of congestive heart failure (CHF) are present even at rest. With any physical activity, increased discomfort is experienced.
>
> From Criteria Committee, New York Heart Association, Inc. (1964). *Diseases of the heart and blood vessels: Nomenclature and criteria for diagnosis* (6th ed.) (p. 114). Boston: Little, Brown & Co.

Digitalis preparations have been a staple treatment for heart failure for over a century, but the mechanisms by which digitalis exerts its effects and the long-term effects of its use are still under study. Studies already completed have shown that digoxin improves symptoms, quality of life, functional capacity, and exercise tolerance (Packer & Cohn, 1999).

CHF often follows a stormy, erratic course. Patients' symptoms wax and wane, sometimes for known reasons (e.g., he can't stay away from sausage and potato chips, she hates to take her diuretic, there's been a new infarction), but sometimes for no discernible reason.

Death may follow a slow progressive decline, occur with an exacerbation of symptoms, or happen suddenly because of arrhythmia. Data from the Study to Understand Prognoses and Preferences for Outcomes and Risks of Treatment (SUPPORT) showed that end-stage patients were given surprisingly optimistic prognoses up to the day of death (Applefeld et al., 1998; Berry, Zeri, & Egan, 1997).

For decades, the New York Heart Association Functional Classification of heart failure patients has been useful in helping researchers and clinicians to compare the severity of the condition between groups of patients or to compare a single patient's functioning at different times. Patients in the palliative care setting are mostly Class III or IV, but the entire classification is given in Box 8-1 for completeness.

## ■ ETIOLOGY AND PATHOPHYSIOLOGY

Conditions leading to heart failure include both ischemic conditions, such as atherosclerosis, and nonischemic conditions, such as cardiomyopathies, congenital defects, valvular abnormalities, and rhythm disturbances.

- Atherosclerosis: Arterial atherosclerosis is a common cause of coronary artery disease, ischemic heart disease, angina, heart attacks, strokes, aneurysms, and peripheral vascular disease. It is frequently associated with a positive family history, diabetes, male sex, hypertension, hyperlipidemia, and smoking. Coronary artery disease is the cause of heart failure in about two-thirds of the patients with left ventricular systolic dysfunction (Packer & Cohn, 1999). Ischemic heart disease is the most common cause for acute heart failure and sudden cardiac death. In an elderly patient or a patient with diabetes, a myocardial infarction (MI) can cause acute heart failure and present as pulmonary edema rather than chest pain (Applefeld et al., 1998).

- Hypertension: Over the last 40 years, the improved diagnosis and treatment of hypertension has reduced this condition from a major to a minor cause of left ventricular hypertrophy and CHF (Ho, Anderson, Kannel, Grossman, & Levy, 1993).

- Diabetes Mellitus: In contrast to hypertension, the aging and fattening of the population has caused increased diabetes mellitus (DM). Diabetes is often associated with diastolic rather than the more common systolic dysfunction (Bonow & Udelson, 1992).

- Cardiomyopathies: The various cardiomyopathic diseases, in which the heart muscle is affected directly, are less common. Cardiomyopathy may be caused by viral, bacterial, or parasitic infection; alcohol or cocaine; chemotherapy; nutritional deficiencies of thiamine, selenium, carnitine, or taurine; hypocalcemia, hypothyroidism, or hyperthyroidism; or radiation. Inborn errors of metabolism like hemochromatosis, collagen vascular disorders, or sarcoidosis can cause cardiomyopathy through deposits of substances in the heart tissue. Some of these causes, such as the vitamin deficiencies and thyroid abnormalities, can be treated and reversed if diagnosed in time (Kubo & Cohn, 1996).

- Congenital Defects and Valvular Disease: Some congenital defects, such as Tetralogy of Fallot, transposition of the great vessels, or coarctation of the aorta may lead to end-stage cardiovascular disease if they have not been repaired or if the repair was not completely successful. End-stage cardiac disease due to valvular disease is much less common now than in the past. The use of penicillin for Group A beta-streptococcal infections prevents rheumatic heart disease and subsequent mitral valve damage. Almost all significantly abnormal valves are now surgically replaced with animal or artificial valves. Valvular heart failure can also strike in old age when a stenotic aortic valve becomes increasingly calcified and reaches a critically small diameter.

- Rhythm Disturbances: The routine implantation of pacemakers has made rhythm disturbances an infrequent diagnosis in end-stage cardiac disease. Abnormalities of the intrinsic electrical system of the heart, such as sick sinus syndrome, can be completely corrected by a pacemaker.

## Associated Symptoms

The cardinal symptoms of CHF are dyspnea and fatigue. If a patient has dealt with CHF for a long time, he or she may be skillful in exact reporting of symptoms. But other patients may not be and their histories must be elicited through careful inquiry. How far can you walk now? Have you fallen? How are you sleeping? How many times are you getting up at night?

Some of the symptoms in the following list, such as cough, labored breathing, and hemoptysis, can also be observed as signs. The most common symptoms of end-stage heart disease are:

- Dyspnea: the sensation of increased work of breathing
- Orthopnea: the occurrence of dyspnea on recumbency
- Paroxysmal nocturnal dyspnea: being wakened from sleep by acute dyspnea
- Dyspnea on exertion
- Fatigue
- Nocturia
- Insomnia
- Weakness
- Decreased activity tolerance
- Anxiety

  Less common symptoms are:
- Palpitations
- Cough
- Hemoptysis
- Nausea, vomiting, or anorexia
- Right upper quadrant pain
- Chest pain/angina

Although end-stage cardiac disease is usually painless, ischemic heart disease, one of its causes, can be extremely painful. As long as the blood supply to heart muscle is reduced but barely adequate, a patient will continue to have angina. When the blood supply is completely cut off, the tissue dies and is replaced by scar tissue, ending the pain.

Even in end-stage disease, some painful compromised heart tissue can remain, with the potential for a further heart attack. Pain can also occur if heart failure is complicated by a pulmonary embolus or emboli (Applefeld et al., 1998).

## ■ HISTORY AND PHYSICAL EXAMINATION

The normal heart, a four-chambered muscular pump controlled by an intrinsically timed electrical system, responds perfectly to increased demands for circulation to the tissues, whether from exercise, acute illness, or emotional arousal. In end-stage cardiac disease, the heart cannot provide for the needs of the body even at rest, so it is usual to find both tachycardia and tachypnea inappropriate to the level of activity.

The cardinal manifestation of fluid retention in CHF causes several of the signs observed. Frequent signs of CHF include:

- Edema, most commonly lower-extremity, but also presacral or even anasarca

- Pulmonary rales and/or wheezing
- Dullness to chest percussion due to pulmonary effusions
- Cyanosis due to poor tissue perfusion
- Distended neck veins
- Enlarged, tender liver
- Abnormal heart sounds (S3, S4, and murmurs)
- A displaced point of maximum impulse (PMI) due to cardiomegaly

Signs found less frequently include (Council on National Cardiac Education for Registered Nurses, 1997; Kubo & Cohn, 1996):

- Syncope, delirium, or dementia (from decreased brain perfusion and oxygenation)
- Diaphoresis, increased sweating
- Ascites, increased abdominal girth
- Narrow pulse pressure
- Cachexia, profound weight loss

The cardiac nurses' improvement program (Council on National Cardiac Education for Registered Nurses, 1997) suggests a basic five-point rapid clinical evaluation that includes vital signs, fluid status, report of dyspnea, pulmonary examination, report of energy level, and appetite.

The vital signs should include sitting and standing blood pressure, heart rate, respiratory rate, and weight. Fluid status is evaluated by checking for edema and neck vein distention. Pulmonary examination evaluates the use of auxiliary muscles and lung sounds.

## ■ DIAGNOSTICS

The most effective general measure for care of end-stage cardiac disease is close attention and follow-up (Packer & Cohn, 1999). If palliative care is to support the individual patient's best quality of life, each decision must be mutual between patient and clinician, with many aspects of care agreed to on a provisional basis. Howard Brody, MD, has stated that for patient-health provider relationships to accomplish a "right and good healing action" the participants must write the same story of the patient's illness (Brody, 1987). In other words, they must agree on the problem, the goal of care, and the plan to reach that goal, all of which may change over time.

The clinician, for instance, needs to know the patient's wishes ahead of time in the case of an acute event. Would the patient wish to go to the hospital if he or she experienced severe chest pain? Would the patient wish to undergo diagnosis and be treated for whatever might be found—whether a heart attack, pulmonary embolus, aneurysm, or ulcer? Or has the patient reached a stage where he or she desires not to undergo any diagnostic testing or therapeutic procedures but only to have his or her pain and symptoms controlled?

For some CHF patients and their families, the changeover from care designed for long-term survival to care for comfort and short-term functioning may be confusing, and the particulars will need to be discussed more than once. Many CHF patients will be taking an ACE inhibitor. Several large studies have shown that this class of medication improves survival and reduces relapse hospitalizations; patients have been urged to take it even if it doesn't improve their symptoms and even if they have annoying but tolerable side effects, such as a cough (Packer & Cohn, 1999). For these patients, it might be reasonable to discontinue the ACE inhibitor.

Patients with atrial fibrillation or dilated cardiomyopathy may be taking warfarin (Coumadin), and this too can be reevaluated. Warfarin use carries a risk of bruising and bleeding and requires frequent blood tests, so a patient may decide to discontinue its use.

Some patients who are unhappy with taking a large number of medications may see palliative care as a license to discontinue them. These patients are usually people under treatment for diabetes, hypertension, arthritis, or hypothyroidism, as well as CHF and may be taking fifteen or more medicines. Patients certainly have the right to stop medications, but they usually come to see that at least some of the drugs, such as diuretics and pain medicines, do contribute to comfort. Conversely, other patients are just the opposite, afraid to stop taking any medication they have been told to take, and may continue taking diuretics even when dehydrated or antihypertensives even with low blood pressure.

Patients may either accept or reject the use of nonpharmacologic interventions. Some patients may be accustomed to a low-sodium diet and have no problem with it, while others may feel terribly oppressed by dietary restrictions. Some patients may still be trying to follow the advice to give up alcohol and cigarettes and lose weight, while others may just not want to hear about it anymore.

Some patients may want to exercise but are afraid, and others may have been encouraged to exercise and refuse. For patients who want it, cardiac rehabilitation may be a wonderful palliative care modality, offering individual evaluation and care and a group setting with other patients.

In standard care, close follow-up instructions have included: "The patient must weigh daily." In palliative care, if this is something a patient wants to do, with the diuretic dose adjusted for weight gains and losses, fine. If not, the patient's fluid status must be evaluated by other means.

Patients diagnosed with end-stage cardiac disease have usually had multiple diagnostic studies (e.g., electrocardiograms, myocardial perfusion scintigraphy, echocardiograms, cardiac catheterizations) to document decreased ejection fraction, arrhythmias, valve status, and cardiac dilatation. It is unlikely any such testing would need to be performed in end-stage disease. Clinical status remains the principal measure of disease progression in heart failure (Packer & Cohn, 1999).

Because anything that increases the demand on the heart will worsen symptoms, it seems prudent to protect the patient from infections, including influenza and pneumonia, by immunization. Also, if the patient agrees, hypertension should be treated. Thyroid disorders, hypovolemia, and dehydration are other possibly stressful and treatable conditions. Laboratory tests for CHF usually show:

- Hypoxemia
- Elevated red cell counts
- Hyponatremia
- Increased blood urea nitrogen and creatinine from decreased kidney perfusion

Few of these measurements are helpful in caring for the patient with end-stage disease. An exception is hypoxemia, which can be measured noninvasively in the case of increased dyspnea. Supplemental oxygen can sometimes correct the hypoxemia and help relieve any associated dyspnea.

The challenge of caring for a patient with end-stage cardiac disease calls for compassion, clinical acumen, and knowledge of the best of current care recommendations. To accompany a patient and those who care about and care for the patient during the last days, weeks, months, or years of life is a tough but rewarding job for those who choose to undertake it.

## References

APPLEFELD, M., Calkins, H., Creager, M.G., O'Gara, P., & Rubenfire, M. (1998). Cardiovascular medicine. In J. H. Holbrook (Ed.), *Medical knowledge self-assessment program* (pp. 927-1028). Philadelphia, PA: American College of Physicians.

BERRY, P., Zeri K., & Egan, K. (1997). *The hospice nurse's study guide: A preparation for the CRNH candidate* (2nd ed.). Pittsburgh, PA: Hospice Nurses Association.

BONOW, R. O., & Udelson, J. E. (1992). Left ventricular diastolic dysfunction as a cause of congestive heart failure: Mechanisms and management. *Annals of Internal Medicine, 117,* 502-510.

BRODY, H. (1987). *Stories of sickness* (p. 185). Chelsea, MI: Yale University Press.

COLUCCI, W. S., & Grossman, W. (1997). Clinical aspects of heart failure. In E. Braunwald, (Ed.), *Heart disease* (5th ed.) (pp. 450-456). Philadelphia: W.B. Saunders.

COUNCIL on National Cardiac Education for Registered Nurses (CONCERN). (1997). *Cardiac nurses: Improving the standards of heart failure care.* New York: Accel Healthcare Communications.

CRITERIA Committee, New York Heart Association, Inc. (1964). *Diseases of the heart and blood vessels: Nomenclature and criteria for diagnosis* (6th ed.) (p. 114). Boston: Little, Brown & Co.

HO, K. K. L., Anderson, K. M., Kannel, W. B., Grossman, W. & Levy, D. (1993). Survival after the onset of congestive heart failure in Framingham Heart Study subjects. *Circulation, 88,* 107-115.

KUBO, S. H., & Cohn, J. N. (1996). Long-term treatment of the ambulatory patient with heart failure. In T. W. Smith. (Ed.), *Cardiovascular therapeutics* (pp. 224). Philadelphia: W. B. Saunders.

PACKER, M., & Cohn, J. (1999). Consensus recommendations for the management of chronic heart failure. *The American Journal of Cardiology, 83*(2A), 1A-38A.

SUPPORT Principal Investigators. (1995). A controlled trial to improve care for seriously ill hospitalized patients: The study to understand prognoses and preferences for outcomes and risks of treatments (SUPPORT). *Journal of the American Medical Association, 274,* 1591-1603.

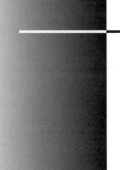

# CHAPTER 9

# *Pulmonary Disease*

PATRICIA H. BERRY

**W**hile chronic, nonmalignant lung disease is the fourth leading cause of death in the United States and affects approximately 10% percent of the population, the literature on care of these persons at the end of life is remarkably sparse. As with most noncancerous end-stage illnesses, research regarding symptom management, especially at the end of life, is sorely lacking.

As you may know, there is clinical lore about the chronic obstructive pulmonary disease (COPD) "personality." Making the transition from curative or life-prolonging care to palliative care is difficult with any disease, but especially so for persons with pulmonary disease and their families. Persons with this illness often bring years of struggle with the health care system and the disability and social service system, while often enduring discord in their family and close relationships. Lung diseases, especially those due to smoking, often cause guilt and blame issues, which, long buried, may resurface at the end of life. Recall the discussion of helping relationships in Chapter 1. It is essential to put preconceived notions about patients and families aside as you approach an often complex situation in the context of end-stage pulmonary disease.

## ■ ETIOLOGY AND PATHOPHYSIOLOGY

Lung diseases commonly seen in end-of-life care fall into the two main categories: (1) obstructive pulmonary disease and (2) restrictive pulmonary disease. While they present a similar symptomatic picture at the end of life, their etiologies and physical findings are often dissimilar.

### Obstructive Pulmonary Disease

*Obstructive pulmonary disease* is defined as a progressive respiratory disease marked by a decrease in airflow, caused by a narrowing or blockage of the airways and one or more of the following conditions. While most persons have a combination of the following pathologies, one of them usually predominates (Kopac, 1996):

1. Emphysema—Results from the trapping of air within the lung and alveolar tissue and permanent destruction of the alveolar tissue.

**137**

Emphysema is further characterized by the following (Uphold & Graham, 1994):

- Airway obstruction
- Hyperinflation
- Loss of lung elastic recoil
- Destruction of the alveolar-capillary interface and thus a progressive decrease in gas exchange

2. Chronic bronchitis—An inflammatory process of the bronchi accompanied by the increased production of mucus. Chronic bronchitis is further defined as the presence of a cough with sputum production occurring on most days for at least a 3-month period during 2 consecutive years and is further characterized by the following (Uphold & Graham, 1994):

- Thickened bronchial walls
- Hyperplastic and hypertrophied mucus glands
- Mucosal inflammation in the bronchial walls—first in the large central airways and later, as the disease progresses, in the smaller airways

3. Bronchoconstriction—The tightening of the smooth muscles of the bronchi, which can result in wheezing, chest tightness, and shortness of breath.

The cause of obstructive pulmonary disease is often unknown, although it is epidemiologically linked with cigarette smoking and exposure to chemical or environmental irritants. Chronic respiratory infections, allergies, heredity, and increased age also predispose persons to chronic obstructive pulmonary disease. An alpha$_1$ protease inhibitor deficiency is suspected as a predisposing factor in younger patients with an onset of the disease under the age of 35 years.

## Restrictive Pulmonary Disease

*Restrictive pulmonary disease* decreases the amount of air that is inhaled, because there is a decrease in the elasticity or amount of lung tissue due to muscle weakness or decreased lung compliance. Pectus excavatum, myasthenia gravis, diffuse idiopathic interstitial fibrosis, and space-occupying lesions (e.g., effusions, tumors) are examples of restrictive lung diseases (Berry, Zeri, & Egan, 1997; Hanson-Flaschen, 1997).

## Overall Disease Progression

The progression of lung disease includes gradually progressive exertional dyspnea and overall gradual decline punctuated with acute exacerbations that are often caused by infection. As with all end-stage illnesses, discussion with the patient and family regarding their understanding of the disease process and desire for treatments—including, but not limited to, resuscitation and artificial ventilation—should be undertaken early in the therapeutic relationship. This is especially important with patients with lung disease because a discussion with them about advance directives and other issues is less likely to occur than with patients with similar prognoses—those with cancer or acquired immunodeficiency syndrome (AIDS), for example (Wachter, Luce, Hearst, & Lo, 1989).

Several markers are helpful in determining if the patient with lung disease is appropriate for palliative treatment. These include:
- Advanced age and a forced expiratory volume ($FEV_1$) of less then 30% predicted and/or a gradual decline in the $FEV_1$ (National Hospice Organization, 1996; Von Gunten & Twaddle, 1996)
- Unresponsiveness to bronchodilators (National Hospice Organization, 1996)
- Pulmonary hypertension, cor pulmonale, or right-sided heart failure attributable to lung disease (Von Gunten & Twaddle, 1996)
- Signs and symptoms of progressive respiratory failure, including low $PO_2$ and high $PCO_2$, which leads to chronic fatigue, very limited exertional tolerance, and a profound feeling of breathlessness (Berry, Zeri, & Egan, 1997; National Hospice Organization, 1996)
- Resting heart rate greater than 100 beats/minute
- Overall decline in performance status and quality of life (Von Gunten & Twaddle, 1996)
- Weight loss greater than 10% of the body weight in the preceding 6 months (Von Gunten & Twaddle, 1996)

### Associated Symptoms

Associated symptoms include (Hanson-Flaschen, 1997; Kopac, 1996; Von Gunten & Twaddle, 1996):
- Dyspnea—Nearly all persons with end-stage lung disease experience dyspnea at the end of life.
- Cough—A cough is sometimes accompanied with increased sputum production with obstructive lung disease; a dry cough is common with restrictive lung disease.
- Pain—In particular, pain can result from rib or vertebral compression fractures related to chronic corticosteroid use.
- Fatigue—The increased work needed to breathe can result in fatigue.
- Insomnia—Retained respiratory secretions, nocturnal hypoxemia, obstructive apnea, dyspnea, anxiety, and depression can contribute to sleeplessness.
- Depression, dysphoria, and anxiety—These symptoms are often related to general disease progression, decreasing functional status, and dyspnea.

## ■ HISTORY AND PHYSICAL EXAMINATION

The history and physical examination of a patient with end-stage lung disease must be approached with an unhurried and calm attentiveness. Eliciting information regarding functional status, insomnia, anxiety, depression, and dyspnea requires patience and attention to subtle yet important changes. Ask the patient and family to provide you with insight into how these symptoms have impacted their own quality of life and functional status. Queries regarding levels of understanding regarding disease progression, the shifting of the goals of care, and the level of support available from family and close others are essential in planning present and future care needs.

There are two types of obstructive lung disease, each with its own unique presentation (Kopac, 1996):

- Type A chronic obstructive pulmonary disorder (COPD); emphysema; sometimes referred to as a "pink puffer":
  - Thin stature; visible muscle wasting
  - Absent central cyanosis
  - Use of accessory muscles for breathing
  - "Barrel chest" appearance
  - Decreased ability to cough effectively
  - Hyperresonance on percussion
  - Distant, diminished breath sounds
  - Clubbed fingers
  - Dyspnea at rest
- Type B COPD; chronic bronchitis; sometimes referred to as a "blue bloater":
  - Typically overweight
  - Central cyanosis is present
  - Minimal use of accessory muscles
  - Resonance on percussion
  - Adventitious breath sounds, typically wheezes
  - Cyanotic clubbed fingers
  - Dyspnea at rest

The history and physical examination findings for patients with restrictive lung disease include the following:

- Distal digital clubbing
- In some interstitial diseases, relapsing infiltrates with fever
- Adventitious breath sounds; end inspiratory crackles, described as "velcro" or "cellophane" in character—typical in pulmonary fibrosis
- Dyspnea with activity

Pulmonary hypertension and cor pulmonale, caused by chronic hypoxemia, are also common in COPD. Severe end-stage COPD can also cause left-sided heart failure (Uphold & Graham, 1994). Refer to the cardiovascular disease discussion earlier in this chapter for further information about cardiovascular disease management.

## ■ DIAGNOSTICS

As with all end-stage illnesses, the overall goals of care should temper the number and extent of diagnostic tests ordered. Ask yourself, as you consider a diagnostic test: "Will the results of this test change the treatment plan?" "Will this test place an undue amount of burden on the patient and family?" "What are the patient's and family's expectations regarding diagnostic testing?" Keeping in mind the goals of care at this stage of illness are most likely palliative, the following diagnostic tests may provide helpful information in achieving these goals:

- Sputum culture—to determine the cause of infection and most appropriate treatment.
- Arterial blood gases—may be helpful in justifying the use of oxygen for comfort or determining when other means to abate dyspnea may be in order.

Always be mindful that persons with lung disease and their families bring a unique history of treatments, experiences, and issues with them to the palliative care setting. The effective management of end-stage pulmonary disease lies in a thorough and comprehensive assessment with attention to detail, aggressive management of symptoms, and an appreciation and acceptance of what this particular disease process means to the person who is ill and his or her family or close others.

## References

BERRY, P., Zeri K., & Egan, K. (1997). *The hospice nurse's study guide: A preparation for the CRNH candidate* (2nd ed.). Pittsburgh, PA: Hospice Nurses Association.

HANSON-FLASCHEN, J. (1997). Advanced lung disease: Palliation and terminal care. *Clinics in Chest Medicine, 18,* 645-655.

KOPAC, C. A. (1996). Respiratory diseases. In C. A. Kopac & V. L. Millonig (Eds.), *Gerontological nursing certification review guide for the Generalist, Clinical Specialist, and Nurse Practitioner.* Potomac, MD: Health Leadership Associates.

NATIONAL Hospice Organization. (1996). *Medical guidelines for determining prognosis in selected noncancer diseases* (2nd ed.). Arlington, VA: National Hospice Organization.

UPHOLD, C. R., & Graham, M. V. (1994). *Clinical guidelines in adult health.* Gainesville, FL: Barmarrae Books.

VON GUNTEN, C. F., & Twaddle, M. L. (1996). Terminal care for noncancer patients. *Clinics in Geriatric Medicine, 12,* 348-349.

WACHTER, R. M., Luce, J. M., Hearst, N., & Lo, B. (1989). Decisions about resuscitation: inequities among patients with different diseases but similar prognoses. *Annals of Internal Medicine, 111,* 525-532.

# CHAPTER 10

# *Gastrointestinal Disease*

PAMELA SUE SPENCER

T he gastrointestinal (GI) system includes the esophagus, stomach, small intestine, large intestine, colon, rectum, gallbladder, biliary tract, liver, and pancreas—organs and tissues that have richly diverse forms and functions. This chapter discusses end-stage gastrointestinal diseases, specifically hepatic failure.

## ■ ETIOLOGY AND PATHOPHYSIOLOGY

Cirrhosis represents the final common pathway of many hepatic disorders characterized by chronic cellular destruction. An intervening stage of increased fibrosis is followed by formation of parenchymal regenerative nodules. It is the nodular distortion of the lobules and vascular network that defines cirrhosis and ultimately plays a critical part in the development of portal hypertension. The cellular and biochemical events leading to this altered growth response and resulting architectural distortion are not well characterized (Yamada, 1998).

### Causes of Cirrhosis

#### Common
- Ethanol
- Chronic hepatitis C
- Chronic hepatitis B with or without hepatitis D

#### Infrequent
- Primary biliary cirrhosis
- Primary sclerosing cholangitis
- Secondary biliary cirrhosis
- Autoimmune hepatitis
- Hemochromatosis
- Cryptogenic cirrhosis

#### Rare
- Wilson's disease
- $\alpha_1$-Antitrypsin deficiency

- Small bowel bypass
- Methotrexate
- Amiodarone
- Methyldopa
- Cystic fibrosis
- Sarcoidosis
- Glycogen storage disease
- Hypervitaminosis A

End-stage liver disease includes malignancy—often potentiated by the risk factors of hepatitis B, C, chronic hepatitis B infection, cirrhosis, hemochromatosis, and ingestion of estrogens and androgens. The progression of disease occurs by direct extension within or from around the liver. Tumors typically alter blood flow within the liver, resulting in rapid spread of tumor. In advanced disease, pneumonia, hepatic failure, and hemorrhage are the causes of death. Tamponade can occur within the liver and lead to necrosis and rupture and finally hemorrhage. If untreated, death occurs in 6 to 8 weeks.

Hepatic failure may also take the form of a rejected transplant. Obviously, these patients and families come to palliative care with unique issues. While the end-stage symptoms of cirrhosis and liver failure are the same, the meaning of the illness for the patient and family is important to explore, recognize, and incorporate into the individual plan of care.

## Associated Symptoms

Clinical manifestations of end-stage liver disease are the same for all types, regardless of cause. Early indications are vague but usually include gastrointestinal symptoms (e.g., anorexia, indigestion, nausea, vomiting, constipation, diarrhea) and dull stomachache. Major symptoms, which develop later as a result of hepatic insufficiency and portal hypertension, may include the following (Isselbacher & Podolsky, 1991):

- Respiratory—Pleural effusion and limited thoracic expansion due to abdominal ascites interfering with efficient gas exchange and leading to hypoxia
- CNS—Progressive symptoms of hepatic encephalopathy: lethargy, mental changes, slurred speech, asterixis, peripheral neuritis, paranoia, hallucinations, extreme obtundation, and coma
- Endocrine—Testicular atrophy, menstrual irregularities, gynecomastia, and loss of chest and axillary hair
- Skin—Severe pruritus, extreme dryness, poor tissue turgor, abnormal pigmentation, spider angiomas, palm erythema, and possibly jaundice
- Hepatic—Jaundice, hepatomegaly, ascites, edema of legs, hepatic encephalopathy, and hepatorenal syndrome, comprising the other major effects of full-fledged cirrhosis
- Miscellaneous—Musty breath, enlarged superficial abdominal veins, muscle atrophy, pain in right abdominal quadrant that worsens when

the patient sits up or leans forward, palpable liver or spleen, and temperature of 101° to 103° F. Bleeding from esophageal varices results from portal hypertension, thus increasing the likelihood of hemorrhage.

# ■ HISTORY AND PHYSICAL EXAMINATION

A comprehensive patient history is paramount when evaluating patients with gastrointestinal complaints at any stage of the disease (Bates, 1979). A clear chronologic account of the patient's problems should include the onset of the problem, the setting in which it developed, and its manifestations. Identification of factors that alleviate or exacerbate the patient's symptoms is helpful. The patient's past medical history detailing illnesses, surgeries, injuries, habits, and family illnesses is valuable. Because many drugs have been found to cause GI injury, a patient medication history is also essential information.

The patient's general appearance and vital signs may suggest clues to his or her overall condition and stability. Inspection of the abdomen may disclose signs of abdominal inflammation, scars, abdominal bulges, or hernias. The liver and spleen are measured and abdominal percussion identifies the amount of air in the stomach and bowel. Percussion also identifies the presence of abdominal masses and ascites.

# ■ DIAGNOSTICS

The diagnosis of end-stage liver disease is often confirmed before the patient seeks palliative care. However, some diagnostics may be appropriate and guide interventions that enhance patient comfort. Plasma ammonia levels are often markedly elevated in end-stage liver disease (Bain, 1998).

Human illness results from a complex interplay of clinical, biologic, psychologic, and sociologic variables. The clinician's understanding of these diverse yet interacting variables is critical for appropriate treatment of end-stage liver disease (Yamada, 1998). The clinician aids in giving realistic prognostic information and facilitating exchange of information with every patient when discussing appropriate diagnostics in relationship to the goals of care.

Many symptoms suffered by patients with end-stage gastrointestinal disease have a number of possible causes and in some cases there are multiple causes in effect. In each situation, the patient needs all the information available to make decisions regarding treatment. Then the goal of the clinician, as with any health care professional, is to support whatever decision and treatment choices are decided upon by the patient in regards to the quantity and quality of life remaining.

It is also important to support cohesion of the family by initiating and promoting interaction, communication, cooperation, and emotional support.

This is a critical role that assists patients through the process. Because end-stage disease is a condition that affects every aspect of the patient's life, being able to identify emotional, spiritual, and social support systems for families and patients is crucial.

## References

BAIN, V. G. (1998). Jaundice, ascites, and hepatic encephalopathy. In D. Doyle, G. Hanks, & N. MacDonald (Eds.), *Oxford textbook of palliative medicine* (pp. 557-571). New York: Oxford University Press.

BATES, B. (1979). *A guide to physical examination* (2nd ed.). Philadelphia: J. B. Lippincott Company.

ISSELBACHER, K. J., & Podolsky, D. K. (1991). Approach to the patient with gastrointestinal disease. In J. D. Wilson et al (Eds.), *Harrison's principles of internal medicine*. New York: McGraw-Hill.

YAMADA, T. (1998). *Handbook of gastroenterology.* Philadelphia: Lippincott-Raven.

# CHAPTER 11

# Renal Disease

KIM K. KUEBLER

**T**his chapter describes the care and management of patients diagnosed with chronic renal failure and end-stage renal disease (ESRD). Renal function exists on a continuum from normal renal function to renal impairment, renal insufficiency, and finally renal failure (Parker, 1995). Chronic renal failure (CRF) occurs when there is a substantial reduction in the glomerular filtration rate—the result of an insufficient amount of active filtrating nephrons within the kidney. A reduction in glomerular filtration rate that has persisted for years or decades produces permanent kidney damage or ESRD. Frequently up to 80% of renal function may be lost before the condition is discovered. Chronic renal failure may progress to ESRD, which mandates dialysis or kidney transplantation (Parker, 1995). Patients with stable renal impairment may not necessarily be diagnosed with CRF but are considered to have progressive renal insufficiency. These patients typically have a serum creatinine of less than 3.0 mg/dL (265 $\mu$mol/L) (American College of Physicians, 1998). Table 11-1 describes the progression of renal disease.

## Diabetes Mellitus and Hypertension

The progression of renal impairment depends on the underlying pathology that contributes to nephron loss. Chronic diseases such as diabetes mellitus (Type I contributes to 40% and Type II contributes to 60% of renal disease) and primary hypertension both interfere with nephron filtration. These two diseases are also largely accountable for 60% of the 250,000 cases of ESRD reported in the United States (American College of Physicians, 1998). Minority patients—especially African Americans, Mexican Americans and Native Americans—constitute a disproportionately large percentage of patients with ESRD, probably because of the higher incidence and severity of diabetes and hypertension in these groups.

Over time, the glomeruli become sclerotic with an excessive accumulation of the extracellular matrix, limiting the glomerules' efficacy of filtration and absorption. The progressive nature of ESRD obliterates the glomerular capillaries—prompting progressive renal destruction involving the extraglomerular interstitium (Parker, 1995).

## TABLE 11-1

### Summary of the Progression of Renal Failure

| Stage | Clinical Finding | Alteration |
|---|---|---|
| Normal | Asymptomatic | Glomerular Filtration Rate (GRF): Normal, 125 mL/min |
| Renal impairment | | GFR: 50 mL/min<br>Serum creatinine: <2<br>BUN: Higher than normal |
| Renal insufficiency | Nocturia, polyuria, nausea, weakness, fatigue, anorexia, weight loss | GFR: 15-40 mL/min<br>Mild anemia<br>Mild azotemia |
| | Occurs over time, decreased urinary output, volume retention, hypertension | |
| Renal failure (acute/chronic) | | GFR: <15 mL/min<br>Serum creatinine: >5 mg/dL |
| | Involves total body systems, manifestations of uremia | Azotemia, anemia, electrolyte imbalance, hyperkalemia, hypocalcemia, hyperphosphatemia |
| End-stage renal disease (nonfunctioning kidney) | | GFR: <5 mL/min<br>Creatinine and BUN: Marked increase<br>Electrolyte imbalances, acidosis |

From Parker, K. (1995). *Management of the patient with renal problems* (Unpublished educational handout). Atlanta, GA: Nell Hodgson Woodruff School of Nursing, Emory University; Price, C. (1992). Issues related to the care of critically ill patients with end-stage renal failure. *AACN Clinical Issues in Critical Care Nursing 3*(3), 585-596.

## Other Causes

The other leading causes of ESRD are glomerulonephritis, polycystic kidney disease, and tubulointerstitial renal diseases. Of these conditions, tubulointerstitial diseases offer the best opportunity for the prevention of ESRD (Seney, Burns, & Silva, 1990). Polycystic kidney disease is the most common genetic cause of ESRD and affects 500,000 Americans (American College of Physicians, 1998).

## Malignancy

Renal failure in advanced malignancy is a common occurrence and is associated with various other etiologic factors (Bower, Brazil, & Coombes, 1998). Malignancy-produced renal failure occurs as a result of tumor infiltration, fluid imbalance, and electrolyte imbalances caused by tumor lysis, hypercalcemia, hypernatremia, and various hematologic factors that occur in myeloma, myelomonocytic leukemia, pancreatic adenocarcinoma, and leiomyosarcoma. Failure may also result from urinary tract obstruction, iatrogenic causes (e.g., chemotherapy, radiotherapy), and paraneoplastic causes (e.g., carcinomas, Hodgkin's disease, non-Hodgkin's lymphoma) (Bower, Brazil, & Coombes, 1998).

CRF is often characterized by the elevation in the serum creatinine concentration as the glomerular filtration rate decreases. Patients are considered to have reached ESRD when the glomerular filtration rate is below 15 mL/min (Parker, 1995). The major causes of CRF, in order of prevalence, are:

- Diabetes
- Hypertension
- Chronic glomerulonephritis
- Urologic disorders
- Cystic kidney diseases
- Unknown

### Associated Symptoms

#### Uremia
Uremia may be considered a systemic disorder affecting multiple organ systems. Renal failure results in the accumulation of potentially toxic substances, yet no single element can be distinguished as the precipitating uremic toxin. Persons diagnosed with renal disease have a propensity to retain what are called *middle molecules*. Their specific nature and pathophysiologic role are not understood. Table 11-2 summarizes other clinical manifestations of chronic renal failure.

## ■ HISTORY AND PHYSICAL EXAMINATION

Patients with a diagnosis of renal disease may present in various ways. The classic signs and symptoms of flank pain, gross hematuria, edema, hypertension, and signs of uremia may not always be present. History and physical examination includes obtaining subjective symptoms from the patient and careful objective evaluation of (Bower, Brazil, & Coombes, 1998; Parker, 1995; Rose & Black, 1988; Shoop, 1994):

- Blood pressure in bilateral arms, both sitting and standing
- Skin color changes or the skin conditions such as dry, scratchy skin; petechiae; or ecchymosis
- Periorbital edema; changes or alterations in the optic fundi; hearing loss
- Breath that smells like acetone or ammonia
- Stomatitis
- Distended neck veins; carotid bruits
- Cardiac murmurs, rubs, and S3 sounds

## TABLE 11-2

### Clinical Manifestations of Chronic Renal Failure

| | |
|---|---|
| Fluid electrolyte and acid-base signs and symptoms | ■ Fluid retention<br>■ Hypernatremia or hyponatremia<br>■ Hyperkalemia<br>■ Hyperphosphatemia<br>■ Hypocalcemia |
| Metabolic signs and symptoms | ■ Carbohydrate intolerance<br>■ BUN accumulation<br>■ Inadequate amino acid metabolism<br>■ Hypertriglyceridemia |
| Neurologic signs and symptoms | ■ Headache, fatigue, apathy, drowsiness, or insomnia<br>■ Behavioral irritability, emotional lability, depression, decreased libido, or seizures<br>■ Paresthesias of periphery, dysesthesias, decreased deep tendon reflexes, changes in gait, foot drop, asterixis, or myoclonus<br>■ Lack of responsiveness to the baroreceptors |
| Cardiovascular signs and symptoms | ■ Hypertension (volume dependent)<br>■ Pericarditis with pain, fever, and a pericardial friction rub or effusion (not necessarily associated with pericarditis)<br>■ Increased risk of coronary artery disease |
| Pulmonary signs and symptoms | ■ Increased susceptibility to infections<br>■ Pulmonary edema<br>■ Pneumonitis (uremic lung)<br>■ Pleuritis<br>■ Pleural effusion |
| Dermatologic signs and symptoms | ■ Dry scaly skin<br>■ Pruritus<br>■ Uremic frost<br>■ Darkened skin due to excess pigmentation<br>■ Ecchymosis or purpura<br>■ Thin, brittle, pitted nails |
| Gastrointestinal signs and symptoms | ■ Anorexia, nausea, or vomiting<br>■ Diarrhea or constipation<br>■ Bad taste in mouth—metallic or salty<br>■ Gingival bleeding |
| Musculoskeletal signs and symptoms | ■ Phosphate and calcium loss, secondary hyperparathyroidism, and bone disease<br>■ Metastatic calcification in soft tissue<br>■ Osteitis fibrosa, osteomalacia, or osteoporosis |
| Hematologic signs and symptoms | ■ Anemia or decreased production of erythropoietin<br>■ Decreased life span of red blood cells<br>■ Bone marrow suppression<br>■ Vitamin, mineral, and iron deficiencies<br>■ Chronic blood loss<br>■ Fatigue and weakness<br>■ Dyspnea on exertion<br>■ Cold intolerance |

From Parker, K. (1992). Nephrology. In L. Burrell (Ed.), *Adult nursing in hospital and community settings.* Charlotte, NC: Appleton-Lange; Parker, K. (1995). *Management of the patient with renal problems* (Unpublished educational handout). Atlanta, GA: Nell Hodgson Woodruff School of Nursing, Emory University; Shoop, K. (1994). Pruritus in end-stage renal disease. *ANNA Journal, 21*(2), 147-153.

- Pulmonary changes; diminished lung sounds; rubs; rales
- Enlargement of the liver or kidney
- Peripheral edema; anascara
- Joint pain; arthritis; bone pain; muscle weakness
- Changes in cognition; asterixis

## ■ DIAGNOSTICS

Before deciding which diagnostics to use in a patient population it is important for the clinician to understand individual patients' comprehension of their chronic illnesses and how they want to carry out the rest of their lives. Chronic renal insufficiency can be an insidious disorder without symptoms until it is far advanced. Once established, it usually progresses to renal failure in spite of excellent care. The patient experiencing renal failure then has choices of dialysis (peritoneal dialysis versus hemodialysis), renal transplantation, or death without treatment (American College of Physicians, 1998).

A clinician may provide palliative care for patients in any of the following settings. A patient in a rural setting may be under the care of a nephrologist in a city many miles away with which the local clinician can practice in palliative collaboration. This patient may be traveling to an intermediate location several times a week for hemodialysis or performing peritoneal dialysis at home. The patient who is waiting and hoping for a transplant or has had a transplant that functioned for years and then failed will also benefit from palliative interventions.

The patient may also be one for whom renal failure is only one of several debilitating chronic conditions and who has opted for no extraordinary means of treatment. The patient may have been through several renal replacement therapies and then made the decision to end them.

For any of these conditions, the clinician and patient can work together to fulfill the patient's goals of treatment. In one patient, this may be careful control of all factors to slow the progression of the disease as much as possible so that he or she can live long enough to have a transplant or see an anniversary, graduation, wedding, or baby's birth. In another, time may be insignificant but quality of life is dependent on being able to still ride a motorcycle, eat and drink what he or she wants, and spend as little time and thought on the disease as possible.

Let us present two patients: Patient A and Patient B. Patient A wants to live as long as possible with the best quality of life obtainable by maximum medical care. Patient B just wants to live comfortably to the end and defines the good life as T-bone steaks, no blood tests or needle sticks of any kind (e.g., erythropoietin is a subcutaneous injection), no urine collections, and no medications—at least no new medications. None of the diagnostics for this patient would be necessary or possible.

Even for Patient B, however, some symptoms may be so distressing that he or she will consider some interventions. Patient B may be willing to take diuretics to control edema. If headaches are severe, the patient may allow blood pressure to be taken, and if it is elevated, may be willing to try an angiotensin-converting enzyme (ACE) inhibitor to get relief. If profoundly weak and pale, but still wishing to get up and around to do things, he or she may submit to blood tests and a transfusion for anemia (since this patient is not waiting for a transplant, transfusions are not contraindicated).

## Creatinine

For Patient A, it will be very important to monitor blood creatinine levels and creatinine clearance at fairly frequent intervals (every 2 to 3 months on a routine basis) or whenever there is a clinical change, such as an infection or elevation in blood pressure. These levels of creatinine clearance determine the dosage amounts and schedules for all medications excreted by the kidney, such as digoxin.

## Phosphate

Monitoring the following levels is important in determining the need for phosphate-binding agents, such as calcium carbonate and supplemental vitamin D and calcium to preserve bone density:
- Calcium
- Phosphorus
- Intact parathyroid hormone (PTH) or N-terminal PTH (not the inactive C-terminal PTH)
- Vitamin D

## Anemia

Anemia should be ruled out. If the hematocrit falls below 30% and other causes of anemia—such as GI bleeding, iron or folate deficiency, and hemolysis—can be eliminated, anemia can be assumed to be caused by erythropoietin deficiency in renal disease (except in cystic disease). Although erythropoietin therapy is very effective, it is expensive and carries a 30% risk of raising blood pressure (American College of Physicians, 1998). Therefore, hemoglobin and hematocrit should be monitored.

In addition to blood pressure, the clinician should monitor the following for those patients receiving erythropoietin treatment:
- Iron stores
- Hematocrit

These values must be followed to assess adequate iron to generate red blood cells and to be sure that the rise in the hematocrit is not too rapid, which would carry a risk of blood clots.

## Protein

Although Patient A will avoid excessive protein, potassium, or sodium intake, the diet should still include 0.6 to 0.8 grams of protein per kilogram of ideal body weight, 2 grams of potassium, and 2 grams of sodium. This patient's intake can also include unlimited fluid until or unless edema, heart failure, or hyponatremia occur (Kopple, 1996). Monitor:

- Serum albumin
- Potassium
- Sodium

Note that if Patient A is a transplant recipient and is receiving immuno-suppressive drugs, the clinician must be alert for other problems and complications, such as opportunistic infections with viruses (e.g., Epstein-Barr virus [EBV], cytomegalovirus [CMV]) or fungi. Other complications include skin and lymphoid cancers, gout, and heart disease. Patients receiving steroids may develop cataracts or aseptic necrosis of the hips and knees.

## Urinalysis

The review of the patient's urinalysis is a major noninvasive procedure to help in the determination of renal disease. The best specimen is obtained by a clean-catch, first-morning void. Determination of the following is essential:

- Color
- Odor
- Clarity
- Specific gravity—normal urine specific gravity is 1.004 to 1.036
- pH
- Protein
- Red blood cells (RBCs)
- White blood cells (WBCs)
- Bilirubin
- Urobilinogen
- Glucose
- Ketones
- Nitrate

### Important Laboratory Values

Important values include the following (Levine, 1983; Price, 1992):

- Creatinine clearance: Every 2 to 3 months, or after a clinical change (e.g., elevated blood pressure, infection)
- Complete blood count (CBC)
- Comprehensive metabolic profile
- PTH
- Vitamin D: Determine the need for phosphate binding agents (e.g., calcium carbonate, supplemental vitamin D and calcium)
- Serum albumin

### Radiologic Studies

If appropriate within the patient's prognosis:

- Kidney, ureter, and bladder (KUB)
- Intravenous pyelogram (IVP) (Levine, 1983; Price, 1992)

- Ultrasound and computed tomography (CT)
- Radionuclide studies (for thromboembolism)
- Renal arteriography (renal mass)
- Pyelography (obstruction) (Parker, 1995)

ESRD affects every dimension of the patient's life. Pharmacologic and dietary treatment options and the compensatory involvement of other body systems become a daily reminder for the patient experiencing this disease (Price, 1992). Because ESRD is a condition for which much research has been done and many options exist, there exists an impressive array of support systems: national organizations, specialized social workers, literature, and internet groups.

The stress of deciding among other options may be appropriate for the patient near the end of life. Patients and families may still have difficult decisions to make or they may be second-guessing themselves for decisions made in the recent or remote past. Spiritual and psychologic support to address this type of suffering may provide much relief.

## ■ ADDITIONAL INFORMATION

Renal Net: Management of Kidney Disease and End-Stage Renal Disease
http://www.renalnet.org/renalnet/renalnet.cfm

Pyelonephrosis Demonstration Case: Case Studies
http://www.brighamrad.harvard.edu/cases/bwh/heache/4/full.html

Hypertension, Dialysis and Clinical Nephrology, Renal Disease Electronic Journal
http://www.hdcn.com/

Kidney Disease
http://www.cde.com/diabetes.world/kidney.htm

## References

AMERICAN College of Physicians. (1998). *Medical knowledge self-assessment program: Nephrology and hypertension*. Philadelphia: Author.

BOWER, M., Brazil, L., & Coombes, R. (1998). Endocrine and metabolic complications of advanced cancer. In D. Doyle, G. Hanks, & N. MacDonald (Eds.), *Oxford textbook of palliative medicine* (2nd ed.). New York: Oxford University Press.

KOPPLE, J. (1996). Dietary consideration in patients with advanced chronic renal failure, acute renal failure and transplant. In R. Schriener & C. Gottschalk (Eds.), *Diseases of the kidney* (6th ed.). Boston: Little & Brown.

LEVINE, D. (1983). *Care of the renal patient*. Philadelphia, PA: W. B. Saunders.

PARKER, K. (1992). Nephrology. In L. Burrell (Ed.), *Adult nursing in hospital and community settings*. Charlotte, NC: Appleton-Lange.

PARKER, K. (1995). *Management of the patient with renal problems* (Unpublished educational handout). Atlanta, GA: Nell Hodgson Woodruff School of Nursing, Emory University.

PRICE, C. (1992). Issues related to the care of critically ill patients with end-stage renal failure. *AACN Clinical Issues in Critical Care Nursing, 3*(3), 585-596.

ROSE, B., & Black, R. (1988). *Manual of clinical problems in nephrology.* Boston: Little & Brown.

SENEY, F. D., Burns, D. K., & Silva, F. G. (1990). Acquired immunodeficiency syndrome and the kidney. *American Journal of Kidney Diseases, 16*(1), 1-13.

SHOOP, K. (1994). Pruritus in end-stage renal disease. *ANNA Journal, 21*(2), 147-153

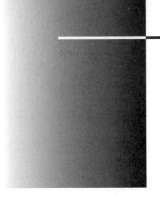

CHAPTER **12**

# *Neurologic Disease*

DEBRA E. HEIDRICH

## ■ ETIOLOGY AND PATHOPHYSIOLOGY

The two basic categories of neurologic diseases seen as primary diagnoses in palliative care settings are: cerebral vascular accidents (CVAs) and degenerative neurologic diseases. The summary of poor prognostic factors for many of these diagnoses, identified by the National Hospice and Palliative Care Organization (NHPCO) (1996), can assist hospice programs in identifying patients appropriate for hospice care. In general, persons with neurologic diseases are most likely to be appropriate for hospice admission if one of the following clinical factors exists (NHPCO, 1996):

- Poor functional status (Karnofsky score: <50%)
- Poor nutritional status
- Age >70 years
- Medical complications—Aspiration pneumonia, upper urinary tract infection, sepsis, refractory Stage III-IV pressure ulcers, or recurrent fever after antibiotics

### Cerebral Vascular Accidents

Approximately 500,000 persons in the United States have CVAs each year, and 150,000 of them die (Luckmann, 1997), making this condition the third leading cause of death in the United States. CVAs tend to be more disabling than fatal (Sacco, 1995), and persons who do not die with the acute event of a CVA tend to stabilize during hospitalization. Those persons who show continuous decline have a poor prognosis and are candidates for palliative care (NHPCO, 1996).

CVAs may be caused by occlusion of the arteries supplying the brain (occlusive stroke) or a rupture in a blood vessel (hemorrhagic stroke). Either mechanism leads to ischemia of brain tissue and has the potential for permanent cell damage. Almost all elderly persons have some degree of blockage of the arterial supply to the brain, mostly due to arteriosclerotic plaques in one or more feeder arteries. The plaque activates the clotting mechanism, leading to clot formation and blockage of the artery. Hemorrhagic strokes most often result from high blood pressure, which causes a blood vessel in the brain to burst (Guyton & Hall, 1996a). Occlusive strokes account for approximately 70% to 80% of all CVAs and are less likely to cause death than hemorrhagic strokes (Luckmann, 1997; Sacco, 1995). Risk factors for CVAs include hypertension, smoking, hypercholesterolemia, cardiovascular disease, and diabetes mellitus (Luckmann, 1997). Death generally results from respiratory compromise, depression of the vital centers of the medulla, or brain stem failure.

## Alzheimer's Disease

Alzheimer's disease is an irreversible form of senile dementia that is characterized by atrophy of the cerebral cortex. It affects 10% to 15% of persons at age 65 and close to 50% of persons over the age of 85. Persons with Alzheimer's disease exhibit a slowly progressive loss of memory, a decline in intellectual function, and disturbances in speech (Luckmann, 1997; Mayeux & Chun, 1995). The prognosis depends on the stage at which the disease is diagnosed. Most persons live for 4 to 10 years after the diagnosis of Alzheimer's, but some will live up to 20 years or more (Mayeux & Chun, 1995). Persons with severe cognitive impairment, limb rigidity, and urinary and fecal incontinence are most likely found in end-of-life care settings.

Only about 10% of cases can be attributed to a genetic abnormality; the rest are considered idiopathic. With Alzheimer's disease, excessive numbers of senile plaques and neurofibrillary tangles occur within the neurons of the cortex, hippocampus basal ganglia, thalamus, and even the cerebellum (Guyton & Hall, 1996b). While most elderly persons have some of these plaques and tangles, persons with Alzheimer's have a much higher number (Luckmann, 1997; Mayeux & Chun, 1995). Biochemically, there is a 50% to 90% reduction in the activity of choline acetyltransferase, the biosynthetic enzyme of acetylcholine. The severity of the cognitive losses with Alzheimer's disease is roughly proportional to the loss of choline acetyltransferase (Mayeux & Chun, 1995).

## Amyotrophic Lateral Sclerosis

Amyotrophic lateral sclerosis (ALS) is a degenerative disease that leads to progressive weakness of skeletal muscles. The prevalence of this disease in the United States is 4 to 6 per 100,000 persons. The cause is unknown, but some 5% to 10% of cases appear to have a genetic link (Luckmann, 1997). Only about 10% of cases are diagnosed before the age of 40. The incidence then increases with age, with a decline noted after the age of 80 (Rowland, 1995). The course of ALS is relentless, without remissions, relapses, or even stable plateaus. Death usually occurs within 2 to 5 years of diagnosis, usually due to respiratory complications. Two factors are associated with a shorter life expectancy: older age at onset and early bulbar symptoms (Luckmann, 1997).

ALS leads to changes within both the central and peripheral nervous systems. Centrally, neurons are replaced by fibrous astrocytes, resulting in gliosis. Peripherally, there is a reduction of large myelinated fibers of the ventral roots, axonal degeneration and atrophy, loss of end plate terminals, decreased choline acetyltransferase and acetylcholinesterase, and depletion of muscarinic, cholinergic, and glycinergic receptors in the spinal cord (Luckmann, 1997). The result is a degeneration of both upper and lower motor neurons. Upper motor neuron degeneration causes hyperactive tendon reflexes, Babinski's reflex, and clonus. Lower motor neuron disease leads to weakness, muscle wasting, and muscle fasciculations (Rowland, 1995). Interestingly, the following functions are not affected by ALS: cognition, sensation, bladder and bowel control, autonomic function, and extraocular movements (Luckmann, 1997; Rowland, 1995).

## Multiple Sclerosis

Multiple sclerosis (MS) is another progressive, degenerative neurologic disease. MS affects the myelin sheath of neurons in the central nervous system, causing demyelination and glial scarring (Luckmann, 1997; Sadiq & Miller, 1995). The prevalence rate varies, with an increase in number of cases at higher latitudes in both northern and southern hemispheres (Sadiq & Miller, 1995). There are approximately 250,000 to 300,000 cases in the United States. While there is no cure for MS, the course tends to include relapses and remissions. The more chronic and progressive type of MS will lead to steady decline. Survival is usually 25 to 35 years after onset of symptoms. Death from MS itself is rare (Sadiq & Miller, 1995). When death does occur from MS, it usually results from infection, respiratory compromise, or severe debilitation (Luckmann, 1997).

There is no known cause of MS. Approximately 15% of cases appear to have a genetic link. Other potential causes include viral infection and autoimmune mechanisms (Luckmann, 1997; Sadiq & Miller, 1995). Plaques form along the myelin sheath of nerves in the central nervous system, leading to demyelination. Inflammation, edema, and death of the myelin-producing cells occur over time. Remissions are probably due to reformation of some myelin, but progressive decline occurs due to scarring and destruction of the nerve axons.

Nerve demyelination and axon scarring causes motor changes (e.g., weakness, spasticity, hyperreflexia) and sensory impairment (e.g., impaired vibration and position sense; impaired perception of pain, temperature, or touch; and moderate to severe pain). When nerves of the cerebellum are involved, the patient experiences ataxia, tremors, nystagmus, and dysarthria. Visual disturbances, bulbar signs, and vertigo occur when the cranial nerves or brain stem are affected. Changes in autonomic functioning may cause bowel incontinence, neurogenic bladder, or sexual dysfunction. Persons with MS are also at risk for depression and cognitive abnormalities (Sadiq & Miller, 1995).

## Parkinson's Disease

Parkinson's disease is an idiopathic syndrome with six cardinal features: tremor at rest, muscle rigidity, bradykinesia, flexed posture, loss of postural reflexes, and autonomic dysfunction. Only two of these features, with at least one being tremor at rest or bradykinesia, are needed for a diagnosis (Fahn, 1995). The etiology of Parkinson's disease is unknown. Like most degenerative neurologic diseases, a small percentage of cases appear to be of genetic etiology. The prevalence rate of Parkinson's disease is about 150 per 100,000 persons, with about 20 per 100,000 persons being diagnosed each year (Fahn, 1995; Luckmann, 1997). There is no cure for this very slowly progressive disease. End-stage Parkinson's disease is identified when the patient no longer has an adequate response to levodopa (Fahn, 1995).

The underlying pathophysiology appears to be a decrease in dopaminergic neurotransmission in the basal ganglia (Fahn, 1995). There is widespread destruction of the substantia nigra that sends dopamine-secreting nerve fibers to caudate nucleus and putamen (all of these structures are part of the basal ganglia). It is believed that dopamine has an inhibitory effect on these areas of the brain and this lack of inhibition leads to continuous output of excitatory signals to the motor control system, resulting in muscle rigidity. Oscillation of feedback circuits causes tremor (Guyton & Hall, 1996c). The deterioration of the basal ganglia leads to a declining ability to initiate movement, control posture, maintain muscle tone, and engage in automatic movements, such as swinging arms while walking and eye blinking (Luckmann, 1997).

The bradykinesia is exhibited in a slow, shuffling gait, a loss of spontaneous facial expression (i.e., a masklike face), drooling from failure to swallow spontaneously, and stooped posture. The tremors are coarse movements at rest which disappear with intentional movement. Muscles become rigid with increased muscle tone. Autonomic dysfunction results in diaphoresis, seborrhea, constipation, urinary hesitancy or retention, and heat intolerance (Luckmann, 1997). Behaviorally, the patient with Parkinson's disease may have a reduced attention span, visuospatial impairment, and personality change. Approximately 15% to 20% of persons with Parkinson's disease have a profound dementia (Fahn, 1995).

## ■ ASSOCIATED SYMPTOMS
### Cerebral Vascular Accidents

The manifestations of CVAs are determined by the location and extent of the infarction and can include decreased level of consciousness, hemiparesis, hemiplegia, numbness, speech impairment, visual disturbance, cranial nerve abnormalities, and coordination difficulties. Complications include atelectasis, pneumonia, pulmonary emboli, seizures, deep vein thrombosis, and hypothalamic syndromes, including inappropriate antidiuretic hormone syndrome, diabetes insipidus, and hyperthermia (Luckmann, 1997).

## Alzheimer's Disease

Persons with Alzheimer's disease are prone to potentially disruptive—sometimes dangerous—behaviors. Wandering, feeling lost, or searching for something; agitation; and overreaction to minor stress are common in even the early stages of the disease (Luckmann, 1997). These behaviors can place a great deal of both physical and emotional stress on the caregivers and may eventually lead to institutionalization of the patient.

Up to 25% of persons with Alzheimer's disease become clinically depressed (Mayeux & Chun, 1995). However, depression may be difficult to diagnose due to the cognitive and functional changes associated with the disease. A trial of antidepressant therapy may be helpful for some patients.

## Amyotrophic Lateral Sclerosis

Muscle cramps, most likely due to hypersensitivity of the denervated muscles, are a common cause of discomfort in persons with ALS (Rowland, 1995). Persons with the bulbar symptoms have both swallowing and speaking difficulties. Aspiration can be a problem, leading to choking or aspiration pneumonia. Losing the ability to talk will require some other form of communication. As the intercostal muscles and diaphragm weaken, dyspnea and respiratory compromise result. Some persons with ALS elect to use a portable mechanical ventilator, which prolongs life but does not prevent this disease from being fatal.

## Multiple Sclerosis

Many of the symptoms associated with MS are discussed above. Patients will likely experience impaired mobility; activity intolerance due to fatigue; alterations in comfort due to neuropathic pain syndromes and muscle spasm pain; alterations in bowel and bladder functioning; potential for falls due to weakness, ataxia, and visual disturbances; impaired nutrition; and risk for aspiration pneumonia due to impaired swallowing. The chronic nature of MS may lead to a breakdown in coping skills and wearing down of social support over time.

## Parkinson's Disease

Episodes of bradykinesia appear to "break through" toward the end of the medication dosing intervals. Careful monitoring of patterns related to medication doses, schedules, and symptom breakthrough can assist in modifying treatment schedules. Sleep disturbances are common with Parkinson's disease and may be caused by muscle activity, alterations in circadian rhythms, disorganized breathing, or variations in dopamine receptor activity (Luckmann, 1997). Some persons with Parkinson's disease have akathisia (an inability to sit still) and "restless leg syndrome." Akathisia is present most of the day and responds to levodopa. "Restless leg syndrome" appears to develop late in the day and sometimes responds to opioids (Fahn, 1995).

# ■ HISTORY AND PHYSICAL EXAMINATION

## History

When obtaining the history, it is important to consider the ability of the patient to provide accurate and complete information. Some neurologic diseases impair mentation, resulting in less than reliable responses from patients. A family member can assist in providing important details. Be careful to not suggest symptoms (Luckmann, 1997). It is important to assess the following:

- History of the neurologic disease to date: presenting symptoms, diagnosis, and changes since diagnosis
  - Mentation status:
    - Language skills—ability to read, speak, and understand spoken words; for persons who have lost the ability to speak, any form of meaningful communication
    - Memory losses: short-term or long-term
    - Difficulty concentrating or making decisions
- Functional ability:
  - Weakness, tremors, or abnormal movements
  - Balance problems
  - Difficulty chewing or swallowing
  - Difficulties with self-care activities
- Sensory perception:
  - Changes in ability to see, smell, hear, or taste
  - Abnormal sensations or pain, such as burning, numbness, tingling, or aching
- Bowel and bladder function:
  - Urinary or bowel incontinence
  - Urinary retention or hesitancy
  - Constipation
- Breathing difficulties
- Psychosocial impact of disease:
  - Signs of anxiety, fear, or depression
  - Patient and family assessment of coping
  - Strength of social support network

## Physical Assessment

The physical assessment identifies the patient's status on the initial visit and is used as a baseline to compare changes over time. In end-of-life care, it is anticipated that the disease will progress and documentation of these changes is important for monitoring the patient's status. Because documentation of declining patient status is required for maintaining hospice support for some patients, even subtle changes are significant. However, not all of the following data are important to monitor in all patients:

- Mental status:
  - Level of consciousness
  - Orientation
  - Mood and affect
- Motor function:
  - Muscle strength of major muscle groups:
    - Use a strength scale:
      - 5 = Full strength
      - 4 = Movement against gravity and some resistance
      - 3 = Movement against gravity but not against resistance
      - 2 = Movement but not against gravity
      - 1 = Trace movement
      - 0 = No movement
  - Muscle groups:
    - Upper extremity: finger abductors, wrist extensors, wrist flexors, biceps, triceps, and deltoids
    - Lower extremity: hip flexors, quadriceps, hamstrings, foot dorsiflexors, and foot plantar flexors
  - Muscle tone: any rigidity, spasticity, or flaccidity; any signs of muscle wasting
- Cranial nerve functioning:
  - Babinski's reflex
  - Any akinesia, dystonia, myoclonus, or tremors
- Ability to speak
- Signs of respiratory compromise
- Sensory function:
  - Ability to sense light touch, pain (pin-prick), and vibration
  - Ability to identify numbers traced in the palm of patient's hand (graphesthesia) and ability to identify objects by feel (stereognosis)
  - Sensory extinction or inattention
- Muscle strength reflexes:
  - Use a rating scale:
    - 0 = Absent response
    - 1 = Barely perceptible response
    - 2 = Average response
    - 3 = Exaggerated or brisk response
    - 4 = Hyperreflexia with clonus
- Tendons to check:
  - Brachioradial
  - Patellar
  - Triceps
  - Biceps
  - Achilles

# ■ DIAGNOSTICS

Magnetic resonance imaging (MRI) or computed tomography (CT) scans may be done to monitor location and severity of cerebral bleeds. This may provide important information for determining if the patient fits the admission criteria of hospice programs. However, after the extent of a CVA has been documented, it is rarely important to use scans to monitor for changes over time in the palliative care setting. If a new CVA or progressive hemorrhage is suspected, the health care team must assess the effect any new information from a scan might have on the overall plan of care. In situations where this information does not change the overall plan, scans are not necessary.

## References

FAHN, S. (1995). Parkinsonism. In L. P. Rowland (Ed.), *Merritt's textbook of neurology* (9th ed.) (pp. 713-730). Baltimore: Williams & Wilkins.

GUYTON, A. C., & Hall, J. E. (1996a). Cerebral blood flow, the cerebrospinal fluid, and brain metabolism. In A. C. Guyton & J. E. Hall (Eds.), *Textbook of medical physiology* (9th ed.) (pp. 783-789). Philadelphia: W. B. Saunders Company.

GUYTON, A. C., & Hall, J. E. (1996b). States of brain activity—sleep; brain waves; epilepsy; and psychosis. In A. C. Guyton & J. E. Hall (Eds.), *Textbook of medical physiology* (9th ed.) (pp. 761-768). Philadelphia: W. B. Saunders Company.

GUYTON, A. C., & Hall, J. E. (1996c). The cerebellum, the basal ganglia, and overall motor control. In A. C. Guyton & J. E. Hall (Eds.), *Textbook of medical physiology* (9th ed.) (pp. 715-731). Philadelphia: W. B. Saunders Company.

LUCKMANN, J. (1997). Caring for people with neurologic disorders. In J. Luckmann, (Ed.), *Saunders' manual of nursing care* (pp. 651-741). Philadelphia: W. B. Saunders Company.

MAYEUX, R., & Chun, M. R. (1995). Dementias. In L. P. Rowland (Ed.), *Merritt's textbook of neurology* (9th ed.) (pp. 677-685). Baltimore: Williams & Wilkins.

NATIONAL Hospice and Palliative Care Organization. (1996). *Medical guidelines for determining prognosis in selected noncancer diseases* (2nd ed.). Arlington, VA: Author.

ROWLAND, L. P. (1995). Hereditary and acquired motor neuron diseases. In L. P. Rowland (Ed.), *Merritt's textbook of neurology* (9th ed.) (pp. 742-749). Baltimore: Williams & Wilkins.

SACCO, R. L. (1995). Pathogenesis, classification, and epidemiology of cerebrovascular disease. In L. P. Rowland (Ed.), *Merritt's textbook of neurology* (9th ed.) (pp. 227-243). Baltimore: Williams & Wilkins.

SADIQ, S. A., & Miller, J. R. (1995). Multiple sclerosis. In L. P. Rowland (Ed.), *Merritt's textbook of neurology* (9th ed.) (pp. 804-825). Baltimore: Williams & Wilkins.

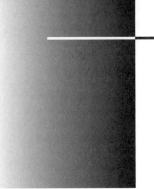

CHAPTER **13**

# *Malignancies*

DEBRA E. HEIDRICH

## ■ ETIOLOGY AND PATHOPHYSIOLOGY

The term *cancer* refers to a group of diseases characterized by uncontrolled growth of abnormal cells, with local tissue invasion and systemic metastasis. It is estimated that 1,268,000 Americans will be diagnosed with cancer in the year 2001 and 553,400 persons—approximately 1,500 a day—are expected to die of malignant disease. Cancer is the second leading cause of death in the United States, accounting for 1 out of every 4 deaths (Greenlee, Hill-Harmon, Murray, & Thun, 2001).

Metastasis is the process by which malignant cells are released from the primary tumor and travel to regional or distant sites where they adhere and grow. Metastasis is the leading cause of both treatment failure and death for most patients who die of cancer (Lydon, 1995; Pfeifer, 1993). Common sites of metastasis are the lymph nodes, bone, brain, liver, and lungs.

Cancer diagnoses that lead most often to terminal illness are those that metastasize early and therefore are diagnosed at advanced stages. The six leading causes of death due to cancer are discussed in the following section. Table 13-1 outlines the metastatic patterns of these diseases.

### Lung Cancer

Accounting for 28% of all cancer deaths, lung cancer is the predominant cause of cancer deaths across all race, gender, and ethnic groups in the United States. In 2001, an estimated 157,400 Americans will die from lung cancer (Greenlee et al., 2001). Squamous cell lung cancers (about 30% of all lung cancers) tend to remain more localized than the other cell types and thus have the best chance for surgical cure. The other cell types—adenocarcinoma, large-cell, and small-cell lung cancers—tend to metastasize early and frequently (Elpern, 1993; Ginsberg, Vokes, & Raben, 1997; Ihde, Pass, & Glatstein, 1997; Lydon, 1995; Shell, Bulson, & Vanderlugt, 1997).

In addition to the common sites of metastasis as outlined in Table 13-1, all cell types of lung cancer are highly likely to metastasize to mediastinal lymph nodes. Other potential sites of metastasis include the pericardium and the pancreas. Lung cancers may also lead to the following paraneoplastic

**TABLE 13-1**

*Common Metastatic Site by Cancer Diagnosis*

| Cancer Diagnosis | Lung | Pleura | Brain | Bone | Liver | Adrenals | Lymph Nodes | Skin | Bone Marrow |
|---|---|---|---|---|---|---|---|---|---|
| **LUNG** | | | | | | | | | |
| Squamous | — | | | X | X | X | X | | |
| Adenocarcinoma | — | XX | XX | XX | XX | XXX | XX | | |
| Large-cell | — | XXX | X | XX | XX | XXX | XXX | | |
| Small-cell | — | XXX | X | XX | XXX | XXX | XXX | | |
| **COLORECTAL** | XX | | X | X | XXX | | XXX | | |
| **BREAST** | XXX | XX | XX | XXX | XXX | XX | XXX | X | |
| **PROSTATE** | XXX | | | XXX | X | | XXX | | |
| **PANCREAS** | XX | XX | X | XX | XXX | XX | XXX | | |
| **NON-HODGKIN'S LYMPHOMA** | XX | X | XX | X | XX | XX | — | X | XX |

XXX, Seen in almost all persons with advanced disease; XX, seen in most persons with advanced disease; X, seen in many persons with advanced disease. From Cohen, A. M., Minsky, B. D., & Schilsky, R. L. (1997). Cancer of the colon. In V. T. DeVita, S. Hellman, & S. A. Rosenberg (Eds.), *Cancer: Principles and practice of oncology* (5th ed., Vol. 1) (pp. 1144-1197). Philadelphia: Lippincott-Raven; Evans, D. B., Abbruzzese, J. L., & Rich, J. A. (1997). Cancer of the pancreas. In V. T. DeVita, S. Hellman, & S. A. Rosenberg (Eds.), *Cancer: Principles and practice of oncology* (5th ed., Vol. 1) (pp. 1054-1087). Philadelphia: Lippincott-Raven; Ginsberg, R. J., Vokes, E. E., & Raben, A. (1997). Non-small-cell lung cancer. In V. T. DeVita, S. Hellman, & S. A. Rosenberg (Eds.), *Cancer: Principles and practice of oncology* (5th ed., Vol. 1) (pp. 858-911). Philadelphia: Lippincott-Raven; Harris, J. R., Morrow, M., & Norton, L. (1997). Breast cancer. In V. T. DeVita, S. Hellman, & S. A. Rosenberg (Eds.), *Cancer: Principles and practice of oncology* (5th ed., Vol. 2) (pp. 1557-1616). Philadelphia: Lippincott-Raven; Hoskin, P. & Makin, W. (1998). *Oncology for palliative medicine.* New York: Oxford University Press; Ihde, D. C., Pass, H. I, & Glatstein, E. (1997). Small-cell lung cancer. In V. T. DeVita, S. Hellman, & S. A. Rosenberg (Eds.), *Cancer: Principles and practice of oncology* (5th ed., Vol. 1) (pp. 911-949). Philadelphia: Lippincott-Raven; Lydon, J. (1995). Metastasis part I: biology and prevention. In S. M. Hubbard, M. Goodman, & M. T. Knobf (Eds.), *Oncology nursing: Patient treatment and support,* 2(5). Philadelphia: Lippincott-Raven; Oesterling, J. E., Fuks, Z., Lee, C. T., & Scher, H. I. (1997). Cancer of the prostate. In V. T. DeVita, S. Hellman, & S. A. Rosenberg (Eds.), *Cancer: Principles and practice of oncology* (5th ed., Vol. 1) (pp. 1322-1386). Philadelphia: Lippincott-Raven; Shipp, M. A., Mauch, P. M., & Harris, H. L. (1997). Non-Hodgkin's lymphomas. In V. T. DeVita, S. Hellman, & S. A. Rosenberg (Eds.), *Cancer: Principles and practice of oncology* (5th ed., Vol. 2) (pp. 2165-2220). Philadelphia: Lippincott-Raven.

syndromes (Bower, Brazil, & Coombes, 1998; Hoskin & Makin, 1998; Ihde et al., 1997; Shell et al., 1997):

- Hypercalcemia occurs secondary to parathyroid hormone–related protein production and is most common with squamous cell lung cancer.
- The syndrome of inappropriate antidiuretic hormone (SIADH) develops due to ectopic arginine vasopressin and is most common with small-cell lung cancer.
- Eaton-Lambert syndrome occurs due to a reduction in acetylcholine released at motor nerve terminals. This syndrome is most common with small-cell lung cancer. Symptoms include proximal muscle weakness, diplopia, bulbar symptoms, dry mouth, impotence, and constipation.
- Ectopic adrenocorticotropic hormone leads to Cushing's syndrome and is seen in small-cell lung cancer. Symptoms include muscle weakness, edema, hypertension, mental changes, glucose intolerance, and weight loss.

The pattern of early and frequent metastasis in lung cancer often translates into patients being diagnosed only when the disease has reached an advanced stage. Indeed, 47% of whites and 51% of blacks are diagnosed with distant metastasis. The 5-year survival rate for individuals diagnosed with distant metastasis is only 2% (Greenlee et al., 2001). Therefore, most patients should be considered for palliative care from the time of diagnosis.

Essentially all chemotherapy for advanced lung cancer is palliative in that cure is not the aim. Survival may be prolonged with chemotherapy, but the potential for increased length of life must be balanced against the effect on quality of life, toxicity of the chemotherapy, and costs of treatment (Grilli, Oxman, & Julian, 1993; Marino, Pampallona, Preatoni, Cantoni, & Invernizzi, 1994). Several promising newer chemotherapy protocols currently under study have both the potential to increase survival and improve quality of living (Gridelli, 2001; Hejna et al., 2000; Rodriguez et al., 2000). It is important to note that persons who respond best to chemotherapy are those who have not been previously treated with chemotherapy and who have a good performance status. Persons who have disease progression while receiving chemotherapy, relapse soon after completion of chemotherapy, or have a compromised performance status have a much lower potential for favorable outcomes from chemotherapy.

## Colorectal Cancer

Colorectal cancer is the second leading cause of total cancer deaths (in the overall population) in the United States. An estimated 56,700 will die of colorectal cancer in 2001, accounting for 10% of all cancer deaths. Across ethnic groups in the United States, blacks are more likely to die from colorectal cancer (23 per 100,000) than other ethnic groups (Greenlee et al., 2001). Sites of metastasis, in order of frequency, include the lymph nodes, liver, lung, brain, bone, and adrenals. Lymph node involvement is evident on diagnosis in approximately 50% of cases; liver metastasis is found in 25% of cases at the time of diagnosis and in up to 70% of cases as the disease progresses (Cohen, Minsky, & Schilsky, 1997; Hampton, 1993; Lydon, 1995; Murphy, 1997).

Colorectal cancer may cause pain involving the abdomen, perineum, and sacrum. It is common for this visceral pain to radiate to the back. In addition, mesenteric involvement by tumor may lead to abdominal pain, which radiates to one or both feet (Hoskin & Makin, 1998). These tumors are also likely to cause (1) obstruction of the bowel, leading to nausea and vomiting and abdominal distension; (2) obstruction of the ureter, causing flank pain, hydronephrosis, and renal failure; and (3) obstruction of the urethra, leading to urinary retention and risk of bladder infection.

Colorectal tumors are resistant to most antineoplastic agents (Hampton, 1993; Murphy, 1997). Therefore, once the disease has metastasized beyond a localized area of the bowel there are few treatment options available.

## Breast Cancer

In the United States, breast cancer is the third leading cause of all cancer deaths (in the overall population) and will be the cause of death for an estimated 40,600 persons in 2001. It is the most common cause of cancer in women and the second leading cause of cancer deaths in women across all ethnic groups (Goodman & Chapman, 1993; Greenlee et al., 2001).

While the lymph nodes are the most frequent site of metastasis, others include the bone, lung, liver, pleura, adrenals, kidney, brain, skin, and chest wall (Crane, 1997; Harris, Morrow, & Norton, 1997; Hoskin & Makin, 1998; Lydon, 1995). Due to the proximity of tumors to the skin surface, breast tumors may cause skin lesions that can progress to fungating tumor wounds.

Metastatic disease is not considered curable (Crane, 1997; Harris et al., 1997; Hoskin & Makin, 1998), but many treatments are available to control metastasis and prolong life considerably. Hormone therapy may be used as an adjuvant in early breast cancer; in later stages of the disease, hormonal therapy may be used for palliation of symptoms. Although hormone therapy is quite effective, the results may not be apparent for several weeks and, indeed, may lead to an initial worsening of symptoms (i.e., "flare response") (Crane, 1997). Therefore, it is not appropriate to initiate hormonal therapy in the final weeks of life.

Women who receive chemotherapy following surgery in early-stage disease demonstrate delayed recurrence and improved overall survival compared to those who do not receive chemotherapy (Crane, 1997). However, its benefit in late-stage disease is not completely clear. Improved survival and symptom control may be possible with combination chemotherapy, even in women who have previously received chemotherapy (Berruti et al., 2000; Kourousis et al., 1998; Nagourney, Link, Blitzer, Forsthoff, & Evans, 2000). No Phase III studies are available at this time to compare these promising survival benefits to standard treatment and best supportive care, especially in women with widely metastatic disease. Study criteria generally require subjects have a high performance status. Women with fewer metastatic sites achieve a better response to chemotherapy. Therefore, when considering treatment for a woman with advanced breast cancer, the APN must evaluate performance status and number of metastatic sites. The beneficial effect of chemotherapy, when given for symptom control, should be apparent by the second or third treatment. If the symptom being treated is not improving, the chemotherapy should be stopped (Hoskin & Makin, 1998).

## Prostate Cancer

Cancer of the prostate is the fourth leading cause of cancer deaths in the United States, and approximately 31,500 men will die of prostate cancer in 2001. It is the second leading cause of cancer deaths in white, black, American-Indian, and Hispanic men. In Asian/Pacific Islanders, prostate cancer is the third leading cause of cancer deaths in men, following lung cancer and colorectal cancer (Greenlee et al., 2001).

Most men are diagnosed with advanced disease, either with local spread within the pelvis (Stage D1) or distant metastasis (Stage D2). Local spread of prostate cancer to the pelvic and abdominal lymph nodes, seminal vesicles, bladder, and peritoneum is common. Frequent sites of metastasis beyond the pelvis are bone, lungs, and liver (Hoskin & Makin, 1998; Lind, Kravitz, & Greig, 1993; Lydon, 1995; Oesterling, Fuks, Lee, & Scher, 1997; Parzuchowski & Wallace, 1997). Men with prostate cancer are at risk for developing urinary outflow obstruction, leading to urinary frequency, hesitancy, and nocturia, which may progress to urinary retention. They are also at risk for urethral obstruction, causing bladder dilatation, hydronephrosis, and impaired renal function.

Prostate cancers are often androgen dependent. Most of these tumors (70% to 85%) will respond to hormonal manipulation, with responses lasting 1 to 3 years. These tumors are also radiosensitive. Systemic irradiation (e.g., Strontium 89) may be helpful for managing bone pain, but does not tend to improve survival. Until recently, chemotherapy did not play a role in the management of prostate cancer. The combination of mitoxantrone and prednisone is now recognized as an established treatment for palliation of symptoms, especially pain, in men with hormone-resistant tumors (Beedassy & Cardi, 1999; Millikan, 1999). Keep in mind that most study subjects showing a good response were less symptomatic and had a good performance status at the initiation of treatment.

## Pancreatic Cancer

Although pancreatic cancer ranks twelfth in incidence of cancers in the United States, it is the fifth leading cause of cancer deaths. In 2001, an estimated 28,900 person will die from this malignancy. The prognosis for persons with pancreatic cancer is poor. The 5-year survival rate is just 4% (Greenlee et al., 2001).

The disease generally does not display early symptoms. By the time pain becomes significant enough for an individual to seek medical evaluation (usually due to pancreatic ductal obstruction), pancreatic cancer is likely to have metastasized. The most common cell type is ductal adenocarcinoma (Daniel, 1997a; Evans, Abbruzzese, & Rich, 1997; Frogge, 1993).

Regional metastatic sites include the regional lymph nodes, major vessels, celiac nerve plexus, duodenum, stomach, bile duct, retroperitoneum, spleen, kidney, adrenals, and colon. Distant metastasis occurs most often to the liver. Jaundice due to biliary obstruction is common. Additional metastatic sites include lung, bone, and brain (Daniel, 1997a; Evans et al., 1997; Frogge, 1993; Hoskin & Makin, 1998). Persons with pancreatic cancer may develop a sudden onset of diabetes due to destruction of the islet cells.

Treatment options are limited. If the disease is localized (which occurs in 7% of cases), surgery offers the only potential for cure. Most often, however, surgery is used for palliation of symptoms by relieving obstructions (or potential obstructions) of the biliary duct and duodenum. The role of radiation therapy is also limited. Palliative uses include relief of intestinal obstruction or unresectable biliary obstruction. Chemotherapy does appear to modestly improve survival and to palliate some symptoms (Burris et al., 1997; Palmer et al., 1994; Glimelius et al., 1996). Patients in clinical trials with gemcitabine demonstrated less pain, improved functional ability, and weight gain (Evans et al., 1997). Patients showing the best responses to chemotherapy are treated soon after diagnosis, having not previously received chemotherapy, and have a good performance status.

## Non-Hodgkin's Lymphoma

Non-Hodgkin's lymphoma will be diagnosed in approximately 56,200 persons in 2001 and 26,300 will die of this disease, making it the sixth leading cause of cancer deaths. The 5-year survival rate is 52% (Greenlee et al., 2001). Persons with AIDS account for some of the increased incidence and mortality seen in non-Hodgkin's lymphoma over the past 6 to 7 years (McFadden, 1993).

There are many different histologic types of non-Hodgkin's lymphoma, and the cell type has a significant influence on prognosis. Of the several different classification systems for lymphoma, most divide the non-Hodgkin's lymphomas into three categories: (1) indolent/low-grade lymphomas; (2) aggressive/intermediate-grade lymphomas; and, (3) highly aggressive/high-grade lymphomas (Daniel, 1997b; McFadden, 1993; Shipp, Mauch, & Harris, 1997). Examples of cell types for these three categories are outlined in Box 13-1, including the median life expectancy if the disease is *not* treated.

Most patients (80%) present with advanced disease, either with regional or distant metastasis (McFadden, 1993). Abdominal lymphadenopathy may be present as palpable masses and cause pain, anorexia, nausea and vomiting, bleeding, diarrhea, and obstruction. Hilar and mediastinal lymphadenopathy causes cough, dyspnea, chest pain, pleural effusion, and superior vena cava syndrome. Skin metastasis presents as red or purplish nodules, usually in the head and neck region. Metastatic processes vary with the type of lymphoma. Follicular cell types tend to metastasize to the bone marrow;

> ### Categories of Non-Hodgkin's Lymphomas Cell Types Based on Disease Aggressiveness
>
> **INDOLENT (MEDIAN LIFE EXPECTANCY MEASURED IN YEARS)**
> - Small lymphocytes
> - Follicular center
> - Mantle cell
> - Nodal marginal zone B-cell
> - Lymphoplasmacytic
> - Cutaneous T-cell
>
> **AGGRESSIVE (MEDIAN LIFE EXPECTANCY MEASURED IN MONTHS)**
> - Anaplastic large cell
> - Diffuse large B-cell
> - Diffuse immunoblastic
> - Peripheral T-cell
>
> **HIGHLY AGGRESSIVE (MEDIAN LIFE EXPECTANCY MEASURED IN WEEKS)**
> - Diffuse small noncleaved cell (Burkitt's)
> - Diffuse small noncleaved cell (non-Burkitt's)
> - Lymphoblastic
> - Adult T-cell leukemia/lymphoma
>
> From McFadden, M. E. (1993). Malignant lymphomas. In S. L. Groenwald, M. H. Frogge, M. Goodman, & C. H. Yarbro (Eds.), *Cancer nursing principles and practice* (3rd ed.) (pp. 1200-1228). Boston: Jones & Bartlett Publishers; Shipp, M. A., Mauch, P. M., & Harris, H. L. (1997). Non-Hodgkin's lymphomas. In V. T. DeVita, S. Hellman, & S. A. Rosenberg (Eds.), *Cancer: Principles and practice of oncology* (5th ed., Vol. 2) (pp. 2165-2220). Philadelphia: Lippincott-Raven.

diffuse cell types disseminate to the brain, bone, and gastrointestinal (GI) tract (Daniel, 1997b; McFadden, 1993; Shipp et al., 1997).

Many patients will receive treatment with curative intent upon diagnosis. Patients with indolent lymphoma who relapse may be retreated with the same or second-line therapy for symptomatic relief. Patients with relapsed intermediate-grade or high-grade lymphomas rarely achieve remission with conventional doses of salvage chemotherapy. Peripheral stem cell or bone marrow transplantation may be an option for some patients (Daniel, 1997b; McFadden, 1993).

## ■ COMMON SYMPTOMS OF ADVANCED CANCERS

As noted in Table 13-1, persons with advanced cancers may have multiple sites of metastasis. Keep in mind that almost all cancers can metastasize to almost any site; the sites identified on the chart are the more common metastatic sites. The symptoms commonly experienced by persons when cancer invades these sites are outlined in the following section.

In addition to the following symptoms, all persons with cancer are at risk for pain due to compression of tissues by the tumor itself, leading to local ischemia, nerve compression, and obstruction of organ systems. Tumors may also invade local blood vessels. Oozing from small vessels may cause anemia; invasion of a major vessel may lead to death from exsanguination. Another common symptom of many advanced cancers is cachexia and anorexia.

## Lymph Node Metastasis

Lymph node metastasis causes pain from inflammation and swelling. When lymph flow is blocked by a tumor, lymphedema results and the affected area is at risk for infection, massive edema, and pain. Enlarged lymph nodes can also compress organs and surrounding tissues, leading to a risk for superior or inferior vena cava syndrome, spinal cord compression, nerve plexus compression, and obstruction of the bowel, urinary tract, or esophagus.

## Bone Metastasis

Bone metastasis causes sharp pain that ranges from moderate to severe in intensity. Bone destruction leads to hypercalcemia and risk for pathologic fractures. Persons with extensive bone metastasis are also at great risk for spinal cord compression from vertebral collapse.

## Brain Metastasis

Brain metastasis puts the individual at risk for increased intracranial pressure and its accompanying symptoms—headache, vomiting, and change in level of consciousness. Depending on the area of the brain involved, personality changes are possible. Persons with brain metastasis are also at risk for seizure activity.

## Liver Metastasis

Liver metastasis interferes with the functioning of the liver, leading to impaired drug metabolism, disturbances in hemostasis, malabsorption, pruritis, anorexia, ascites, jaundice, and hepatic encephalopathy. Pain along the right rib margin is caused by the enlarging liver and is often referred around to the back.

## Lung Tumors and Metastasis

Lung tumors, whether primary or metastatic, put the individual at risk for cough from irritation; dyspnea from effusion, atelectasis, and pneumonia; and wheezing from bronchospasm and obstruction. Hemoptysis results when tumor erodes blood vessels in the lung. Large tumors can compress local organs and tissues. If the esophagus is compressed, the individual experiences dysphagia; neuropathic pain occurs if there is pressure on the brachial plexus.

## Adrenal Metastasis

Adrenal metastases are often asymptomatic until the tumor size is at least 5 cm. With increasing tumor size, the individual experiences abdominal or back pain, as well as the gradual onset of weakness, lethargy, and anorexia. Hyperpigmentation is observed, especially in buccal mucosa, skin creases, and sites of friction. Nausea, vomiting, and postural hypotension are late signs of adrenal metastasis.

### Bone Marrow Involvement

Bone marrow involvement by tumor leads to infections related to neutropenia, bleeding resulting from thrombocytopenia, and fatigue and dyspnea from anemia.

## ■ HISTORY AND PHYSICAL EXAMINATION

A complete history and physical of the individual with advanced cancer is essential for disease and symptom treatment planning.

### General Assessment

Identify and evaluate anorexia/cachexia, weight loss, fatigue level, functional status, pain, and temperature.

### Cardiac Assessment

Evaluate pulse rate and rhythm, heart sounds, and blood pressure.

### Respiratory Assessment

- Assess respiratory rate, effort, and patient reports of dyspnea.
- Auscultate the lungs to identify any wheezing, rales, crackles, pleural rub, decreased breath sounds, or distant breath sounds.
- Percuss the lungs, noting any dullness over effusions or atelectasis.
- Observe sputum for hemoptysis and evaluate the color and consistency for signs of infection.
- Observe the color of nail beds and mucous membranes for signs of cyanosis.

### Skin/Mucous Membrane Assessment

- Identify erythema, skin breakdown, dryness or lesions of mucous membranes, bruising/petechiae, jaundice, hyperpigmentation, or signs of itching.
- Evaluate any tumor nodules or wounds.

### Abdominal Assessment

- Assess bowel status, bowel patterns, and any problems with nausea or vomiting.
- Auscultate bowel sounds and percuss the abdomen to identify air, fluid, or consolidation.
- Palpate lightly to identify presence of lymphadenopathy or enlargement or tenderness of the liver, spleen, and kidneys.
- Look also for signs of bleeding—frank bleeding of upper or lower GI tract, melena, and coffee ground emesis.

## Genitourinary Tract Assessment

- Assess urinary output and observe the concentration and color of the urine.
- Evaluate for hematuria and dysuria.
- Identify any difficulties with urinary retention.

## Musculoskeletal Assessment

- Evaluate range of motion and muscle strength.
- Note any lymphedema or sign of infection.
- It is also important to identify the potential for pathologic fracture.

## Neurologic Assessment

- Assess motor strength and coordination.
- Evaluate changes in sensation and mental status.
- Identify signs of increased intracranial pressure—headache, wide pulse pressure, increased blood pressure, and bradycardia.

# ■ DIAGNOSTICS

Diagnostic testing should be considered if the identification or confirmation of the underlying cause of uncomfortable symptoms will influence the course of action. If, for example, superior vena cava syndrome is suspected but the patient is clearly close to death, interventions to promote comfort (e.g., corticosteroids to reduce inflammation, opioids to treat dyspnea) can be instituted without confirmation of the diagnosis with an x-ray study or computed tomography (CT) scan. Likewise, serum aspartate aminotransferase (AST) and alanine aminotransferase (ALT) levels, while supplying chemical evidence of liver dysfunction, are not necessarily helpful in managing symptoms.

- Chest x-ray studies identify bronchial obstruction, atelectasis, pneumonia, pleural effusion, and superior vena cava syndrome.
- CT scans may show metastasis to brain, liver, lungs, adrenal glands, and abdomen; pleural effusion; superior vena cava syndrome; and spinal cord compression.
- Bone scans show sites of bone metastasis.
- Sputum culture and sensitivity tests assist in selecting the appropriate antiinfective interventions if pulmonary infection recurs or is persistent after empiric antibiotic treatment.
- Blood count and serum chemistries, including complete blood count, calcium, sodium, and glucose, identify bone marrow deficiencies and chemical imbalances.

# ■ INTERVENTIONS PARTICULAR TO METASTATIC DISEASE

All of the symptoms addressed in Unit IV are potential complications of advanced cancer. The APN is encouraged to refer to Unit IV for interventions to manage these symptoms. In addition, the following section presents interventions specifically helpful for symptom management in advanced cancer. These interventions are to be considered in combination with the interventions in Unit IV.

## Bone Metastasis

The pain associated with bone metastasis often requires a combination of opioid and non-steroidal antiinflammatory drugs (NSAIDs). Radiation therapy is also very helpful for the pain of bone metastasis. It appears that there is no difference in pain relief using high-dose single fractions versus fractionated schedules (Pinover & Coia, 1998). Consider that high-dose single fractions are less disruptive to daily living. Systemic radiopharmaceuticals (e.g., Strontium 89) may be considered if widespread bone metastasis and patient has a prognosis of at least 3 months. In addition, if the primary tumor is breast or prostate, consider hormonal manipulation.

## Brain Metastasis

The symptoms of increased intracranial pressure and sometimes behavioral changes due to brain tumors improve with corticosteroid treatment. Loading doses of corticosteroids (dexamethasone or methylprednisolone) are followed by a maintenance dose at the lowest effective dose. A frequently cited initial dose of dexamethasone is 4 mg qid (Caracini & Martini, 1998). Taper the dose by 2 mg every 2 to 3 days to the minimum dose required for symptom management. The median survival on steroids alone is 4 weeks, which may be the only action necessary for symptom management if the prognosis is short. A short course (1 to 2 weeks) of radiation therapy may be helpful if the tumor is radiosensitive and the patient has a prognosis of months.

It is also helpful to restrict parenteral or enteral fluids. However, it is generally not beneficial to restrict oral fluids due to natural decline in oral intake with advanced cancer. In the event of sudden increase in intracranial pressure with risk of herniation—and if reversal of this condition is in the patient's interest—consider admission to an intensive care unit for assisted ventilation, administration of hyperosmolar agents (mannitol), and administration of high-dose intravenous corticosteroids. These intensive measures are rarely appropriate in the palliative care setting because reversal of the disease process is not possible.

## Liver Metastasis

If the pain associated with liver metastasis persists despite maximal pharmacological management, consider a celiac plexus block. If the underlying disease process is small-cell lung cancer, chemotherapy may by appropriate after careful evaluation. Before initiating chemotherapy, the individual's previous response to chemotherapy, length of time from last treatment to disease progression, and functional status must be considered.

Corticosteroids are sometimes helpful for anorexia and malaise associated with liver metastasis, and cholestyramine is helpful for pruritus. Treat encephalopathy as a terminal event; do not institute unpleasant therapies (e.g., magnesium sulphate enemas and lactulose).

## Pleural Effusions

Thoracentesis provides relief of the dyspnea and discomfort associated with pleural effusions. In the presence of recurrent effusions, consider instillation of a sclerosing agent, such as doxycycline, bleomycin, or talc (Pass, 1997; Robinson & Ruckdeschel, 1998).

## Compression/Obstruction due to Tumor or Lymphadenopathy

Consider using corticosteroids to decrease inflammation and relieve compression. Radiation therapy is helpful if the tumor is radiosensitive and the individual has a prognosis of months. A surgical procedure to debulk the tumor or bypass the obstruction is an option if the patient is a good surgical candidate. Placement of stints is helpful to maintain the patency of ureters and the biliary duct.

The care of the person with advanced cancer and his or her family requires a combination of in-depth knowledge of the underlying disease process and probable symptom progression and expertise in symptom management. As with all persons at the end of life, cancer patients and their families have often experienced years of tiresome and perhaps ineffective treatment, uncomfortable symptoms (many of which are not adequately controlled), and an increasing burden on their caregivers. Oftentimes patients and families have lost faith in the health care system. In addition to expertise related to the disease process and progression, the APN needs to establish and maintain a relationship based on mutual trust and respect.

## References

Beedassy, A., & Cardi, G. (1999). Chemotherapy in advanced prostate cancer. *Seminars in Oncology, 26,* 428-438.

Berruti, A., Sperone, P., Bottini, A., Gorzegno, G., Lorusso, V., Brunelli, A., Botta, M., Tampellini, M., Donadio, M., Mancarella, S., DeLena, M., Alquati, P., & Dogliotti, L. (2000). Phase II study of vinorelbine with protracted fluorouracil infusion as a second- or third-line approach for advanced breast cancer patients previously treated with anthracycline. *Journal of Clinical Oncology, 18,* 3370-3377.

Bower, M., Brazil, L., & Coombes, R. C. (1998). Endocrine and metabolic complications of advanced cancer. In D. Doyle, G. W. C. Hanks, & N. MacDonald (Eds.), *Oxford textbook of palliative medicine* (2nd ed.) (pp. 709-725). New York: Oxford University Press.

Burris, H. A., Moore, M. J., Andersen, J., Green, M. R., Rothenberg, M. L., Modiano, M. R., Cripps, M. C., Portenoy, R. K., Storniolo, A. M., Tarassoff, P., Nelson, R., Door, F. A., Stephens, C. D., & Von Hoff, D. D. (1997). Improvements in survival and clinical benefits with gemcitabine as first-line therapy for patients with advanced pancreas cancer: A randomized trial. *Journal of Clinical Oncology, 15,* 2403-2413.

CARACINI, A., & Martini, C. (1998). Neurologic problems. In D. Doyle, G. W. C. Hanks, & N. MacDonald (Eds.), *Oxford textbook of palliative medicine* (2nd ed.) (pp. 727-749). New York: Oxford University Press.

COHEN, A. M., Minsky, B. D., & Schilsky, R. L. (1997). Cancer of the colon. In V. T. DeVita, S. Hellman, & S. A. Rosenberg (Eds.), *Cancer: Principles and practice of oncology* (5th ed., Vol. 1) (pp. 1144-1197). Philadelphia: Lippincott-Raven.

CRANE, R. (1997). Breast cancers. In S. E. Otto (Ed.), *Oncology nursing* (3rd ed.) (pp. 81-123). St. Louis: Mosby.

DANIEL, B. T. (1997a). Gastrointestinal cancers. In S. E. Otto (Ed.), *Oncology nursing* (3rd ed.) (pp. 140-163). St. Louis: Mosby.

DANIEL, B. T. (1997b). Malignant lymphoma. In S. E. Otto (Ed.), *Oncology nursing* (3rd ed.) (pp. 347-365). St. Louis: Mosby.

ELPERN, E. H. (1993). Lung cancer. In S. L. Groenwald, M. H. Frogge, M. Goodman, & C. H. Yarbro (Eds.), *Cancer nursing principles and practice* (3rd ed.) (pp. 1174-1199). Boston: Jones & Bartlett Publishers.

EVANS, D. B., Abbruzzese, J. L., & Rich, J. A. (1997). Cancer of the pancreas. In V. T. DeVita, S. Hellman, & S. A. Rosenberg (Eds.), *Cancer: Principles and practice of oncology* (5th ed., Vol. 1) (pp. 1054-1087). Philadelphia: Lippencott-Raven.

FROGGE, M. H. (1993). Gastrointestinal cancer: Esophagus, stomach, liver, and pancreas. In S. L. Groenwald, M. H. Frogge, M. Goodman, & C. H. Yarbro (Eds.), *Cancer nursing principles and practice* (3rd ed.) (pp. 1004-1043). Boston: Jones & Bartlett Publishers.

GINSBERG, R. J., Vokes, E. E., & Raben, A. (1997). Non–small-cell lung cancer. In V. T. DeVita, S. Hellman, & S. A. Rosenberg (Eds.), *Cancer: Principles and practice of oncology* (5th ed., Vol. 1) (pp. 858-911). Philadelphia: Lippincott-Raven.

GLIMELIUS, B., Hoffman, K., Sjoden, P. O., Jacobsson, G., Sellstrom, H., Enander, L. K., Linne, T., & Svensson, C. (1996). Chemotherapy improves survival and quality of life in advanced pancreatic and biliary cancer. *Annals of Oncology, 7,* 593-600.

GOODMAN, M., & Chapman, D. D. (1993). Breast cancer. In S. L. Groenwald, M. H. Frogge, M. Goodman, & C. H. Yarbro (Eds.), *Cancer nursing principles and practice* (3rd ed.) (pp. 903-958). Boston: Jones & Bartlett Publishers.

GREENLEE, R. T., Hill-Harmon, M. B., Murray, T., & Thun, M. (2001). Cancer statistics, 2001. *CA: A Cancer Journal for Clinician, 51,* 15-36.

GRIDELLI, C. (2001). The ELVIS Trial: A phase III study of single-agent vinorelbine as first-line treatment in elderly patients with advanced non–small-cell lung cancer. *Oncologist, 6*(Suppl 1), 4-7.

GRILLI, R., Oxman, A. D., & Julian, J. A., (1993). Chemotherapy for advanced non–small-cell lung cancer: How much benefit is enough? *Journal of Clinical Oncology, 11,* 1866-1872.

HAMPTON, B. (1993). Gastrointestinal cancer: Colon, rectum, and anus. In S. L. Groenwald, M. H. Frogge, M. Goodman, & C. H. Yarbro (Eds.), *Cancer Nursing principles and practice* (3rd ed.) (pp. 1044-1064). Boston: Jones & Bartlett Publishers.

HARRIS, J. R., Morrow, M., & Norton, L. (1997). Breast cancer. In V. T. DeVita, S. Hellman, & S. A. Rosenberg (Eds.), *Cancer: Principles and practice of oncology* (5th ed., Vol. 2) (pp. 1557-1616). Philadelphia: Lippincott-Raven.

HEJNA, M., Kornek, G., Raderer, M., Ulrich-Pur, H., Fiebinger, W. C., Marosi, B., Greul, R., & Scheithauer, W. (2000). Treatment of patients with advanced non–small-cell lung cancer using docetaxel and gemcitabine plus granulocyte-colony stimulating factor. *Cancer, 89,* 516-522.

HOSKIN, P. & Makin, W. (1998). *Oncology for palliative medicine.* New York: Oxford University Press.

IHDE, D. C., Pass, H. I, & Glatstein, E. (1997). Small-cell lung cancer. In V. T. DeVita, S. Hellman, & S. A. Rosenberg (Eds.), *Cancer: Principles and practice of oncology* (5th ed., Vol. 1) (pp. 911-949). Philadelphia: Lippincott-Raven.

KOUROUSIS, C., Kakolyris, S., Androulakis, N., Heras, P., Vlachonicolis, J., Vamvakas, L., Vlata, M., Hatzidaki, D., Samonis, G., & Georgoulias, V. (1998). Salvage chemotherapy with paclitaxel, vinorelbine, and cisplatin (PVC) in anthracycline-resistant advanced breast cancer. *American Journal of Clinical Oncology, 21,* 226-232.

LIND, J., Kravitz, K., & Greig, B. (1993). Urologic and male genital malignancies. In S. L. Groenwald, M. H. Frogge, M. Goodman, & C. H. Yarbro (Eds.), *Cancer nursing principles and practice* (3rd ed.) (pp. 1258-1315). Boston: Jones & Bartlett Publishers.

LYDON, J. (1995). Metastasis part I: Biology and prevention. In S. M. Hubbard, M. Goodman, & M. T. Knobf (Eds.), *Oncology nursing: Patient treatment and support, 2*(5). Philadelphia: Lippincott-Raven Publishers.

MARINO, P., Pampallona, S., Preatoni, A., Cantoni, A., & Invernizzi, F. (1994). Chemotherapy versus supportive care in advanced non–small-cell lung cancer: Results of a metaanalysis of the literature. *Chest, 106,* 861-865.

McFADDEN, M. E. (1993). Malignant lymphomas. In S. L. Groenwald, M. H. Frogge, M. Goodman, & C. H. Yarbro (Eds.), *Cancer nursing principles and practice* (3rd ed.) (pp. 1200-1228). Boston: Jones & Bartlett.

MILLIKAN, R. E. (1999). Chemotherapy in advanced prostatic carcinoma. *Seminars in Oncology, 26,* 185-191.

MURPHY, M. E. (1997). Colorectal cancers. In S. E. Otto (Ed.), *Oncology nursing* (3rd ed.) (pp. 124-139). St. Louis: Mosby.

NAGOURNEY, R. A., Link, J. S., Blitzer, J. B., Forsthoff, S., & Evans, S. S. (2000). Gemcitabine plus cisplatin repeating doublet therapy in previously treated, relapsed breast cancer patients. *Journal of Clinical Oncology, 18,* 2245-2249.

OESTERLING, J. E., Fuks, Z., Lee, C. T., & Scher, H. I. (1997). Cancer of the prostate. In V. T. DeVita, S. Hellman, & S. A. Rosenberg (Eds.), *Cancer: Principles and practice of oncology* (5th ed., Vol. 1) (pp. 1322-1386). Philadelphia: Lippincott-Raven.

PALMER, K. R., Kerr, M., Knowles, G., Cull, A., Carter, D. C., & Leonard, R. C. (1994). Chemotherapy prolongs survival in inoperable pancreatic carcinoma. *British Journal of Surgery, 81,* 882-885.

PARZUCHOWSKI, J., & Wallace, M. (1997). Genitourinary cancers. In S. E. Otto (Ed.), *Oncology nursing* (3rd ed.) (pp. 164-195). St. Louis: Mosby.

PASS, H. I. (1997). Malignant pleural and pericardial effusions. In V. T. DeVita, S. Hellman, & S. A. Rosenberg (Eds.), *Cancer: Principles and practice of oncology* (5th ed., Vol. 2) (pp. 2586-2598). Philadelphia: Lippincott-Raven.

PFEIFER, K. A. (1993). Pathophysiology. In S. L. Groenwald, M. H. Frogge, M. Goodman, & C. H. Yarbro (Eds.), *Cancer nursing principles and practice* (3rd ed.) (pp. 1-20). Boston: Jones & Bartlett Publishers.

PINOVER, W. H., & Coia, L. R. (1998). Palliative radiation therapy. In A. M. Berger, R. K. Portenoy, & D. E. Weissman (Eds.), *Principles and practice of supportive oncology* (pp. 603-626). Philadelphia: Lippincott-Raven.

ROBINSON, L. A., & Ruckdeschel, J. C. (1998). Management of pleural and pericardial effusions. In A. M. Berger, R. K. Portenoy, & D. E. Weissman (Eds.), *Principles and practice of supportive oncology* (pp. 327-352). Philadelphia: Lippincott-Raven.

RODRIGUEZ, J., Cortes, J., Calvo, E., Azinovic, I., Fernandez-Hildago, O., Martinez-Monge, R., Garzon, C., de Irala, J., Martinez-Aguillo, M., y Cajal, T. R., & Brugarolas, A. (2000). Paclitaxel, cisplatin, and gemcitabine combination chemotherapy with a multidisciplinary therapeutic approach in metastatic non–small-cell lung carcinoma: A phase II study. *Cancer, 89,* 2622-2629.

SHELL, J. A., Bulson, K. R., & Vanderlugt, L. F. (1997). Lung cancers. In S. E. Otto (Ed.), *Oncology nursing* (3rd ed.) (pp. 312-346). St. Louis: Mosby.

SHIPP, M. A., Mauch, P. M., & Harris, H. L. (1997). Non-Hodgkin's lymphomas. In V. T. DeVita, S. Hellman, & S. A. Rosenberg (Eds.), *Cancer: Principles and practice of oncology* (5th ed., Vol. 2) (pp. 2165-2220). Philadelphia: Lippincott-Raven.

# HIV- and AIDS-Related Disease

JAMES DESHOTELS, KIM K. KUEBLER

**H**uman immunodeficiency virus (HIV) infection has received international attention because of its global impact on health and health care. The World Health Organization projected HIV to infect 40 to 100 million persons worldwide by the year 2000, 90% of which are in developing countries and 50% of which are women (American College of Physicians, 1991; Andreoli, Bennett, Carpenter, & Plum, 1997).

Like other chronic diseases, HIV displays a continuum from the initial seroconversion to terminal stages, characterized by overwhelming opportunistic infection. Statistics reveal that in the absence of therapy, this slowly progressive disease has an average course of 10 to 14 years.

The Centers for Disease Control (CDC) classification system defines AIDS as a $CD_4$ cell count of less than 200 cells per microliter, with or without an opportunistic illness or malignancy. Probably the most functional assessment of HIV disease progression is the $CD_4$ cell count, which is the basis for disease staging and many therapeutic recommendations. End-stage or late HIV disease is usually defined by $CD_4$ cell counts between 50 and 200 cells per microliter (American College of Physicians, 1991; De Vicenzi, 1994).

The immune suppression occurring in the late stages of HIV disease results in an increased incidence of opportunistic infections. Common opportunistic infections found in patients with a $CD_4$ cell count less than 200 per microliter include:

- *Mycobacterium avium* complex (MAC)
- Cryptococcal meningitis
- Cytomegalovirus (CMV)
- Progressive multifocal leukoencephalopathy (PML)
- Aspergillosis
- Disseminated histoplasmosis
- Coccidioidomycosis
- Disseminated bartonellosis

The advent of protease inhibitors has drastically changed the face of HIV disease, particularly in its advanced stages. Determining when a patient has entered the terminal stage of HIV disease is based on assessment of clinical status, continuing therapy, or the absence of specific therapies for various infections. A shift to palliative care—where the focus of interventions is the provision of comfort rather than specific treatment—is preferable when the patient has entered the terminal stage of the disease (Canadian Association of Nurses in AIDS Care, 1996).

# ■ ETIOLOGY AND PATHOPHYSIOLOGY

The causative agent of HIV disease, HIV-1, was identified between 1983 and 1984. At that time, retrospective studies of stored serum specimens revealed that HIV had been present in areas of Central Africa for some 20 years. Since 1981, the HIV epidemic has become a worldwide pandemic.

HIV disease is primarily transmitted though heterosexual intercourse. Though first recognized in homosexual men and intravenous drug users in the USA, HIV is rapidly becoming a disease of poor women and children, particularly those of color. In 1996, women accounted for 20% of new HIV cases. A major cause of this epidemiologic shift is intravenous drug use and sexual contact with drug users, who tend to be concentrated in inner cities of larger metropolitan areas. HIV appears in both semen and cervicovaginal secretions and can be transmitted to and from both males and females during sexual activity (Andreoli, Bennett, Carpenter, & Plum, 1997). Partners can also be infected and reinfected with multiple strains or mutations of the virus.

Prior to 1985, blood transfusions accounted for nearly 3% of AIDS cases in the United States but because of antibody screening of donated blood and treatment of blood factors before administration to hemophiliacs, this incidence is now quite rare.

# ■ ASSESSMENT AND MEASUREMENT

HIV disease is usually described as having four stages (Andreoli et al., 1997; Ungvarski & Flaskerud, 1999).

## Asymptomatic Stage

- Acute primary HIV infection
- Asymptomatic condition and/or persistent generalized lymphadenopathy

## Early Symptomatic Stage

- $CD_4$ and T cell counts drop to approximately 500 cells per microliter
- HIV viral load copy count increases to 10,000 to 100,000 per ml
- Patients present with clinical conditions such as:
  - Oropharyngeal and vulvovaginal candidiasis
  - Cervical dysplasia
  - Herpes zoster
  - Pelvic inflammatory disease (PID)

- Listeriosis
- Peripheral neuropathy

## Late Symptomatic Stage

- $CD_4$ and T cell counts are less than 200 cells per microliter
- HIV viral load becomes greater than 100,000 copies per ml
- Opportunistic infections or a diagnosis of a malignancy that meets the criteria for the Centers for Disease Control (CDC) definition of AIDS:
  - Kaposi's sarcoma
  - Pneumocystis carinii pneumonia (PCP)
  - Other opportunistic infections listed previously
  - HIV encephalopathy
  - HIV wasting syndrome (cachexia)
  - Pulmonary tuberculosis
  - Recurrent bacterial pneumonia
  - Invasive cervical cancer

## Advanced HIV Disease

- $CD_4$ counts are less than 50 cells per microliter
- Severe opportunistic infections and malignant lesions occur
- Prognosis is usually 1 year

Clinical manifestations of end-stage HIV disease include, but are not limited to, the following: generalized lymphadenopathy, hepatomegaly, splenomegaly, cachexia, failure to thrive, oral candidiasis, recurrent diarrhea, parotitis, cardiomegaly, hepatitis, nephropathy, CNS disease, lymphoid interstitial pneumonia, recurrent invasive bacterial infections, opportunistic infections, and specific malignancies (Canadian Association of Nurses in AIDS Care, 1996).

Symptomatology of end-stage AIDS may include, but is not limited to, the following: pain, diarrhea, nausea and vomiting, dehydration, urinary incontinence, fever, respiratory symptoms (e.g., chest pain, cough, hypoxemia, dyspnea), decubitus ulcers, delirium and dementia, wasting, depression, anxiety, fear, and fatigue.

Despite the use of protease inhibitors, the incidence of metabolic complications in HIV disease has increased, including emerging diabetic symptoms and "buffalo humps," now understood to be adverse effects of protease inhibitors. The clinician should understand that these complications of protease inhibitor therapy can generally be classified into disorders of glucose utilization, lipid metabolism, and fat distribution (Swindells, 1999). Until more prospective research is done to understand the metabolic disorders occurring in patients receiving protease inhibitors, it is important to obtain periodic measurements of fasting serum glucose and lipid levels in the patients who continue to receive these medications.

With the advent of protease inhibitors and the use of combination antiretroviral therapies, more persons with HIV disease can expect to remain on antiretroviral therapy for the remainder of their lives. Discontinuation of such regimens should occur when the risks, discomfort, adverse effects, or other costs of further treatment would outweigh any benefit. A patient with advanced AIDS who is no longer responding to any available regimen, experiencing severe toxicity, and is not a candidate for any clinical trials should consider discontinuing antiretroviral therapies (Starr, 1999).

## ■ HISTORY AND PHYSICAL EXAMINATION

As with any case of immune system depletion, the clinician should perform a comprehensive baseline history and physical examination on the patient with HIV infection and as comprehensive an examination as indicated when the patient is symptomatic. If the patient presents with a predominant symptom of fever, the multitude of possible causes and associated signs and symptoms should be explored (Walsh-D'Epiro, 1999). Assessment of fever, for instance, may include assessment of the following: medications (for medication-related fever), tick exposure, animal contact, myalgias, headache, mental confusion, cardiovascular accident, nonproductive cough, vision changes or ocular pain, fatigue, abdominal pain, back pain, and neck pain.

## ■ DIAGNOSTICS

Significant diagnostic studies include $CD_4$, $CD_8$, and viral load counts. Plasma HIV-1 RNA titers and $CD_4$ cell counts will offer the clinician the most trustworthy appraisals of the patient's overall health status and prognosis. The $CD_4$ cell count predicts end-organ damage and the risk of opportunistic infections. Studies associated with the detection of opportunistic infections and symptomatology include:
- Complete blood count (CBC) (with or without platelet count)
- Comprehensive metabolic profile
- Hepatic panel
- Culture and sensitivity tests
    The use of mental status examinations, as well as depression and anxiety scales, may also be indicated. A specific discussion of recommended studies, their indications, and scheduling is summarized in Table 14-1.

## ■ INTERVENTION AND TREATMENT

When the AIDS epidemic was first identified in the early 1980s, many patients did not feel that hospice programs met their needs. The emphasis on symptom control versus disease control—which often meets the needs of persons with advanced cancer—was not the most effective strategy for the care of persons with late-stage AIDS. Palliative care models have been reevaluated to provide services specific for the management of advanced AIDS. In Australia, designated palliative care services provide flexibility to meet the needs of the patient. This service is consultative and often assists the pri-

## TABLE 14-1

### Recommended Studies in HIV Disease

| Test | Purpose | Comments |
|------|---------|----------|
| T cell subsets | Staging and prognosis | Every 3-6 months when $CD_4$ cell count is 200-300 cells/$\mu$l; optional when cell counts are below 100 cells/$\mu$l |
| Complete blood count (CBC) with platelets | Detection of anemia, leukopenia, thrombocytopenia | As indicated by symptomatology or pharmacology |
| Chemistries | Detection of renal disease, chronic viral hepatitis, polyclonal gammopathy, infiltrative liver disease, fluid and electrolyte status | As indicated by symptomatology or pharmacology |
| VDRL and RPR tests | Syphilis screening | Yearly in sexually active patients |
| Toxoplasma IgG | Detect risk of cerebral toxoplasmosis | Every 2-3 years or as indicated by symptoms |
| PPD skin test | Tuberculosis screening | Yearly, unless anergic for 2 years |

*VDRL,* Venereal Disease Research Laboratory; *RPR,* rapid plasma reagin; *IgG,* immune globulin G; *PPD,* purified protein derivative. From Hecht, F., & Solovay, B. (1994). *HIV infection: A primary care approach.* Boston: Massachusetts Medical Society.

mary care team, general practitioner, and community nurse or hospital staff in providing continuity in patient care.

This framework of care can be compared to the British Macmillan nurse model, in which the nurse acts as a palliative care consultant for the specific patient population. Disease-specific antimicrobials or other treatments are now often used predominately as the best way to relieve symptoms (Glare & Cooney, 1996; Hecht & Solovay, 1994; Rakel, 1998).

Shifting the focus of care away from curing the disease and prolonging survival toward meeting the patient's needs and improving quality of life should direct the clinician to the appropriate interventions in end-stage HIV disease. This includes the use of antibiotic prophylaxis for opportunistic infections in clients with $CD_4$ cell counts of less than 200 cells per microliter. As with all other palliative interventions, the use of antibiotics may relieve symptoms and optimize quality of life.

Symptom control is a crucial component in effective treatment of end-stage AIDS and will become paramount as death nears. Of significant concern are:

- Pain
- Diarrhea
- Nausea and vomiting

- Dehydration
- Urinary incontinence
- Fever
- Dyspnea
- Cough
- Decubitus ulcers
- Delirium
- Dementia
- Cachexia
- Depression
- Anxiety and fear

Some symptoms of end-stage HIV disease may require interventions not traditionally associated with hospice care. Particular issues of concern may include the provision of long-term intravenous therapy for symptom control (e.g., ganciclovir or foscarnet to prevent blindness in CMV retinitis), periodic transfusions to correct anemias and their symptomatic effects, or continuation of suppressive medications for specific HIV-related opportunistic diseases (Ungvarski & Flaskerud, 1999).

## ■ EVALUATION AND FOLLOW-UP

Evaluation and follow-up care for advanced HIV disease may become a daily task for the primary provider. This may occur in the home setting and require home visits or may necessitate final placement in an AIDS hospice or similar setting where comprehensive care can be provided. Open communication, attention to symptoms and signs of diseases or of treatment failure, and the need for medication adjustment are key functions of the primary provider and the entire care team, including family and volunteers. Ultimately, follow-up will include whatever postmortem care and support are available, indicated, or requested by the family and significant others. The involvement and availability of counselors, clergy, and support groups may be crucial for patient, family, and caregivers alike.

## ■ PATIENT AND FAMILY EDUCATION

By the time HIV disease reaches the terminal stage, education should focus on the dying process and the current needs of the patient and family. Knowing what to expect in terms of the disease process and the patient's behavior can assuage significant amounts of fear and anxiety for all concerned.

Crucial issues for patient and family education include the social, cultural, psychologic, and existential implications of HIV disease. Persons infected with HIV are often stigmatized for having a disease associated with homosexuality, promiscuity, and drug addiction or abuse, even if their exposure was occupational, prenatal, or by an infected blood transfusion. It is a hard fact of life in our culture that a child living with HIV may be "picked on" by other children and abandoned in school and social activities because of unfounded fears of HIV disease transmission. It is important for the clinician to serve as educator and advocate for the patient in this setting.

Psychological and existential issues specific to HIV infection may include those of lifestyle and sexual orientation. The person may face guilt, stigma, or recrimination on the part of family, significant others, or significant groups, especially if there is a history of high-risk behaviors. The clinician can play a key role in educating the patient and family about these issues and may be able to help mediate such conflicts and facilitate reconciliation between the client, significant others, and institutions.

The care and management of persons with AIDS can be extremely complex, requiring a deep and broad understanding of continuously changing medication regimens, drug interactions, and complex serologic findings, as well as pathophysiology. Appropriate physician collaboration and use of specialty resources is crucial to obtaining optimal outcomes in this area of infectious disease. For example, there may be multiple possible causes of fever, pneumonia, or failed antibiotic therapy. Patients experiencing these complications should be referred when possible.

When a patient tests positive for tuberculosis (TB), the local Public Health Department must be contacted; the clinician is obligated to inform the public health system of identified cases of TB. In many areas of the world, TB and HIV occur together in epidemic proportions. A negative purified protein derivative (PPD) skin test does not always preclude TB exposure or infection in advanced HIV disease. Detection of acid-fast bacteria on a smear of deep pulmonary secretions is considered diagnostic of TB. Immune suppression and similarity of symptomatology complicate symptomatic evaluation and clinical diagnosis in concomitant TB and HIV disease. Conducted before referral, meticulous evaluation can save the patient from needless expense, wasted time, and worries.

## References

AMERICAN College of Physicians (1991). *Medical knowledge self-assessment program IX: Infectious disease medicine.* Philadelphia, PA: Author.

ANDREOLI, T. E., Bennett, J. C., Carpenter, C. C. J., & Plum, F. (Eds.). (1997). *Cecil essentials of medicine* (4th ed.). Philadelphia: W. B. Saunders.

CANADIAN Association of Nurses in AIDS Care. (1996). *A comprehensive guide for the care of persons with HIV disease.* Toronto, Ontario, Canada: Author.

DE VICENZI, I. (1994). European study group on heterosexual transmission of HIV. *New England Journal of Medicine, 331,* 341-346.

GLARE, P., & Cooney N., (1996). HIV and palliative care. *Medical Journal of Australia, 164*(10), 612-615.

HECHT, F., & Solovay, B. (1994). *HIV infection: A primary care approach.* Boston, MA: Massachusetts Medical Society.

RAKEL, R. (1998). *Essentials of family practice* (2nd ed.). Philadelphia, PA: W. B. Saunders.

STARR, C. (1999, March). The latest recommendations for antiretroviral therapy. *Patient care for the nurse practitioner: Infectious diseases* [special report], 28-39.

SWINDELLS, S. (1999). Metabolic complications of HIV disease. *The Nurse Practitioner, 24,* 125-129.

UNGVARSKI, P. & Flaskerud, J. (1999). *HIV/AIDS: A guide to primary care management.* Philadelphia, PA: W. B. Saunders.

WALSH-D'EPIRO, N. (1999). HIV disease, persistent fever, nonresolving pneumonia, tuberculosis. *Patient Care for the Nurse Practitioner, 2*(3), 20-40.

# PART FOUR

## Clinical Practice Guidelines

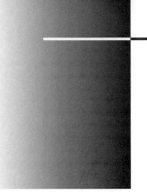

CHAPTER **15**

# *Ascites*

DEBRA E. HEIDRICH

## ■ DEFINITION AND INCIDENCE

Ascites is the accumulation of fluid in the abdomen. The majority of persons with ascites have advanced liver disease—usually cirrhosis (von Gunten & Twaddle, 1998). Other nonmalignant diseases associated with ascites include portal vein thrombosis, congestive heart failure, tuberculosis, hepatic venous obstruction, nephrotic syndrome, pancreatitis, and bowel perforation (Bain, 1998). Approximately 10% of persons with ascites have a malignancy as the primary cause (von Gunten & Twaddle, 1998). About 6% of patients entering hospices have ascites (Waller & Caroline, 2000).

Dyspnea and orthopnea may occur with advanced ascites due to pressure on the diaphragm and leakage of ascites fluid into the pleural space (Bain, 1998). Persons with cirrhosis and ascites have higher variceal pressure than those without ascites and thus are at greater risk for variceal bleeding, which is associated with a high mortality rate (Kravetz et al., 2000). The presence of malignant ascites is a poor prognostic sign, with a one-year survival of 40% and a mean survival of less than 4 months (Bain, 1998; Maxwell, 1993; von Gunten & Twaddle, 1998).

## ■ ETIOLOGY AND PATHOPHYSIOLOGY

Several mechanisms lead to the development of ascites. It is most likely due to a combination of sodium retention, mediated by hormonal and neural mechanisms, and portal hypertension. As the disease progresses, the kidneys are no longer able to compensate for the increased sodium, leading to an increase in total body sodium and water. Portal hypertension develops because of cirrhotic changes in the liver, which causes restriction of normal blood flow in the venous and lymphatic systems. This increase in portal pressure, along with decreased oncotic pressure from defective hepatic protein synthesis, causes the excess fluid to leak through the outer surface of the liver and transude from the portal vascular system, accumulating in the peritoneal cavity (Bain, 1998; Guyton & Hall, 1996; von Gunten & Twaddle, 1998).

Malignant ascites occurs with intraperitoneal spread of tumor and is common with ovarian cancer, breast cancer, gastrointestinal malignancies, and liver metastases (Marincola & Schwartzentruber, 1997; Maxwell, 1993;

Twycross, 1998; von Gunten & Twaddle, 1998). Tumor cells on the peritoneal surface interfere with normal venous and lymphatic drainage, causing fluid to leak into the abdominal cavity. This fluid contains tumor cells that can induce additional fluid accumulation via secretion of vasoactive substances (Bain, 1998; Maxwell, 1993). Portal hypertension may be present in persons with liver cancer, contributing to the development of ascites. In addition, a decrease in oncotic pressure due to hypoalbuminemia, common with cancer anorexia and cachexia, contributes to an increase in fluid accumulation in the peritoneum (Bain, 1998; Luckmann, 1997). Obstruction or invasion of lymphatic channels by tumors may lead to chylous ascites.

# ■ ASSESSMENT AND MEASUREMENT

The physical appearance of a large abdomen is a somewhat late sign of ascites. It has been estimated that 2 liters of ascitic fluid must be present before bulging is appreciated on physical examination (Tabbarah & Casciato, 1990). The earliest signs of ascites are often patient complaints of bloating, abdominal discomfort or pain, and increasing weight or waist size (e.g., clothes don't fit). Patients may also complain of fatigue, inability to sit upright, heartburn, nausea, early satiety, and constipation. As the ascites becomes more pronounced, dyspnea and orthopnea may occur. Edema of the legs is also possible with progressive ascites (Bain, 1998; Twycross, 1998; von Gunten & Twaddle, 1998).

# ■ HISTORY AND PHYSICAL EXAMINATION

The presence of liver disease, heart disease, renal disease, or cancer may help determine the underlying pathophysiology of the ascites. The patient should be asked about the presence, onset, and severity of the following symptoms:

- Weight gain, which can be as much as 50 to 60 pounds (Maxwell, 1993)
- Increasing abdominal girth
- Indigestion, nausea, and early satiety
- Sensation of fullness or bloating
- Ankle swelling
- Dyspnea
- Constipation
- Urinary frequency

   The physical examination of ascites and its complications includes the following:

- Comparison of weight to baseline
- Measurement of abdominal girth
- Assessment of abdomen:
  - Observation for distension with bulging flanks when the patient is supine; may be difficult to discern if the patient is obese or if less than 2 liters of fluid is present (von Gunten & Twaddle, 1998)

- Percussion of abdomen:
  - Note any shifting dullness on percussion with position changes. Generally, you will hear tympany near the umbilicus and dullness as you percuss outward. If the patient turns to one side, the dullness shifts to the dependent areas.
    - Feel for evidence of a fluid wave (e.g., when flank it tapped on one side an impulse is felt on the opposite side). Be sure to block transmission of a wave through subcutaneous fat by having an assistant place the medial edges of both hands firmly down the midline of the abdomen.
  - Observation for stretched skin across abdomen
  - Observation for abdominal venous engorgement
  - Observation for changes in umbilicus; may be flattened or everted
- Assessment of scrotal and/or lower-extremity edema
- Assessment for associated complications:
  - Dyspnea, due to pressure on diaphragm or pleural effusion:
    - Note rate and depth of respiration.
    - Assess for diminished or absent breath sounds.
  - Dehydration or malnutrition due to nausea and early satiety:
    - Assess hydration of mucous membranes.
    - Assess general nutritional status.

## ■ DIAGNOSTICS

Abdominal x-ray studies, ultrasound, and computed tomography (CT) scans do verify the presence of free fluid in the abdomen, but these tests are generally not required after a thorough history and physical examination. In an x-ray study, ascites appears with hazy or ground glass features, distended and separated loops of bowel, and poor definition of abdominal organs (Bain, 1998; von Gunten & Twaddle, 1998).

When paracentesis is performed, the fluid is examined for color, clarity, and the presence of blood. Cytology and examination of the protein concentration of the fluid are tests that assist in determining the cause of ascites. In end-of-life care, the cause is often evident, so these tests are rarely required. More commonly, to select the appropriate antibiotic intervention when infection is suspected, the peritoneal fluid is examined for cell count, gram stain, and culture.

## ■ INTERVENTION AND TREATMENT

Sodium and water restriction and diuretics may be effective for ascites due to cirrhosis or malignant liver involvement (e.g., when portal hypertension plays a role) but is rarely effective for other types of malignant ascites. Sodium is restricted to 100 mmol/day (approximately 2 g/day) or less (Bain, 1998). In end-of-life care, it is important to balance the potential therapeutic effects of sodium restriction with the quality of living benefits of allowing persons to eat whatever foods taste good to them. As the appetite decreases, the appropriateness of a sodium-restricted diet also decreases.

For diuretic therapy, spironolactone is more effective than loop diuretics. However, a combination of spironolactone and loop diuretics (e.g., furosemide) may be even more effective. Twycross (1998) suggests starting with 100 to 200 mg PO of spironolactone per day. If this is not effective after 1 week, the spironolactone may be increased to 200 to 300 mg PO per day and furosemide 40 mg PO may be added. If this regimen is not effective by the second week, the patient should be given spironolactone 200 mg with 80 mg of furosemide by mouth. Potential complications of diuretics, especially overuse of diuretics, include fluid and electrolyte imbalances, postural hypotension, hepatic encephalopathy, and prerenal failure (Bain, 1998).

In addition to monitoring for potential complications of diuretic therapy, the practitioner must also monitor for other burdens of these medications. Persons with fatigue and limited mobility may find that diuretic therapy leads to expenditure of energy (e.g., ambulating to the bathroom, getting out of bed to the bedside commode) that might be better used for other more important activities. Persons experiencing early satiety may find that taking medications leaves little room for the intake of more satisfying food or fluids.

Paracentesis may be helpful to achieve short-term relief of uncomfortable symptoms, such as abdominal discomfort and dyspnea. While it is noted that the removal of more than 1 liter of ascites fluid may lead to hypotension (Luckmann, 1997), it is not uncommon to remove significantly more fluid in patients with tense abdomens. The incidence of hypotension appears to be greater if the paracentesis is used for nonmalignant ascites (von Gunten & Twaddle, 1998). Up to 5 liters may be removed safely at a single session, especially in patients who have malignant ascites or in patients with nonmalignant ascites who have some peripheral edema (Bain, 1998; von Gunten & Twaddle, 1998). Persons with nonmalignant ascites, low serum albumin, and no edema may benefit from the infusion of 40 grams of albumin intravenously, both before and 6 to 8 hours after the removal of more than 2 liters of ascitic fluid (von Gunten & Twaddle, 1998). For patients who cannot tolerate the complete removal of ascitic fluid, relief from symptoms may be obtained after the removal of only 2 liters of fluid (Twycross, 1998).

There is always a risk of infection with paracentesis. Strict sterile technique should be used for the procedure. Other complications include visceral damage and the potential for bleeding. Patients with platelet counts less than 100,000 should not have paracentesis (Luckmann, 1997).

Ascitic fluid often reaccumulates following paracentesis. Repeated removal of fluid can lead to protein deficiencies and electrolyte abnormalities.

The patient's overall physical condition will guide decisions about appropriate monitoring and replacement of electrolytes.

Intracavitary chemotherapy may control ascites and decrease the frequency of paracenteses. However, there are no good prospective studies to demonstrate the true effectiveness of this intervention. Bleomycin, 60 to 120 mg in 100 ml of saline, is often the agent of choice. It is instilled via the peritoneal catheter after paracentesis. The patient must change positions every few minutes for an hour to disperse the medication. Side effects include fever and abdominal tenderness (Waller & Caroline, 2000).

When repeated paracenteses are required, consider placement of a Tenckhoff or Groshong catheter. This allows the patient or family to drain ascitic fluid at home. One retrospective study of indwelling peritoneal catheters for drainage of peritoneal fluid demonstrated the catheters remain functioning for a median of 37 days (Lee, Lau, & Yeong, 2000). The most common cause of catheter-related problems is infection.

A peritoneovenous shunt, using the LeVeen or Denver shunt, provides continuous shunting of ascitic fluid from the abdomen through a one-way, pressure-sensitive valve to a silicone catheter emptying into the superior vena cava. These shunts can be placed under local anesthesia, although some surgeons may prefer general anesthesia. This procedure is an option for persons who may require repeated paracenteses for comfort who can also tolerate a surgical procedure. The life expectancy of the patient helps to determine the appropriateness of a peritoneal drain versus a shunt.

In the past, peritoneovenous shunts have not been recommended for malignant ascites because of concerns about dumping malignant cells into the circulation and the tendency for the shunts to fail because of occlusion (Luckmann, 1997; Twycross, 1998; von Gunten & Twaddle, 1998). However, studies support this procedure is well tolerated and achieves control of ascites in the majority of patients with minimal complications (Tueche & Pector, 2000; Wickremesekera & Stubbs, 1997).

The administration of octreotide, 200 to 400 μg SC per day, is reported to be effective in some cases of intractable ascites (Cairns & Malone, 1999). The true cost-benefit ratio of this intervention has not been adequately evaluated.

In addition to decreasing the fluid in the abdomen, interventions should also include instituting an effective bowel regimen to treat constipation. A stimulant and softener are often necessary.

## ■ EVALUATION AND FOLLOW-UP

- Assess abdominal girth after treatment as a measurement of effectiveness.
- Monitor for signs of reaccumulation of fluid.
- Measure abdominal girth regularly to identify changes.

- Assess for symptoms associated with fluid accumulation.
- Monitor weight.
- Following paracentesis:
  - Monitor for postural hypotension.
  - Monitor the puncture site for leakage.
  - Monitor vital signs for evidence of infection.
- Provide site care if Tenckhoff or Groshong catheter is used.

## ■ PATIENT AND FAMILY EDUCATION

- Teach signs and symptoms to report:
  - Signs of fluid accumulation (e.g., abdominal discomfort or bloating, dyspnea)
  - Signs of infection
- Prepare for paracentesis:
  - Explain the purpose of the paracentesis.
  - Explain the procedure, potential complications, and follow-up care.
  - Explain that reaccumulation of fluid is likely.
- Provide information about diuretic therapy, as appropriate.
- If ascites is caused by liver disease, discuss the "pros and cons" of a low-sodium diet and fluid restriction.
- Teach appropriate use of bowel stimulants and softeners. Encourage to report to the practitioner if there is no bowel movement for more than 2 days.

## ✔ CASE STUDY

Mrs. Sanchez is 58 years old and has advanced ovarian cancer. Over the past month she has noticed an increasing difficulty in fastening the waist closures of pants and skirts. The only pants she can wear now are sweat pants with a draw-string waist. She complains of a poor appetite but has gained about 25 pounds. She states she is always tired and has difficulty lying flat in bed because of shortness of breath but she is able to sleep if she keeps the head of her bed elevated.

On physical examination, the nurse observes a protruding abdomen when Mrs. Sanchez is standing or sitting and bulging flanks when the patient is lying. The skin across the abdomen is tight with prominent veins. With percussion, tympany is noted over the umbilicus and dullness at the flanks when Mrs. Sanchez is lying on her back. When the patient lies on her left side, the nurse notes tympany on the right (upper) side and dullness on the left (dependent) side. Her abdominal girth is measured at 144 centimeters.

With the diagnosis of ovarian cancer, the cause of ascites is evident and no diagnostic tests are ordered at this time. Because sodium/fluid restrictions and diuretics are of little value with malignant ascites, a paracentesis at the out-patient clinic is performed. About 4 liters of yellow, turbid fluid are removed. Mrs. Sanchez tolerates the procedure well with no signs of postural hypoten-sion. She experiences immediate relief of dyspnea and the generalized ab-dominal discomfort. Her abdominal girth after the procedure is measured at 105 centimeters. Markings are placed on her abdomen so that her caregiver can monitor the abdominal girth at home. A bowel regimen of docusate sodium 100 mg with casanthranol 30 mg (Peri-Colace) PO is initiated.

Over the next 4 weeks, Mrs. Sanchez's abdominal girth gradually in-creases to 124 centimeters and the uncomfortable symptoms return. As re-peat paracenteses are anticipated, a Tenckhoff catheter is placed and 3 liters of yellow, turbid ascitic fluid is removed. The caregiver is taught to provide daily dressing changes around the catheter, using sterile technique, and to monitor the site for redness, swelling, or drainage. The caregiver is also taught how to attach a drainage bag to the stopcock on the catheter and drain up to 2 liters of fluid whenever Mrs. Sanchez complains of abdominal fullness.

Over the next month, the caregiver reports a decreased need to drain fluid to keep Mrs. Sanchez comfortable. She is eating and drinking very little and is now completely bedbound. Mrs. Sanchez dies at home 5 days later with no abdominal distension, no abdominal discomfort, and no dyspnea.

## References

BAIN, V. G. (1998). Jaundice, ascites, and hepatic encephalopathy. In D. Doyle, G. W. C. Hanks, & N. MacDonald (Eds.), *Oxford textbook of palliative medicine* (2nd ed.) (pp. 557-571). New York: Oxford University Press.

CAIRNS, W. & Malone, R. (1999). Octreotide as an agent for the relief of malignant ascites in palliative care patients. *Palliative Medicine, 13*, 429.

Guyton, A. C., & Hall, J. E. (1996). The liver as an organ. In A. C. Guyton & J. E. Hall (Eds.), *Textbook of medical physiology* (9th ed.) (pp. 883-888). Philadelphia: W. B. Saunders.

KRAVETZ, D., Bildozola, M., Argonz, J., Romero, G., Korula, J., Munoz, A., Suarez, A., & Terg, R. (2000). Patients with ascites have higher variceal pressure and wall tension than patients without ascites. *The American Journal of Gastroenterology, 95*, 1770-1775.

LEE, A., Lau, T. A., & Yeong, K. Y. (2000). Indwelling catheters for the management of malignant ascites. *Supportive Care in Cancer, 8*, 493-499.

LUCKMANN, J. (1997). *Saunders manual of nursing care*. Philadelphia: W. B. Saunders.

MARINCOLA, F. M. & Schwartzentruber, D. J. (1997). Malignant ascites. In V. T. DeVita, S. Hellman, & S. A. Rosenberg (Eds.), *Cancer: Principles and practice of oncology* (5th ed., Vol. 2) (pp. 2598-2606). Philadelphia: Lippincott-Raven.

MAXWELL, M. B. (1993). Malignant effusions and edemas. In S. L. Groenwald, M. H. Frogge, M. Goodman, & C. H. Yarbro (Eds.), *Cancer nursing principles and practice,* (3rd ed.) (pp. 675-695). Boston: Jones & Bartlett Publishers.

TABBARAH, H. J. & Casciato, D. A. (1990). Malignant effusions. In C. M. Haskell (Ed.), *Cancer treatment* (pp. 815-825). Philadelphia: W. B. Saunders.

TUECHE, S. G., & Pector, J. C. (2000). Peritoneovenous shunt in malignant ascites. The Bordet Institute experience from 1975-1998. *Hepato-Gastroenterology, 47,* 1322-1324.

TWYCROSS, R. (1998). *Symptom management in advanced cancer* (2nd ed.) Abington, UK: Radcliffe Medical Press, Ltd.

VON GUNTEN, C. F. & Twaddle, M. L. (1998). Diagnosis and management of ascites. In A. M. Berger, R. K. Portenoy, & D. E. Weissman (Eds.), *Principles and practice of supportive oncology* (pp. 217-221). Philadelphia: Lippincott-Raven.

WALLER, A. & Caroline, N. L. (2000). *Handbook of palliative care in cancer* (2nd ed.). Boston: Butterworth-Heinemann.

WICKREMESEKERA, S. K., & Stubbs, R. S. (1997). Peritoneovenous shunting for malignant ascites. *New Zealand Medical Journal, 110* (1037), 33-35.

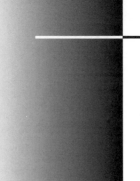

CHAPTER **16**

# *Anxiety*

KIM K. KUEBLER, DEBRA E. HEIDRICH

## ■ DEFINITION AND INCIDENCE

Anxiety is an experience of vague, diffuse apprehension or uneasiness, often accompanied by feelings of uncertainty and helplessness. In nursing diagnosis terminology, the source of anxiety is either nonspecific or unknown; whereas for fear, the source of the uneasiness is known (Carpenito, 2000; Luckmann, 1997; McFarland, 1989). As these two nursing diagnoses overlap in terms of defining characteristics and appropriate interventions, the term anxiety is used here to describe a symptom associated with apprehension and uneasiness. Anxiety may be mild, moderate, severe, or extreme. Whereas mild anxiety can be beneficial—leading persons to seek appropriate information and support—increased or sustained anxiety can be detrimental both physiologically and psychologically.

Studies of incidence rates of anxiety are difficult to interpret as the term is neither defined nor measured consistently. Mild to moderate anxiety is common and expected when facing the physical, psychosocial, emotional, and spiritual issues associated with cancer (Bush, 1998; Payne & Massie, 1998; Vachon, 1998) and terminal illnesses (Breitbart, Chochinov, & Passik, 1998). Many persons possess the necessary coping skills to manage lower levels of anxiety. However, in those with borderline coping skills, mild anxiety may progress to severe anxiety. Thus, even mild anxiety, although expected, must be assessed and addressed. Contrary to some beliefs, a high level of anxiety is not inevitable during the terminal phase of illness and should not be expected or tolerated (Breitbart, Chochinov, & Passik, 1998).

Anxiety disorders are syndromes characterized by anxiety that is beyond the norm in intensity, duration, or behavioral manifestations (Bush, 1998; Luckmann, 1997). There are several *DSM-IV* anxiety disorder diagnoses, including: panic attack, panic disorder, phobias, obsessive-compulsive disorder, posttraumatic stress disorder, and generalized anxiety disorder (American Psychiatric Association, 1994). Anxiety disorders occur in approximately 15% of the general population; women are affected twice as often as men (Luckmann, 1997). The incidence of anxiety disorders appears higher in persons with cancer and those at the end of life (Breitbart, Chochinov, & Passik, 1998; Payne & Massie, 1998;

**199**

Vachon, 1998). Psychiatric disorders, including anxiety, often are unrecognized and untreated in the terminally ill, as a result of several factors (Academy of Psychosomatic Medicine, 1999):

- Difficulty in differentiating symptoms of physical disease from a psychiatric problem
- Belief that many of the symptoms of psychiatric illnesses are normal in the dying process
- Belief that persons at the end of life do not respond to treatment of psychiatric problems
- Barriers associated with accessing trained psychiatrists
- Stigma associated with a psychiatric diagnosis by professionals, family, and patient
- Emphasis on symptom treatment versus a formal palliative diagnosis

## ■ ETIOLOGY AND PATHOPHYSIOLOGY

Anxiety has many causes—physical, psychosocial, emotional, and spiritual. Anxiety can be a manifestation of a medical problem (e.g., hypoxia) or a symptom of physical discomfort (e.g., dyspnea, pain, nausea). Many practitioners have observed that physical discomfort is often perceived as being worse in the presence of anxiety, creating a snowball effect of a symptom, anxiety, worsening of symptom, and worsening of anxiety. In addition, anxiety is sometimes a side effect of medications or a symptom of medication/substance withdrawal.

Cognitive impairment, regardless of the underlying cause, can disrupt both the receiving and the processing of sensory information, resulting in diminished ability to handle stressful situations and creating the sensation of anxiety (Allen, 1999). Unrelieved anxiety has also been implicated as a contributing factor for postoperative delirium (Bowman, 1992). Similar studies linking anxiety with delirium in advanced illness have not been published, but it is prudent for the practitioner to view unrelieved anxiety as a potential cause.

A host of psychologic or emotional concerns may lead to anxiety. Concerns about control of symptoms, addiction to medicines, self-concept and role changes, the dying process, and unresolved family or financial issues are examples of the fears and concerns contributing to anxiety in both patients and caregivers. And certainly anxiety may be a symptom of spiritual distress.

The following illustrate the wide-ranging causes of anxiety (Breitbart, Chochinov, & Passik, 1998; Jackson & Lipman, 1999; Stiefel, Guex, & DelSarte, 1998; Vachon, 1998).

### Anxiety as a Symptom of a Physical Problem

- Any unrelieved distressing symptom such as pain or dyspnea
- An underlying somatic process (hypoxia, sepsis)

- An adverse drug reaction such as akathisia (haloperidol), psychosis (corticosteroids), or toxicity (meperidine)
- Medication/substance withdrawal (alcohol, anticonvulsants, benzodiazepines, nicotine, and opioids)
- A symptom of actual or impending delirium

## Medical Problems Associated with Anxiety Symptoms

- Cardiovascular: angina, arrhythmias, valvular disease, congestive heart failure (CHF), myocardial infarction (MI)
- Fluid and electrolyte imbalances: dehydration, hyponatremia, hyperkalemia, hypercalcemia or hypocalcemia
- Endocrine: hyperthyroidism, hypothyroidism, Cushing's syndrome, Addison's disease, hyperparathyroidism, abnormal glucose levels
- Pulmonary: asthma, chronic obstructive pulmonary disease (COPD), dyspnea, hypercapnia, hypoxia, pneumothorax, pulmonary embolism, sleep apnea
- Neurologic: encephalopathy, vertigo, delirium, cerebrovascular accident (CVA), multiple sclerosis (MS), transient ischemic attacks (TIAs), hematoma
- Hematologic/malignancy: any brain metastasis, anemia, pheochromocytoma
- Nutritional: anemia, folate deficiency, vitamin $B_{12}$ deficiency
- Drug or medication side effects:
  - Medications commonly used in the palliative care setting are likely to contribute to anxiety, including bronchodilators, phenothiazines, corticosteroids, digitalis preparations, and anticholinergics.
  - Central nervous system stimulants are sometimes used to counteract the sedative side effects of opioids; many also lead to anxiety, including caffeine, methylphenidate (Ritalin), and amphetamine

## Anxiety as a Symptom of a Psychosocial, Emotional, or Spiritual Concern

- A normal reaction to a threatening situation
- An indication of an anxiety disorder as defined by *DSM-IV* criteria
- An expression of existential or spiritual suffering

Anxiety leads to activation of the sympathetic nervous system, eliciting the stress or fight-or-flight response. The effects of this mass discharge of the sympathetic nervous system are listed in Box 16-1. The physiologic changes that occur with the stress response are initially adaptive, enhancing the body's ability to perform physically and mentally; however, a sustained stress response can lead to complications associated with continued overstimulation and physiologic exhaustion, including hypertension, palpitations and stress on cardiac functioning, nausea, tissue breakdown, hyperglycemia, impaired psychologic functioning, pulmonary emboli, and immunosuppression.

| BOX 16-1 | *The Stress Response* |
|---|---|

- Increased arterial pressure
- Increased blood flow to skeletal muscles
- Decreased blood flow to gastrointestinal tract and kidneys
- Increased rates of cellular metabolism
- Increased blood glucose level
- Increased glycolysis in the liver and muscles
- Increased muscle strength
- Increased mental activity
- Increased rate of blood coagulation
- Increased number of circulating T lymphocytes

From Guyton, A. C., & Hall, J. E. (1996). The autonomic nervous system: The adrenal medulla. In *Textbook of medical physiology* (9th ed.) (pp. 769-781). Philadelphia: W. B. Saunders.

# ■ ASSESSMENT AND MEASUREMENT

Anxiety is manifested in many ways—subjective experiences, observable signs, and physiologic changes. These symptoms vary with the intensity of the patient's anxiety (Bush, 1998; Carpenito, 2000; McFarland, 1989).

## Subjective Experiences Associated with Anxiety

- Apprehension, uneasiness, fear
- Tension or nervousness
- Irritability
- Restlessness
- Loss of control (feelings of helplessness, angry outbursts)
- Increased attention with mild anxiety, difficulty with concentration with increasing anxiety
- Physical discomforts: headaches; pains in neck, back, or chest; nausea; hot or cold flashes

## Observable Signs of Anxiety

- Tense posture
- Fidgeting with fingers or clothing
- Frequent sighing
- Dryness and licking of dry lips
- Trembling
- Insomnia
- Changes in communication: more quiet or more talkative than usual
- Changes in speech: pitch higher than normal, voice tremors

## Physiologic Signs of Anxiety

- Changes in vital signs: increase in heart rate, respiratory rate, and systolic blood pressure

- Diaphoresis
- Flushing or pallor
- Dry mouth
- Dilated pupils
- Urinary frequency or urgency
- Diarrhea
- Fatigue

The appropriate treatment of anxiety is guided by the severity of this symptom. Although there are several well-researched rating scales for anxiety disorders, there is no good, concise tool for measuring "normal" anxiety. The level of anxiety is inferred on the basis of the severity of the patient's subjective feelings, observable signs, and physical symptoms associated with anxiety. As with other subjective symptoms, asking individuals to rate their anxiety on a numeric scale may be helpful. Table 16-1 is based on selected defining characteristics of mild, moderate, severe, and extreme anxiety as described by McFarland (1989) and is provided as a guide.

It is recommended that individuals with severe or very severe levels of anxiety and those with prolonged anxiety be further screened for a clinical anxiety disorder. Consultation with a psychologist or psychiatrist is recommended for persons with anxiety disorders.

## ■ HISTORY AND PHYSICAL EXAMINATION

Anxiety is characterized by a variety of subjective feelings, observable behaviors, and physiologic changes and has multiple causes; the history and physical examination must include assessment of physical, psychologic, emotional, and spiritual issues. The advanced practice nurse (APN) must evaluate the following:

- General appearance: dress, hygiene, motor activity, facial expression, and speech pattern
- Primary and secondary medical diagnoses, noting those with a potential for complications with anxiety symptoms; for example, bone metastasis and hypercalcemia, lung disease and hypoxia, syndrome of inappropriate antidiuretic hormone (SIADH), and hyponatremia
- Systems review:
  - Cardiovascular: tachycardia, increased systolic pressure, angina, facial flushing or pallor, diaphoresis
  - Respiratory: dyspnea, tachypnea, signs of hypoxia
  - Gastrointestinal: nausea, vomiting, diarrhea
  - Musculoskeletal: muscle tension, trembling
- Presence of pain from any source
- Use of any medications associated with anxiety
- Psychoemotional status:
  - Patient and family's understanding of the advanced illness:
    - Present concerns or worries, including those about the illness itself, the symptoms, or the management of symptoms

## TABLE 16-1

### Levels of Anxiety

| Level of Anxiety | Level of Tension Apprehension/ | Communication | Activity/ Sleep | Problem-Solving/ Learning Ability | Physical Symptoms |
|---|---|---|---|---|---|
| Mild | Mild uneasiness | Repetitive questioning | Restlessness | Enhanced | Usually none |
| Moderate | Slight discomfort Moderate uneasiness Feeling shaky or rattled | Increased verbalization (or more quiet than usual) | Pacing Difficulty sleeping | Narrowed perception—concentrating only on problem Learning is enhanced | Increased pulse and respiration, muscle tension, diaphoresis, and trembling |
| Severe | Severe uneasiness Sense of impending doom Feelings of powerlessness | Difficult or inappropriate communication | Purposeless activity Insomnia | Inability to concentrate/ inability to learn | Moderate symptoms and tachycardia, hyperventilation, nausea, headache, and trembling may be uncontrollable |
| Extreme (Panic) | Extreme uneasiness Extreme sense of helplessness, powerlessness | Unintelligible | Hyperactivity or immobility Sleeplessness | Inability to learn | Severe symptoms and dilated pupils, pallor, and vomiting |

From McFarland, G. K. (1989). Functional health pattern VII: Self-perception, self-concept. In J. M. Thompson, G. K. McFarland, J. E. Hirsch, S. M. Tucker, & A. C. Bowers (Eds.), *Mosby's manual of clinical nursing* (2nd ed.) (pp. 1739-1758). St. Louis: C. V. Mosby.

- Stresses affecting the patient/family: any change in health, marital status, family unit, living arrangements, responsibilities, employment, or financial status
    - Self-appraisal of patient and family adjustment to these changes
- History of substance abuse: alcohol, nicotine, prescription medications, or illicit drugs
- History of an anxiety disorder, depression, or other mental health disorder:
    - Time since diagnosis, treatments, ongoing interventions, current status
- Presence and severity of anxiety at this time:
    - Feelings of uneasiness, tension, or restlessness
    - Presence and severity of observable signs or physiologic changes associated with anxiety
- Resources available to manage anxiety: social support, religion, recreational or social activities, support groups, professional assistance
- Spiritual belief system, including spiritual meaning of experiences, beliefs about an afterlife, and existential concerns and questions

## ■ DIAGNOSTICS

The appropriate use of diagnostic tests is determined by the suspected underlying cause of the anxiety. Should a medical complication, such as hypercalcemia, be a potential cause, blood and chemical assessment may be indicated.

## ■ INTERVENTION AND TREATMENT

Appropriate treatment depends on the underlying cause and level of anxiety. However, because anxiety is typically multidimensional it is helpful to utilize multiple approaches to manage this symptom.

### Treat Physical Causes

- Aggressively treat uncomfortable symptoms, such as pain, dyspnea, and nausea.
- Manage, as feasible and appropriate, medical conditions contributing to anxiety, such as anemia, hypercalcemia, SIADH, and pulmonary compromise.
- Reduce or discontinue medications that may be contributing to anxiety.
- Identify symptoms potentially related to withdrawal:
    - Taper benzodiazepines, rather than discontinuing suddenly if the patient has been taking them for a long period.
    - Consider use of a nicotine patch for patients who have a history of smoking but are physically unable to do so.

### Enhance Coping Skills

For mild-to-moderate anxiety:
- Listen actively to expression of concerns and fears.
- Encourage ventilation of feelings.

- Convey respect for the individual and acceptance of feelings (i.e., feelings are neither right nor wrong; they just are).
- Provide information to clarify misconceptions, answer questions, and alleviate concerns. For example, discussion of the facts about the extremely low incidence of addiction when opioids are used for pain management may significantly decrease anxiety and pain.
- Clarify information and reinforce teaching frequently.
- Teach relaxation techniques:
  - Use complementary therapies, such as music, art, imagery, and massage.
- Assist the individual to identify anxiety-provoking stimuli.
  - Assist in developing strategies to prevent or modify an anxiety-provoking situation, if possible.
  - When a situation cannot be prevented, encourage the patient to recognize the onset of anxiety early and intervene before it escalates.
- Refer to counseling services, as appropriate, such as medical social services, pastoral counseling, and financial/estate planning.
- Consider referral to a support group, as appropriate.
- Encourage the person to accept assistance to reduce stress:
  - Make lists of tasks that can be delegated.
  - Delegate these tasks to available extended family, worship community, and neighborhood or civic group members.

For severe anxiety:

- Provide a safe, calm, nonstimulating environment:
  - Remove as many stressors as possible, including limiting number of persons in the room.
  - Avoid moving the patient from familiar surroundings, if possible.
  - Encourage the physical presence of a trusted person.
- Communicate in short, simple sentences in a calm tone of voice.
- Do not overload the person with information; the ability to concentrate and learn is impaired.
- Avoid asking the individual to make decisions.
- Allow expression of feelings, without probing or confrontation.
- Consider consultation with a clinical psychiatrist.

## Pharmacologic Interventions

Although the interventions to enhance coping skills are effective for mild, and to some degree moderate, anxiety, anxiolytic medications are very important in the treatment of prolonged or severe anxiety. If anxiety is interfering with quality of living, a short course of anxiolytic medication may reduce the unpleasant symptoms associated with anxiety and enable the individual to learn new coping skills. Severe anxiety and anxiety disorders often require ongoing pharmacologic treatment in addition to psychotherapy. Table 16-2 provides dosage ranges for the medications discussed later.

## TABLE 16-2

### Anxiolytics

| Drug | Onset and Dosage | Half-Life* | Comments | Scheduled Drug |
|------|------------------|-----------|----------|----------------|
| **BENZODIAZEPINES** | | | | |
| Lorazepam (Ativan) | 0.5-2.0 mg PO tid-qid | O: 30 min ½: 10-14 hrs | Used for short-term anxiety, preoperative sedation, and reliable bioavailability in IM dosing. Moderately priced | Class IV |
| Alprazolam (Xanax) | 0.25-2.0 mg PO tid-qid | O: 30 min ½: 12-15 hrs | Commonly recommended for both anxiety and panic disorders. Costly | Class IV |
| Diazepam (Valium) | 5-10 mg PO bid-qid | O: 30 min ½: 20-50 hrs | Short-term anxiety, alcohol withdrawal, myoclonus, preoperative sedation, seizures; variable bioavailability with IM dosing | Class IV |
| Clonazepam (Klonopin) | 0.5-2 mg PO bid-qid | O: 1-2 hrs ½: 18-50 hrs | Adjuvant for neuropathic pain, seizure maintenance, panic disorders | Class IV |
| Clorazepate dipotassium (Tranxene) | 15-90 mg PO/day in divided doses (7.5 mg qd to bid in elderly) | O: 15 min ½: 30-100 hrs | Anxiety, alcohol withdrawal, seizures | Class IV |

From Breitbart, W., Chochinov, M., & Passik, S. (1998). Psychiatric aspects of palliative care. In D. Doyle, G. Hanks, & N. MacDonald (Eds.), *Oxford textbook of palliative medicine* (2nd ed.) (pp. 933-954). New York: Oxford University Press; Payne, D. K., & Massie, M. J. (1998). Depression and anxiety. In A. M. Berger, R. K. Portenoy, & D. E. Weissman (Eds.), *Principles and practice of supportive oncology* (pp. 497-511). Philadelphia: Lippincott-Raven; Puzantian, T., & Stimmel, G. (1999). 1999-2000 Review of psychotropic drugs. The Health-System Pharmacy Newsmagazine; Pharmacy Practice News; CNS News Special Edition. New York: AstraZeneca; Skidmore-Roth, L. (2001). *Mosby's 2001 nursing drug reference.* St. Louis: Mosby.

*O, onset; ½, half-life; M, active metabolites.

Continued

**TABLE 16-2**

*Anxiolytics—cont'd*

| Drug | Onset and Dosage | Half-Life* | Comments | Scheduled Drug |
|------|------------------|-----------|----------|----------------|
| **NEUROLEPTICS** | | | | |
| Haloperidol (Haldol) | 0.5-5 PO/SC q2-12h | O: 2-6 hrs ½: 24 hrs | Anxiety with confusion or hallucinations; nonsedating | N/A |
| Thioridazine (Mellaril) | 10-50 mg PO/SC tid | O: 2-4 hrs ½: 26-36 hrs | Anxiety with confusion or hallucinations; sedating | N/A |
| **NONBENZODIAZEPINES** | | | | |
| Buspirone (BuSpar) | 5-20 mg PO tid | O: Single dose, 40-90 min ½: 2-3 hrs | Chronic anxiety; takes 1-2 weeks for therapeutic effect; do not use as prn. Anxiety in persons with severely compromised respiratory status | N/A |
| **ANTIHISTAMINES** | | | | |
| Hydroxyzine (Atarax) | 10-50 PO tid | O: 30 min ½: 3 hrs | More CNS effect than diphenhydramine | N/A |
| Diphenhydramine (Benadryl) | 25-50 PO tid | O: 1-3 hrs ½: 2-7 hrs | | N/A |

From Breitbart, W., Chochinov, M., & Passik, S. (1998). Psychiatric aspects of palliative care. In D. Doyle, G. Hanks, & N. MacDonald (Eds.), *Oxford textbook of palliative medicine* (2nd ed.) (pp. 933-954). New York: Oxford University Press; Payne, D. K., & Massie, M. J. (1998). Depression and anxiety. In A. M. Berger, R. K. Portenoy, & D. E. Weissman (Eds.), *Principles and practice of supportive oncology* (pp. 497-511). Philadelphia: Lippincott-Raven; Puzantian, T., & Stimmel, G. (1999). 1999-2000 Review of psychotropic drugs. The Health-System Pharmacy Newsmagazine; Pharmacy Practice News; CNS News Special Edition. New York: AstraZeneca; Skidmore-Roth, L. (2001). *Mosby's 2001 nursing drug reference*. St. Louis: Mosby.
*O, onset; ½, half-life; M, active metabolites.

**Benzodiazepines.**   The benzodiazepines are the most commonly pre-scribed anxiolytics. These medications work by potentiating gamma-aminobutyric acid (GABA), an inhibitory neurotransmitter in the central nervous system (CNS). The result is CNS suppression, especially at the level of the limbic system (Skidmore-Roth, 2001). The benzodiazepines with a short half-life (e.g., lorazepam) are generally preferred in elderly patients and for short-term management of anxiety. Alprazolam has an intermediate half-life (approximately 14 hours) and is also an effective, widely used anxiolytic. A potential problem with the short-acting benzodiazepines is end-of-dose failure; the medications with a longer half-life, such as clonazepam, may be preferred if breakthrough anxiety is present (Breitbart, Chochinov, & Passik, 1998; Bush, 1998; Payne & Massie, 1998).

Lorazepam, oxazepam, and temazepam are metabolized by conjugation with glucuronic acid in the liver and have no active metabolites, making them the safest for use in individuals who have hepatic disease (Breitbart, Chochinov, & Passik, 1998; Payne & Massie, 1998). All benzodiazepines have the potential to cause drowsiness, dizziness, and ataxia. Therefore, pa-tients must be evaluated and monitored for the potential of falling.

**Neuroleptics.**   The neuroleptic medications are used when the benzodi-azepines are not effective or when confusion or hallucinations accompany the anxiety. (Note: The combination of anxiety with a mental status change is often a sign of delirium.) Haloperidol is used most frequently; thioridazine has been noted to be helpful when insomnia is problematic (Breitbart, Chochinov, & Passik, 1998; Payne & Massie, 1998). These medications work by suppressing the cerebral cortex, limbic system, and hypothalamus and by blocking CNS dopamine receptors (Skidmore-Roth, 2001).

**Other anxiolytics.**   Buspirone is a nonbenzodiazepine anxiolytic. Inhibi-tion of serotonin appears to be the mechanism of action (Skidmore-Roth, 1999). This medication may take 1 to 2 weeks to reach maximal effectiveness and is generally used for chronic anxiety. The practitioner must be cautious when switching to buspirone from a benzodiazepine as buspirone does not block benzodiazepine withdrawal (Breitbart, Chochinov, & Passik, 1998).

Antihistamines have also been used for their anxiolytic properties (Breit-bart, Chochinov, & Passik, 1998; Payne & Massie, 1998). Hydroxyzine ap-pears to depress the CNS more than diphenhydramine, but both have been used. Some practitioners prefer the use of antihistamines if the patient's res-piratory status is extremely compromised and there is a concern about res-piratory depression from benzodiazepines (Payne & Massie, 1998). However, as the antihistamines tend to have a relatively mild anxiolytic effect, a ben-zodiazepine or neuroleptic may be required for moderate to severe anxiety even in the presence of a compromised respiratory system.

## ■ PATIENT AND FAMILY EDUCATION

Providing information is extremely important in the management of anxi-ety, including explaining aspects of symptom management to alleviate the source of some of the anxiety and discussing the recognition and management of anxiety itself. Both the patient and the family are at risk, because anxiety in one person can exacerbate that in another. Thus, it is important to include both patients and caregivers when providing information.

- Teach good symptom assessment and management.
- Provide information to correct misconceptions and fears regarding medications (e.g., addiction, respiratory depression, sedation).
- Assist the individual to identify his or her own signs of anxiety.
- Teach relaxation and other stress management techniques.
- Provide information on anxiety as a symptom that requires treatment and not a sign of weakness.
- Teach the importance of using many approaches to managing anxiety, including counseling.
- Teach appropriate use of anxiolytic medications and potential side effects.

## ■ EVALUATION AND PLAN FOR FOLLOW-UP

Successful intervention for anxiety leads to a resolution or, at least, a decrease in the subjective and objective signs of anxiety. Evaluating the subjective aspects of anxiety includes asking the individual about feelings of uneasiness, apprehension, and helplessness. Use of a numeric scale or anxiety assessment tool as part of the initial assessment makes monitoring and documenting changes in subjective feelings easier. Objective signs of anxiety are also monitored to determine the effectiveness of the interventions.

The potential for anxiety is always present in persons with advanced illness and their caregivers, making ongoing evaluation a necessity. And, as anxiety can change from day to day, the ongoing evaluation process should include not only present anxiety, but any anxiety in the past 24 hours or since the last visit/appointment. Be sure to consider that meeting with a health care professional sometimes increases and sometimes decreases anxiety.

The evaluation process includes monitoring for side effects of any medications ordered for anxiety, making appropriate changes in types of medications, doses, or schedules.

✔ **CASE STUDY** Mrs. White is 58 years old and has a diagnosis of metastatic breast cancer. She had a lumpectomy followed by radiation therapy and chemotherapy 5 years ago. About 2 years ago, she experienced hip and rib pain and was diagnosed with metastatic disease to the bone and liver. Her pain has been well managed by a combination of oxycodone and ibuprofen.

Mr. White is a very caring and supportive spouse. He maintains a full-time job as a factory supervisor. Their daughter, who is married and has two children, ages 4 and 6, is Mrs. White's primary caregiver during the day.

Her family describes Mrs. White as a "worrier," reporting that she has always been "high-strung." Mrs. White states she is "sort of an anxious person by nature" but feels shakier than usual right now. She rates her anxiety as a 5 on a 0 to 10 scale. She also reports occasional palpitations, shortness of breath, and difficulty in sleeping. The nurse notes trembling of hands, rapid pace of speech, and difficulty in sitting still. Vital signs show a heart rate of 78, respiratory rate of 16, and blood pressure of 150/74. When asked about concerns, she expresses that she is a burden to her family and she is concerned that at some point the pain will get out of control. She has stopped playing cards each week with her friends, because she "just can't concentrate" on the game and the conversations.

Mrs. White is exhibiting signs of a moderate level of anxiety. As the anxiety symptoms are distressing to the patient and interfere with her ability to concentrate and sleep, a prescription is written for lorazepam 0.5 mg PO tid, prn. The APN encourages the patient to take the lorazepam in the morning and at bedtime, and, if needed, at midday for a few days, at which time the nurse will talk with her again. The APN also talks with Mrs. White about the use of medications for pain relief and assures her that her pain will continue to be managed effectively. They also have a discussion about the work of caring for a loved one who is ill—work which is often offset by the desires of the family to be with and share their love with the ill person. Although the nurse plans to continue to address emotional issues and concerns, a referral is made for the medical social worker to meet with the patient and family for additional counseling.

After 3 days, Mrs. White reports feeling much better, rating her anxiety as a 0 to 2 on a 0 to 10 scale. She is taking the lorazepam three times a day but says she feels she does not need it as much anymore. Mrs. White and her family have met with the social worker once and plan to meet with her every 2 weeks. The dosing schedule is changed to 0.5 mg at bedtime, and q4-6h prn.

For approximately 3 weeks, Mrs. White took only the lorazepam at bedtime, if she was "having worries" then. As her physical condition deteriorated, she became more weak and required more physical assistance. Her pain escalated, requiring a change in the dosage of opioid. With these changes, there was a return of both subjective and objective signs of anxiety. The lorazepam was restarted at 0.5 mg tid and continued until her death.

## References

ACADEMY of Psychosomatic Medicine. (1999). *Psychiatric aspects of excellent end-of-life care* (Position statement). Chicago: Academy of Psychosomatic Medicine.

ALLEN, L. A. (1999). Treating agitation without drugs. *American Journal of Nursing,* 99(4), 36-41.

AMERICAN Psychiatric Association. (1994). *Diagnostic and statistical manual of mental disorders* (4th ed.) (DSM-IV). Washington, DC: American Psychiatric Association.

Bowman, A. M. (1992). The relationship of anxiety to the development of postoperative delirium. *Journal of Gerontological Nursing,* 18, 24-30.

Breitbart, W., Chochinov, M., & Passik, S. (1998). Psychiatric aspects of palliative care. In D. Doyle, G. Hanks, & N. MacDonald (Eds.), *Oxford textbook of palliative medicine* (2nd ed.) (pp. 933-954). New York: Oxford University Press.

Bush, N. J. (1998). Anxiety and the cancer experience. In R. M. Carroll-Johnson, L. M. Gorman, & N. J. Bush (Eds.), *Psychosocial nursing care* (pp. 125-138). Pittsburgh: Oncology Nursing Press.

Carpenito, L. J. (2000). *Nursing diagnosis: Application to clinical practice* (8th ed.). Philadelphia: J. B. Lippincott.

Guyton, A. C., & Hall, J. E. (1996). The autonomic nervous system: The adrenal medulla. In *Textbook of medical physiology* (9th ed.) (pp. 769-781). Philadelphia: W. B. Saunders.

Jackson, K. C., & Lipman, A. G. (1999). Anxiety in palliative care patients. *Journal of Pharmaceutical Care in Pain & Symptom Control,* 7(4), 23-35.

Luckmann, J. (1997). Caring for people with mental disorders. In *Saunders manual of nursing care* (pp. 1899-1930). Philadelphia: W. B. Saunders.

McFarland, G. K. (1989). Functional health pattern VII: Self-perception, self-concept. In J. M. Thompson, G. K. McFarland, J. E. Hirsch, S. M. Tucker, & A. C. Bowers (Eds.), *Mosby's manual of clinical nursing* (2nd ed.) (pp. 1739-1758). St. Louis: C. V. Mosby.

Payne, D. K., & Massie, M. J. (1998). Depression and anxiety. In A. M. Berger, R. K. Portenoy, & D. E. Weissman (Eds.), *Principles and practice of supportive oncology* (pp. 497-511). Philadelphia: Lippincott-Raven.

Puzantian, T., & Stimmel, G. (1999). *1999-2000 Review of psychotropic drugs.* CNS News Special Edition. New York: AstraZeneca.

Skidmore-Roth, L. (2001). *Mosby's 2001 nursing drug reference.* St. Louis: Mosby.

Stiefel, F., Guex, P., & DelSarte, O. (1998). An introduction to psychooncology with special emphasis on its development in historical and cultural context. In R. Portenoy & E. Bruera (Eds.), *Topics in palliative care* (Vol. 3) (pp. 175-189). New York: Oxford University Press.

Vachon, M. L. S. (1998). The emotional problems of the patient. In D. Doyle, G. Hanks, & N. MacDonald (Eds.), *Oxford textbook of palliative medicine* (2nd ed.) (pp. 883-907). New York: Oxford University Press.

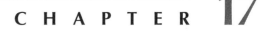

# *Cachexia and Anorexia*

SANDY MCKINNON, KIM K. KUEBLER

## ■ DEFINITION AND INCIDENCE

Most people with advanced cancer (50% to 80%) or acquired immunodeficiency syndrome (AIDS) experience anorexia, defined as a loss of appetite accompanied by poor food intake, and/or cachexia, which is characterized by profound physical wasting and weight loss. Anorexia and cachexia are major factors in causing the death of almost half of all cancer patients (Billingsley & Alexander, 1996).

## ■ ETIOLOGY AND PATHOPHYSIOLOGY

Although the syndrome of weight loss, loss of appetite, and profound weakness has long been recognized in cancer patients, we do not yet have a complete understanding of or agreement on the factors that contribute to its cause. Cachexia was previously thought to be the result of a "metabolic furnace" within the tumor itself, pulling in all of the body's nutritional support while producing toxins that led to anorexia (Walker & Bruera, 1998). Researchers have recently begun to understand that the cachexia and anorexia associated with advanced cancer and AIDS are much more complex. Most current research points to a multifactorial combination or cascade of contributing problems (Jaskowiak & Alexander, 1998; Loprinzi, Goldberg, & Peethambaram, 1998; MacDonald, Alexander, & Bruera, 1995).

Cachexia and anorexia syndrome may include the following contributing problems (Billingsley & Alexander, 1996).

### Psychologic

- Stress
- Altered taste perception
- Learned food aversions

### Cancer Treatment Side Effects

- Nausea
- Stomatitis

- Xerostomia
- Fatigue

## Solid Tumor Effects

- Mechanical obstruction (i.e., bowel obstruction)
- Cytokines produced by tumor
- Lipid mobilizing factors
- Protein metabolism

## Host Related Effects

- Increased energy expenditure at rest
- Autonomic dysfunction (nausea, constipation, etc.)
- Alteration in carbohydrate metabolism
- Cytokines produced by host macrophages

The variants of anorexia and cachexia are directly related to the histologic type of cancer. For example, whereas lung cancer patients may experience weight loss that is marked and early in the disease process, breast cancer patients may not lose any weight. The reasons for this difference are not well understood but may relate to variations in the production of protein cytokines such as tumor necrosis factor (TNF), interleukin 1 (Il-1), and interleukin 6 (Il-6). Cytokines are polypeptide molecules synthesized by macrophages, monocytes, lymphocytes, and tumor cells in response to stimuli such as infection, trauma, stress, and neoplastic growth (Billingsley & Alexander, 1996).

Considerable research attention is being paid to the roles that cytokines play in creating and mediating the metabolic changes leading to cachexia. It is theorized that tumors may act as a catalyst leading to a cascade of cytokines producing multiple metabolic abnormalities (Fainsinger, 1996).

The observation that very small tumors may produce profound cachexia in some types of cancer supports the hypothesis that soluble mediators such as cytokines either arise from the tumor or from the host (patient) in response to the tumor (Billingsley & Alexander, 1996). However, as noted by MacDonald (1998), this theory is not universally accepted as identifying the primary cause of the syndrome. Lipolytic and proteolytic factors produced by the tumor may play the central role in cachexia and anorexia, though many researchers believe that a combination of cytokines and tumor factors will ultimately be found as contributors (MacDonald, 1998). The fact that effective treatments for cachexia remain elusive may be explained in part by our growing appreciation for the complexity of the underlying cause.

## ■ ASSESSMENT AND MEASUREMENT

Patients must be assessed for potentially reversible causes of weight loss or lack of appetite before the diagnosis of cachexia-anorexia syndrome can be made. Consider the following factors (Walker & Bruera, 1998):

- Radiation or chemotherapy treatments
- Severe, untreated pain
- Constipation
- Adjustment disorder, depression, or cognitive failure
- Mechanical obstruction of alimentary canal by tumor
- Oral disorders such as candida infection or poorly fitting dentures
- Appetite reducing medications

Weight may be monitored through the use of scales, although the rapidly falling numbers may be a source of distress to some patients. Appetite is a subjective experience that may be measured by using a visual analog or numerical scale. By asking a patient to indicate a number between 0 and 10, where 10 represents an excellent appetite and 0 means no appetite at all, it is possible to monitor the patient's status and the results of interventions.

## ■ HISTORY AND PHYSICAL EXAMINATION

A thorough history includes the following information:
- Review of current illness including treatments
- Review of past or concurrent illnesses such as diabetes mellitus
- History of weight loss
- Exploration of dietary and fluid intake, taste changes, food aversions and preferences
- Exploration of current symptom profile, including pain, nausea, dysphagia, bowel habits, fatigue
- Review of functional status
- Review of medications
- Psychologic distress, body image

A thorough physical examination includes the following:
- The oral cavity for evidence of fungal, bacteria, or viral infection; stomatitis; mucositis; xerostomia; or direct tumor involvement
- The abdomen for evidence of masses, bowel sounds
- The skin for evidence of dehydration, areas of redness or breakdown

Autonomic dysfunction, common in people with advanced cancer, may be apparent through examination of the cardiovascular system (postural hypotension, history of syncopal episodes, and a fixed heart rate) and the gastrointestinal system (nausea, anorexia, constipation, or diarrhea) (Pereira & Bruera, 1996).

## ■ DIAGNOSTICS

Cachectic patients will probably show evidence of a low serum albumin level, decreased total protein levels, anemia, and increased serum triglyceride level, glucose levels, and lactic acidosis. However, these laboratory investigations are generally considered to be nonspecific, too variable, and not helpful in diagnosing or monitoring anorexia and cachexia in people with a terminal illness (Billingsley & Alexander, 1996; Walker & Bruera, 1998).

Depending on the stage of illness and treatment goals, it may be appropriate to monitor easily reversible problems such as electrolyte and metabolic imbalances (sodium, potassium, magnesium, calcium levels). More elaborate evaluations such as the use of extensive dietary intake monitoring and skinfold thickness measurements should be reserved for clinical trials.

Radiologic investigations may be helpful to rule out treatable problems such as bowel obstruction and constipation.

## ■ INTERVENTION AND TREATMENT

With the palliative care goal of improving quality of life, treatment must be aimed at minimizing symptoms that affect appetite, implementing measures to improve appetite, and educating patients and families about the potential benefits and limits of treatment interventions (Fainsinger, 1998). When we see patients losing weight and family members feeling distress about failing appetites, we must understand that our response cannot be simply to find ways to introduce more nutrients into the person. This approach has not been successful and may actually create harm.

### Preventative Measures

At present, anorexia and cachexia remain part of the total picture in most people with advanced cancer or AIDS, and preventative interventions remain elusive. The prevention of this devastating syndrome will ultimately hinge on our ability to understand its pathophysiologic processes. Because malnutrition has been shown to have a significant effect on psychologic and physiologic well-being as well as survival, further research is critical. There are some intriguing possibilities on the horizon. For example, investigators in several settings are exploring the use of dietary supplements of omega-3 polyunsaturated fatty acids to improve immunologic function and reduce cancer-related anorexia and cachexia (Gogos et al., 1998; Vigano & Bruera, 1996).

### Supportive Measures

- Ensure good mouth care.
- Maintain pleasant surroundings with small meals of favorite foods.
- Refer to a clinical dietitian, if available.
- Choose oral support rather than parenteral intervention.
- Encourage patients and families to think of food as a comfort measure. Advise offering favorite foods without worrying about nutritional value.

### Enteral and Parenteral Supplemental Feeding

Enteral feeding may be considered for some patients (with cancers such as head and neck or esophageal) who have an appetite but are unable to eat as a result of obstruction. Side effects of this method may include aspiration pneumonia and diarrhea.

If the underlying problems in cachexia were simply disorders in the patient's ability to eat enough or absorb what was eaten, then total parenteral nutrition (TPN) would be the answer. However, research has shown that TPN does not improve the overall condition and function. Parenteral feeding is not recommended as a method to treat cachexia and in fact has been associated with high morbidity rates (Loprinzi, Goldberg, & Peethambaram, 1998).

### Pharmacologic Intervention

Research into drug therapy continues, but results have been somewhat disappointing and the medications can be expensive. The following may be considered for patients who wish this intervention (Fainsinger, 1996; Loprinzi, Goldberg, & Peethambaram, 1998):

- Progestational agents: megestrol acetate, 160-800 mg/day, PO. Although there is no clear evidence that this drug improves quality of life, research has shown that it can definitely improve appetite and can increase non-fluid weight in some patients. It is generally well tolerated but may increase the risk of thromboembolic complications, mild edema, vaginal spotting in women, and impotence in men. These medications can be very expensive.
- Corticosteroids: dexamethasone, starting at 4-8 mg/day, PO. This drug has been less effective than megestrol acetate in improving appetite, and benefits may be short lasting. Side effects may include immunosuppression, weakness, and osteoporosis. However, corticosteroids are less expensive than progestational agents.
- Prokinetic agents such as metoclopramide, 10 mg orally before meals may improve gastric emptying and decrease nausea.
- Cannabinoids: derivatives of marijuana have been formulated into oral medications such as dronabinol (in the United States) and nabilone (in Canada). They may be more tolerable for younger patients. Side effects can include altered mentation. Doses are generally 5 to 15 mg/day when taken orally.

## ■ PATIENT AND FAMILY EDUCATION

The symptoms of anorexia and cachexia can be devastating for patients and families, representing a visible sign of illness. The ability to eat is so closely associated with health and well-being that many people have great difficulty accepting that adequate nutrition is no longer possible. It is essential to explain to patients and families that most people with advanced cancer lose weight because of complex metabolic problems that cannot be changed, not because they are not eating (Fainsinger, 1998). Eating more or using enteral or parenteral supplements will not make a difference and may lead to more distress.

## ■ EVALUATION AND PLAN FOR FOLLOW-UP

Regular assessment and coaching of patients and families are essential to support their ability to cope. Helping to keep both the patient and family informed will enable them to make informed decisions about trying the various interventions.

✔ **CASE STUDY**

Upon arriving at the patient's residence, you find Mrs. M. in some distress. She has been cooking and baking, trying to find something that will tempt her husband, Mr. M., into eating. Mr. M. is a 68-year-old retired firefighter and has been diagnosed with non–small-cell lung cancer. He completed a 5-week course of radiation 8 months ago but unfortunately a recent chest radiograph showed evidence of hilar spread, and an ultrasound of his abdomen 1 week ago indicated several liver metastases. In spite of Mrs. M.'s pleas that he "fight with everything he's got," Mr. M. has elected to have no further treatment, knowing that his disease is no longer curable. Mr. M.'s appetite has been waning for the last month or so, and he has obviously lost weight. His clothes are too big for him, and he has begun to look very frail. This has upset Mrs. M. and their two adult children. They have been pressuring Mr. M. to eat more, and neighbors and friends have been preparing casseroles and various kinds of food to try to entice him to eat.

You ask to spend some time alone with Mr. M. and settle into a seat in the living room beside his big easy chair. He tells you that he has been "living" in his chair, and that he doesn't seem to have any energy. He describes tiring easily but adds that he's not surprised, since he hasn't eaten very much. He notes that he got his appetite and energy back "a little bit" after the radiation finished but is just "not interested" in food anymore, although it is "all that Mrs. M. seems to think about." Upon questioning, Mr. M. admits to being nauseated much of the time and adds that "nothing tastes right." His appetite is 1 out of 10, with 0 being the worst it could be. He is able to drink the equivalent of about 1½ to 2 liters per day of water, soup, and weak tea. Constipation is a problem, and he has not had a bowel movement for a week.

A review of medications shows that Mr. M. is taking long-acting oral morphine, 30 mg q12h, with one or two "breakthroughs" each day for abdominal discomfort. He is taking a vitamin supplement at his wife's insistence and using laxatives sporadically. On examination Mr. M. is very thin, with a scaphoid abdomen, a palpable liver edge, and minimal bowel sounds on auscultation. His skin appears dry and his mouth is moist, with no evidence of infection, fungal or otherwise.

using laxatives sporadically. On examination Mr. M. is very thin, with a scaphoid abdomen, a palpable liver edge, and minimal bowel sounds on auscultation. His skin appears dry and his mouth is moist, with no evidence of infection, fungal or otherwise.

You invite Mrs. M. to join you and Mr. M. for a discussion of your findings and plan for care. You explain that although it is normal for Mr. M. to lack an appetite with this illness, you have some suggestions to make. You prescribe metoclopramide 10 mg at meals and prn for its prokinetic and antiemetic properties. You also explain that Mr. M. should be having regular bowel movements in spite of his low oral intake and encourage regular laxatives and arrange for enemas as required. Mrs. M. asks about supplemental feeding, "if it should come to that." Mr. M. winces but appears more settled when you explain that it does not help and in fact can cause harm in some cases. You add that the cancer has changed the way Mr. M.'s body processes the food he eats, and that he would probably continue to lose weight even if he could eat a normal diet. Nevertheless, Mrs. M. is pleased when Mr. M. agrees to try high-calorie drinks. They are also looking forward to a course of megestrol acetate 160 mg tid for 2 weeks to see whether Mr. M.'s appetite can be improved. You explain that rather than arguing about food, it will be better to think of eating in terms of comfort rather than nutrition. Mrs. M. agrees to serve small meals of food that Mr. M. feels like eating.

On a return visit a week later, you are pleased to find that Mr. M.'s appetite has improved to 4 or 5 of a possible 10. Mrs. M. is thrilled that Mr. M. is able to eat more than before and says that she is not "nagging" anymore. She adds that she knows this reprieve is temporary, but she and Mr. M. are still happy about the change.

## References

BILLINGSLEY, K. G., & Alexander, H. R. (1996). The pathophysiology of cachexia in advanced cancer and AIDS. In E. Bruera & I. Higginson (Eds.), *Cachexia-anorexia in cancer patients* (pp. 1-22). New York: Oxford University Press.

FAINSINGER, R. L. (1996). Pharmacological approach to cancer anorexia and cachexia. In E. Bruera & I. Higginson (Eds.), *Cachexia-anorexia in cancer patients* (pp. 128-140). Toronto: Oxford University Press.

FAINSINGER, R. L. (1998). Practical considerations in the management of anorexia/cachexia: What do we say and what do we do? In E. Bruera & R. Portenoy (Eds.), *Topics in palliative care* (Vol. 2) (pp. 141-152). New York: Oxford University Press.

GOGOS, C. A., Ginopoulos, P., Salsa, B., Apostolidou, E., Zoumbos, N. C., & Kalfarentzos, F. (1998). Dietary omega-3 polyunsaturated fatty acids plus vitamin E restore immunodeficiency and prolong survival for severely ill patients with generalized malignancy. *Cancer, 82*(2), 395-402.

JASKOWIAK, N. T., & Alexander, H. R. (1998). The pathophysiology of cancer cachexia. In D. Doyle, G. Hanks, & N. MacDonald (Eds.), *Oxford textbook of palliative medicine* (pp. 534-548). Oxford: Oxford University Press.

Loprinzi, C. L., Goldberg, R. M., & Peethambaram, P. P. (1998). Cancer anorexia/cachexia. In A. M. Berger, R. K. Portenoy, & D. E. Weissman (Eds.), *Principles and practice of supportive oncology* (pp. 133-155). Philadelphia: Lippincott-Raven.

MacDonald, N. (Ed.). (1998). *Palliative care medicine: A case-based manual.* Toronto: Oxford University Press.

MacDonald, N., Alexander, H. R., & Bruera, E. (1995). Cachexia-anorexia-asthenia. *Journal of Pain and Symptom Management, 10*(2), 151-155.

Pereira, J., & Bruera, E. (1996). Chronic nausea. In E. Bruera & I. Higginson (Eds.), *Cachexia-anorexia in cancer patients* (pp. 23-37). Toronto: Oxford University Press.

Vigano, A., & Bruera, E. (1996). Enteral and parenteral nutrition in cancer patients. In E. Bruera & I. Higginson (Eds.), *Cachexia-anorexia in cancer patients* (pp. 110-127). Toronto: Oxford University Press.

Walker, P., & Bruera, E. (1998). Anorexia-cachexia syndrome. In N. MacDonald (Ed.), *Palliative medicine: A case-based manual* (pp. 1-14). Toronto: Oxford University Press.

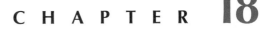

CHAPTER **18**

# *Constipation*

DEBRA E. HEIDRICH

## ■ DEFINITION AND INCIDENCE

A general definition of constipation is slow movement of feces through the large intestine (Guyton & Hall, 1996a), resulting in hard, dry stool that may be difficult to expel. However, constipation has different meanings to different people (Mercadante, 1998). Persons may report constipation if feces are hard and dry; if there is straining, difficulty, or discomfort in expelling stool; or if stools are less frequent than normal for them.

In the normal population the incidence of constipation may range from 5% to 20%. Studies of persons with advanced cancer and other terminal illness indicate the incidence of constipation ranges from 23% to 55% (Conill et al., 1997; Curtis, Krech, & Walsh, 1991; Lichter & Hunt, 1990; Vainio & Auvinen, 1996). However, this is likely an underestimate of the true incidence as constipation is frequently underdiagnosed (Sykes, 1998).

Constipation is uncomfortable and must be treated aggressively. The patient with constipation often experiences abdominal discomfort, cramping, and distension. Unresolved constipation leads to fecal impaction—a large amount of hard, dry feces that accumulates in the rectum and sigmoid colon and cannot be evacuated. Patients who associate constipation with the use of opioids or other medications may discontinue or decrease these medications, leading to uncontrolled symptoms and additional discomfort.

## ■ ETIOLOGY AND PATHOPHYSIOLOGY

Normal bowel function requires the interaction of many body systems to break down food, allow proper absorption and transport of fluids and nutritional elements, and move the remaining food residue through the gastrointestinal tract to form feces for excretion. Alterations in any of these body systems can negatively affect bowel functioning (Basta & Anderson, 1998).

Many factors contribute to constipation in persons with terminal illness, including the following:

- Immobility: Persons with little to no activity cannot maintain normal bowel motility. As defecation requires upright posture and strong abdominal, diaphragmatic, and anal muscles, individuals with generalized

221

fatigue and weakness and those who cannot sit on a toilet or bedside commode are at great risk for constipation (Basta & Anderson, 1998).

- Diet and hydration: Patients with terminal illnesses often find it difficult to eat and drink adequate amounts of food and fluid for a variety of reasons (see Chapter 17, Cachexia and Anorexia). Low-residue diets may lack the necessary bulk to propel the feces through the bowel. The resulting constipation worsens when there is inadequate fluid intake; as a result more water is reabsorbed from the colon and hard, dry stool is produced (Basta & Anderson, 1998).

- Medications: Many medications can contribute to constipation. *Opioids* bind with opioid receptors in the gastrointestinal (GI) tract leading to (1) a decrease in intestinal secretions, (2) a decrease in propulsive movements, and (3) an increase in internal anal sphincter tone. The net effects of stimulation of the GI opioid receptors are a decrease in stool hydration and an increase in transit time in the colon, leading to constipation. *Anticholinergics* and other medications with anticholinergic effects (e.g., tricyclic antidepressants, phenothiazines, some antipsychotics, antiparkinsonian agents) slow peristalsis, increasing the risk of constipation. In addition to these medications, the use of antacids containing calcium or aluminum, iron supplements, diuretics, antihypertensives, or antidiarrheal medications contributes to the incidence of constipation (Basta & Anderson, 1998; Sykes, 1998). Overuse of laxatives can lead to a weakening of the defecation reflexes, inhibiting natural bowel functioning (Guyton & Hall, 1998a). Persons with a history of chronic laxative use often require larger doses or stronger laxatives to achieve an effect (Basta & Anderson, 1998).

- Chemical imbalances: Constipation frequently occurs with hypercalcemia. It is believed that a high serum calcium level depresses the contractility of the muscle walls of the gastrointestinal tract (Guyton & Hall, 1996b). In addition, polyuria with hypercalcemia may lead to dehydration, further contributing to constipation. Hypokalemia can also lead to constipation, or in some situations, paralytic ileus, which probably results from the unresponsiveness of hyperpolarized gastrointestinal smooth muscle (Luckmann, 1997). A common cause of hypokalemia is administration of thiazide diuretics without potassium replacement.

- Pressure/compression of intestines: Cancer patients with abdominal involvement by the tumor require more laxatives than other patients on opioid therapy (Mancini, Hanson, Neumann, & Bruera, 2000). Patients with ascites, abdominal or pelvic tumors, or enlarged lymph nodes are at risk for abnormalities in digestion and elimination. A partial bowel obstruction, from tumor growth inside the intestinal lumen or compression from outside, slows motility, contributing to constipation and potentially leading to a complete obstruction (Basta & Anderson, 1998; Sykes, 1998). Persons with a history of abdominal surgery are also at risk for the development of adhesions. These adhesions can decrease intestinal lumen size, interfering with transit time in the bowel; partial and complete bowel obstruction are possible.

- Changes in the innervation of the GI tract: Constipation has been noted in many patients with motor disorders, such as spinal cord lesions and neurologic diseases. This constipation is likely the result of visceral neuropathy and a disturbance in the nerve supply of the colon, slowing the transit time. In addition, persons who have neurologic diseases may experience failure of the puborectalis and anal sphincter muscles to relax, causing intractable constipation (Mercadante, 2000). The innervation of the intestinal tract can also be interrupted by surgery. A history of abdominal surgery provides helpful information for assessing constipation. Neuropathy is a complication of some cancer chemotherapy agents, in particular the vinca alkaloids, vincristine, and vinblastine. Although constipation is a well-documented side effect of these medications in persons undergoing active treatment, the long-term effects are not clear. Those persons who have received high cumulative doses of the vinca alkaloids may be at risk for long-term side effects (Mercadante, 1998), including persistent constipation. The elderly may experience sensory changes affecting bowel functioning. In particular, rectal insensitivity may lead to a decrease in the urge to defecate (Sykes, 1998). When the urge to defecate is ignored, the anal muscles become weakened, resulting in a risk for constipation and impaction.
- Psychosocial concerns: Under conditions of fear, anxiety, stress, and depression, epinephrine is released as a sympathetic stress response. Epinephrine decreases peristalsis, leading to a risk for constipation. However, the stress response can also increase intestinal mucus formation and cause pain and cramping. Thus some patients, when stressed, have alternating bouts of diarrhea and constipation. Persons who are embarrassed about using bedpans or bedside commodes may ignore the need to defecate to preserve their privacy. And persons who are confused, lethargic, weak, or in pain may not respond to the defecation reflexes. As noted, this inattention to the urge to defecate can result in weakened anal muscles.

## ■ ASSESSMENT AND MEASUREMENT

Constipation is identified via patient report of infrequent or absent bowel movements, difficulty or pain in defecating, incomplete defecation, or hard, dry stool. Although patients may associate symptoms such as abdominal pain, bloating, flatulence, nausea, malaise, and headache with constipation, these symptoms are not specific to constipation (Sykes, 1998). Stool amount, consistency, and frequency and the length of time since the last bowel movement are important assessment data.

It is important to identify the patient's definition of constipation. Some may report constipation if a day passes without a bowel movement despite the lack of other symptoms. This may or may not indicate actual constipation. "Normal" bowel habits can range from a bowel movement one to three times a week to daily or several daily bowel movements.

# ■ HISTORY AND PHYSICAL EXAMINATION

When performing the history and physical examination, be sensitive to the fact that many persons are at least uncomfortable, if not extremely embarrassed, by questioning about bowels and bowel functioning. APNs must maintain an environment as conducive to patient privacy as possible during history taking and examination.

## General Assessment

- Review the patient's medical history and presence of any disease affecting bowel functioning.
- Assess fluid and food intake, including amounts and types of fluids and food.
- Assess hydration status: skin turgor, urinary output.
- Ask about medications, noting any opioids, tricyclic antidepressants, anticholinergics, sedatives, antiemetics, antipsychotics, antacids, and diuretics.
- Evaluate activity level and ability to use a toilet or bedside commode.

## History Related to Complaint of Constipation

- Establish what the patient means by "constipation."
- Establish the date of the last bowel movement, including amount, color, and consistency of stool.
- Ask about any discomfort or bleeding with bowel movements.
- Ask about normal bowel patterns and history of constipation problems.
- Ask what the individual has done to try to relieve constipation—both currently and in the past.
- Identify any medications/enemas and their effects, including side effects.
- Identify manual manipulation, such as application of anal pressure or digital removal of stool.

## GI Assessment

- Evaluate for complaints of abdominal pain or cramping.
- Be aware that constipation is sometimes "treated" with opioids if a complete assessment of the source of a patient's pain is not done (Sykes, 1998).
- Note the presence of any nausea or vomiting.
- Examine the abdomen:
  - Note distension.
- Listen for bowel sounds:
  - Increased activity occurs in early intestinal obstruction.
  - Decreased or absent bowel sounds may indicate ileus or peritonitis.

- High-pitched tinkling sounds indicate fluid and air under tension in a dilated bowel.
- Rushes of high-pitched sounds with abdominal cramping indicate intestinal obstruction (Bickley & Hoekelman, 1999).
- Palpate the abdomen to identify masses and areas of tenderness.
- Percuss, noting any ascites or trapped air.

### Rectal Examination

- Inspect the rectum for fissures, tears, hemorrhoids, fistulas, or tumors.
- Perform a digital examination to identify stool or tumors in the rectum.
- Avoid digital examination if the patient is neutropenic or thrombocytopenic or has known tumors.

### Psychoemotional Assessment

- Assess the patient's ability to maintain privacy for toileting.
- Evaluate the patient's stress/anxiety level.
- Assess for any confusion or dementia.

## ■ DIAGNOSTICS

As with all symptom evaluation in palliative care, radiographic and laboratory procedures should be performed only when confirmation of the underlying problem will change the course of treatment. If the cause of constipation can be identified on the basis of the medical diagnosis, treatments, and combination of other presenting symptoms, confirmation by radiography or blood work may not be necessary to determine an appropriate course of treatment.

- An abdominal film may differentiate between constipation and obstruction (Mercadante, 1998). It is only performed if there is persistent doubt and is rarely necessary (Sykes, 1998).
- Barium studies may be useful in distinguishing between a paralytic ileus and mechanical obstruction (Mercadante, 1998).
- Radiographic studies of colonic transit time, although useful in some settings to determine which areas of the bowel are not functioning, are rarely well tolerated by persons with advanced illness (Mercadante, 1998; Sykes, 1998).
- Serum electrolyte levels will identify hypercalcemia or hypokalemia.

## ■ INTERVENTION AND TREATMENT

### Prophylactic Interventions

The goal in palliative care is to prevent constipation rather than wait for it to develop. The appropriateness of the following interventions to prevent constipation is determined by the individual's performance status, mental status, and ability to eat and drink.

- Increase the activity level to stimulate natural bowel functioning.
- Walk or sit upright after meals, as this helps digestion (Basta & Anderson, 1998).
- Encourage range of motion and isometric exercises to maintain some muscle strength for patients who are unable to get out of bed (Basta & Anderson, 1998).
- Encourage adequate oral fluid intake (at least eight glasses per day).
- Encourage the patient to drink warm fluids (e.g., coffee or tea) with or after meals as they stimulate the bowel.
- Encourage foods high in bulk and fiber for persons with normal appetite:
  - The required increase in fiber to treat constipation is often not tolerated by persons with advanced illness, and dietary changes alone are generally not sufficient. The dietary emphasis for the terminally ill should be on identifying patient likes and desires versus providing fiber and bulk (Sykes, 1998).
- Instruct caregivers to respond quickly to requests to defecate.
- Encourage the use of a toilet or bedside commode so the patient can maintain upright position.
- Allow the patient privacy during toileting.
  - Use of a raised toilet seat and bathroom handrails can increase the individual's independence, promoting safety and privacy (Twycross, 1997).
- Evaluate discontinuation or decreased dosing of medications contributing to constipation.

## Laxatives

Despite maximal use of prophylactic interventions, many persons with terminal illness require laxatives to treat and prevent constipation (Sykes, 1998). There is very little research to guide the appropriate choice of laxatives or combinations of laxatives. Consider the characteristics of the patient's constipation when selecting a laxative: hard stool requires a softener; soft, difficult to pass stool requires a stimulant. Likewise the patient's response to the laxative regimen will guide titration or changes in the doses and types of laxatives used: too much softening leads to fecal leakage and incontinence; too much stimulant causes abdominal cramping (Sykes, 1998).

Patients for whom the cause of constipation cannot be eliminated will require routine use of laxatives. Low doses of laxatives are best given at night; higher doses may need to be divided, usually into morning and evening doses. Persons receiving opioid therapy often require the routine use of a combination of stimulant and softening laxatives.

Laxative agents differ according to active ingredients and mechanism of action. The following discussion outlines the mechanisms of action for the various types of laxatives, examples of each type, and starting doses.

**Softening agents.** Important considerations for softening agents include:

- Lubricant laxatives soften the stool by penetrating the stool and by preventing some absorption of water from the intestinal tract. These agents also lubricate the intestinal wall, making elimination easier (Basta & Anderson, 1998). Lubricant laxatives are less palatable then many other types of laxatives. The onset of action is approximately 6 to 8 hours after administration. Mineral oil (e.g., Fleet Mineral Oil Enema, Liqui-Doss, Milkinol) is the most frequently used lubricant laxative. The oral dose is 15 to 30 ml per day. Mineral oil enemas are generally 4 oz.

- Bulk-forming laxatives provide material that resists bacterial breakdown (nondigestible methylcellulose, psyllium, or polycarbophil), which enhances stool bulk and shortens transit time; these laxatives also provide substrates for bacterial growth, promoting increased transit time via fermentation (Basta & Anderson, 1998; Sykes, 1998). Because of the water binding capacity of these products, persons using bulk-forming laxatives must take them orally with 6 to 8 ounces of water or juice and maintain adequate overall fluid intake—at least 1.5 to 2 liters/day. Bulk-forming laxatives should be avoided if fluid intake is not adequate or if there is a suspicion of intestinal stricture or bowel obstruction (Waller & Caroline, 2000). Most bulk-forming laxatives take 12 to 72 hours to produce results. Examples include the following:
  - Methylcellulose powder (e.g., Citrucel), 3 to 4 g/day PO
  - Psyllium (e.g., Natural Fiberall, Metamucil), 3 to 4 g/day PO
  - Polycarbophil (e.g., Fiberall, FiberCon), 3 to 4 g/day PO

- Emollients/surfactants act as detergents to increase water penetration into fecal matter (Sykes, 1998). They produce softer, moister fecal material. These laxatives are rarely sufficient alone for opioid-induced constipation as the longer transit time caused by the opioids counteracts the benefits of the softeners (Basta & Anderson, 1998). Time to action is 12 to 72 hours after administration. Docusate sodium (Colace) 300 mg/day PO is the most commonly used emollient laxative.

- Osmotic laxatives create an osmotic gradient in the lumen and prevent water absorption from the small intestine. The oral doses required for opioid-induced constipation often lead to bloating, cramping, and diarrhea (Basta & Anderson, 1998; Sykes, 1998). However, glycerin suppositories produce their effect in the colon and have minimal side effects. Oral agents take 12 to 72 hours to work; suppositories stimulate bowel movements in 15 to 30 minutes. Examples include the following:
  - Lactulose (e.g., Cephulac, Duphalac), 15 ml/ bid PO
  - Sorbitol, 30 ml/day PO
  - Glycerin, 1 suppository, per rectum

- Saline laxatives are poorly absorbed and produce an immediate osmotic gradient. In addition to the influx of fluids secondary to osmosis, the magnesium salts may stimulate the secretion of cholecystokinin, which stimulates motility (Basta & Anderson, 1998; Sykes, 1998). Oral preparations take 30 minutes to 3 hours to work. Saline enemas are generally effective within 15 minutes. Examples include the following:

- Magnesium citrate, 120 to 240 ml/day PO
- Magnesium hydroxide (e.g., Milk of Magnesia), 2 to 4 g/day PO
- Sodium biphosphate/sodium phosphate (e.g., Fleet Enema, 1/day per rectum; Fleet Phospho-Buffered Saline Soda, 20 to 30 ml/day PO)

**Stimulant Laxatives.**    The stimulant laxatives increase gastrointestinal motility by stimulating the submucosal nerve plexus of the intestinal smooth muscle (Basta & Anderson, 1998; Sykes, 1998). The absorption of water and electrolytes in the colon is reduced with the use of stimulant laxatives. Stimulants may cause cramping, electrolyte disturbances, and dehydration. As castor oil is a very potent stimulant, often causing these negative side effects, it is rarely used.

Depending on availability, laxatives may be given by mouth as pills or liquids or by rectum as suppositories or enemas. In addition to the effect of the medication being given, the use of the rectal route may initiate defecation by stimulation of the anocolonic reflex (Sykes, 1998).

The rectal route is considered second-line therapy for use when the oral route is insufficient. The rectal route of administration is not pleasant for the patient or the caregivers giving the medication. All effort should be made to maintain routine bowel movements with oral medication. Examples, with starting doses, include the following:

- Senna (Senokot, Senolax), 15 mg/day PO (Senna teas are also available at some health food stores)
- Bisacodyl (Oral: Correctol, Dulcolax, Feen-A-Mint; Suppository: Bisco-Lax, Fleet Laxative), 10 mg/day PO
- Casanthranol/docusate sodium (Docu-K Plus, Genasoft Plus, Peri-Colace), 30 mg/day PO
- Cascara sagrada (Milk of Magnesia-Cascara, Concentrated), 5 ml/day PO
- Castor oil, 15-60 ml/day PO

**Combination Laxatives.**    Combining laxatives with different mechanisms of action produces synergistic effects. A combination of a stimulant and a softener is recommended for patients receiving opioid therapy. Others may benefit from this combination as well. There are several combination laxatives available on the market, although the same effect can be obtained by taking the two medications separately. Examples of combination laxatives include the following:

- Bisacodyl/docusate sodium (Modane Plus)
- Casanthranol/docusate sodium (Docu-K Plus, Genasoft Plus, Peri-Colace)
- Senna/docusate sodium (Senokot-S)

**Other Medications with Laxative Effects.**    Prokinetic agents have been investigated for the treatment of constipation. Cisapride, a prokinetic agent discussed in some texts for treatment of constipation, is no longer available because it has significant side effects. The subcutaneous infusion of metoclopramide is noted to be effective in the treatment of narcotic bowel syndrome

(Bruera, Brenneis, Michand, & MacDonald, 1987). Further investigations comparing metoclopramide with standard laxative therapies are needed to determine its role as an oral laxative.

Opioid-induced constipation has also been treated with the opioid antagonist naloxone, given orally. The opioid effect on the gastrointestinal tract is mediated via peripheral opioid receptors. As a result of first-pass hepatic metabolism there is very little systemic availability of oral naloxone, allowing the naloxone to antagonize the gastrointestinal peripheral opioid receptors without a significant antagonist effect on central opioid receptors. The result is a laxative effect without withdrawal or breakthrough pain (Sykes, 1998). However, a withdrawal response is possible, so patients must be monitored closely for pain and uncomfortable symptoms. The starting dose should not exceed 5 mg; the dose can then be titrated upward for effectiveness, watching carefully for side effects. This intervention has not been rigorously studied and its effectiveness compared to that of other interventions is not clear.

**Guidelines for Using Laxatives.**   Unfortunately there is no "gold standard" for the management of constipation. Each patient situation is different in terms of the factors contributing to constipation, and these contributing factors may change over time in the same patient. The following serves as a logical approach to the treatment of constipation:

1. Rule out obstruction.
2. Disimpact the bowel, if necessary.
3. Initiate a bowel regimen. Persons receiving opioids require a combination of a stimulant laxative and an emollient softener. The initial laxative therapy for other patients with constipation will be based on the history and physical examination findings:
   - If there is soft stool in the rectum that is difficult to eliminate, begin with a stimulant laxative.
   - If there is a small amount of hard, dry stool in the rectum, initiate therapy with an emollient laxative.
   - If there is little to no stool in the rectum, the patient may require a combination of a softener and a laxative.
4. If there is no bowel movement over 2 to 3 days, add an extra stimulant laxative or a mild saline laxative (e.g., magnesium hydroxide):
   - If the extra stimulant works, evaluate adding more softener or stimulant to the routine bowel regimen, on the basis of assessment of the amount and consistency of the stool (see Step 3).
   - If the extra stimulant is not effective, move to Step 5.
5. Use a saline enema to clear the colon of stool:
   - If the enema is effective, evaluate adding more softener and/or stimulant to the daily regimen (as in Step 3).
   - If the enema is not effective, the constipation may be occurring higher up in the bowel. Move to Step 6.

6. Use an oral saline (e.g., magnesium citrate) or osmotic laxative (e.g., lactulose):
   - If this intervention is effective, evaluate adding more softener and/or stimulant to the daily regimen (as in Step 3).
   - If this step is not effective, consider repeating the saline or osmotic laxative (if the patient did not experience cramping or bloating). Nontraditional laxatives, such as metoclopramide, or oral naloxone may be considered.

## ■ PATIENT AND FAMILY EDUCATION

Patients and families require information on the importance of reporting constipation, the appropriate use of the prophylactic interventions, and the appropriate use of laxatives:
- Discuss the importance of reporting bowel functioning, including frequency, amount, and consistency of stools and any discomfort associated with defecation, to the health care team.
- Teach patients who are able to do so to participate in exercise activities or isometric abdominal and pelvic exercises.
- Instruct the patient to take in at least eight glasses of fluid each day and to increase the bulk in the diet, both as tolerated by the patient.
- Encourage the use of warm liquids with meals to stimulate bowel functioning.
- Discuss the importance of responding immediately to the urge to defecate with both the patient and the caregivers.
- Discuss the benefit of maintaining an upright position for defecation; encourage the use of a toilet or bedside commode.
- Caregivers may require instruction on proper transfer techniques for assisting the patient out of a bed or chair to a bedside commode.
- Teach the appropriate dosing and schedule of laxative medications. Those that require 6 hours or longer to work are best dosed at night.
- Encourage the patient and family to report any cramping, bloating, stool leakage, or diarrhea associated with taking the prescribed laxatives.
- Discuss the importance of avoiding the bulk-forming laxatives for persons taking opioids and for those whose fluid intake is limited.

## ■ EVALUATION AND PLAN FOR FOLLOW-UP

The effectiveness of the interventions to manage constipation is determined by reassessing the patient's bowel status. Ask about the frequency, amount, and consistency of stools and about any discomfort or difficulty passing stool. It is also important to ask about the effectiveness of laxatives to determine appropriate changes in the plan of care.

Assessment of bowel status must be a part of the ongoing, routine evaluation of the patient to determine if the prescribed regimen continues to be effective over the course of the patient's care. Persons with advanced illnesses will experience changes in the disease process, fluid intake, activity level, and prescribed medications that will affect the bowels and necessitate modifications in the care plan.

✔ **CASE STUDY**   Mr. Jones has metastatic lung cancer and a history of congestive heart failure. He received treatment with combination chemotherapy 6 months ago, and he tolerated it well. However, the cancer progressed and he was referred for hospice palliative care at home. Mr. Jones weighs 152 pounds, down from his baseline of 200 pounds. He has a poor appetite and states that he feels nauseous if he eats more than a few bites of food. He keeps a 1-quart pitcher of water at his bedside and reports drinking the entire quart over the course of a day. He also drinks a small glass of orange juice with breakfast. He is able to walk to the bathroom with the assistance of his wife. He reports that he has not had a bowel movement in 3 days despite taking Metamucil every day. He is complaining of abdominal bloating and cramping.

Mr. Jones' medications include the following: sustained-release oxycodone 40 mg bid, immediate-release oxycodone 10 mg q1-2h for breakthrough pain or dyspnea, ibuprofen 400 mg qid, furosemide 40 mg qd, and digoxin 0.125 mg qd.

On physical examination, the APN notes that there is no stool in the rectum and that bowel sounds are hyperactive. The nurse discusses the constipating effects of the opioids and the need to use both a stimulant and a softener laxative. She also explains that the bulk-forming laxatives are not a good choice at this time. The patient is instructed to take magnesium citrate, 120 to 240 ml over ice, as tolerated. Two hours later Mr. Jones reports that he has passed a small amount of hard feces and feels there is more stool in the rectum. A bisacodyl (Dulcolax) suppository is administered in order to empty the rectum of stool. The patient is then started on a regimen of casanthranol 30 mg/docusate sodium 100 mg (Peri-Colace) 2 tablets at hs. He also is instructed to take magnesium hydroxide (Milk of Magnesia-Cascara, Concentrated), 30 ml at hs, if more than 2 days pass without a bowel movement.

This regimen works well for Mr. Jones for about a month. Then he reports needing to take the Milk of Magnesia every 2 days. Mrs. Jones also states that the patient gets short of breath walking to the bathroom and, in general, his activity level has decreased. The nurse instructs the patient to increase the Peri-Colace to 3 tablets at hs. On physical assessment the nurse notes that the patient is slightly dehydrated with no peripheral edema and instructs him to discontinue the furosemide. She also discusses the energy-saving benefits of a bedside commode and, with the patient's and wife's permission, orders one for the patient.

*Continued*

Mr. Jones continued to have bowel movements of soft, formed stool every 1 to 2 days up until 3 days ago. He is now bed-bound and taking in only sips of fluids and having some difficulty swallowing pills. The Peri-Colace is discontinued. The APN monitors for bowel sounds, abdominal distension, and the presence of stool in the rectum. The following day some stool is noted in the rectum and the nurse administers a Dulcolax suppository. Mr. Jones dies peacefully 2 days later, with no sign of abdominal distension or discomfort.

## References

BASTA, S., & Anderson, D. L. (1998). Mechanisms and management of constipation in the cancer patient. *Journal of Pharmaceutical Care in Pain & Symptom Control, 6*(3), 21-40.

BICKLEY, L. S., & Hoekelman, R. A. (1999). The abdomen. In L. S. Bickley & R. A. Hoekelman, *Bates' guide to physical examination and history taking* (7th ed.) (pp. 355-386). Philadelphia: Lippincott.

BRUERA, E., Brenneis, C., Michand, M., & MacDonald, N. (1987). Continuous subcutaneous infusion of metoclopramide for treatment of narcotic bowel syndrome. *Cancer Treatment Reports, 28*, 1033-1038.

CONILL, C., Verger, E., Henriquez, I., Saiz, N., Espier, M., Lugo, R., & Garrigos, A. (1997). Symptom prevalence in the last week of life. *Journal of Pain and Symptom Management, 14*(6), 328-331.

CURTIS, E., Krech, R., & Walsh, T. D. (1991). Common symptoms in patients with advanced cancer. *Journal of Palliative Care, 7*(2), 25-29.

GUYTON, A. C., & Hall, J. E. (1996a). Physiology of gastrointestinal disorders. In A. C. Guyton & J. E. Hall, *Textbook of medical physiology* (9th ed.) (pp. 845-851). Philadelphia: W. B. Saunders.

GUYTON, A. C., & Hall, J. E. (1996b). Parathyroid hormone, calcitonin, calcium and phosphate metabolism, vitamin D, bone, and teeth. In A. C. Guyton & J. E. Hall, *Textbook of medical physiology* (9th ed.) (pp. 985-1002). Philadelphia: W. B. Saunders.

LICHTER, I., & Hunt, E. (1990). The last 48 hours of life. *Journal of Palliative Care, 6*(4), 7-15.

LUCKMANN, J. (1997). Caring for people with fluid, electrolyte, and acid-base imbalances. In *Saunders manual of nursing care* (pp. 235-290). Philadelphia: W. B. Saunders.

MANCINI, I. L., Hanson, J., Neumann, C. M., & Bruera, E. D. (2000). Opioid type and other clinical predictors of laxative dose in advanced cancer patients: A retrospective study. *Journal of Palliative Medicine, 3*(1), 49-56.

MERCADANTE, S. (1998). Diarrhea, malabsorption, and constipation. In A. Berger, R. K. Portenoy, & D. E. Weissman (Eds.), *Principles and practice of supportive oncology* (pp. 191-205). Philadelphia: Lippincott-Raven.

SYKES, N. P. (1998). Constipation and diarrhea. In D. Doyle, G. W. C. Hanks, & N. MacDonald (Eds.), *Oxford textbook of palliative medicine* (2nd ed.) (pp. 513-526). New York: Oxford University Press.

TWYCROSS, R. (1997). *Symptom management in advanced cancer* (2nd ed.). Oxon, UK: Radcliffe Medical Press.

VAINIO, A., & Auvinen, A. (1996). Prevalence of symptoms among patients with advanced cancer: An international collaborative study. *Journal of Pain and Symptom Management, 12*(1), 3-10.

WALLER, A., & Caroline, N. L. (2000). *Handbook of palliative care in cancer* (2nd ed.). Boston: Butterworth-Heinemann.

# Cough

PATRICIA H. BERRY

## ■ DEFINITION AND INCIDENCE

Cough is a normal mechanism in the respiratory system designed to protect a person from potential harm (Ahemdzai, 1998). Its purpose is to expel particles and excess mucus from the trachea and main bronchi (Twycross, 1997). As a protective mechanism, cough only demands attention when perceived as excessive. When it occurs in prolonged bouts, it is exhausting and frightening and, in some cases, it can exacerbate dyspnea, and lead to loss of sleep, increased blood pressure, ruptured blood vessels, hemoptysis, nausea and vomiting, musculoskeletal pain, and rib fracture (Kemp, 1997; Twycross, 1997). In addition, cough may have been the symptom that prompted the patient to seek health care, as it is the most common symptom that sends otherwise healthy persons to the physician (Ahemdzai, 1998). Thus the symptom of cough may also be an unwelcome reminder of disease activity (Ahemdzai, 1998). The incidence of cough in end-stage illness is as high as 83%, making it one of the most common symptoms seen in terminally ill persons (Stegman, 1999).

## ■ ETIOLOGY AND PATHOPHYSIOLOGY

Normally cough serves to maintain the cleanliness and patency of the airway. It assists the respiratory cilia to transport mucus, fluids, and inhaled foreign bodies upward, where they can be either swallowed or spit out. Although the origins of cough in persons with advanced illness are diverse, they fall into three physiologic categories: excessive production of bronchial fluids and secretions, inhalation of foreign materials, and abnormal stimulation of receptors in the airways (Ahemdzai, 1998). Clinically the development of a troublesome cough requiring intervention can be attributed to four disease-related categories, which are summarized in Table 19-1.

## ■ ASSESSMENT AND MEASUREMENT

The underlying cause of cough can be identified with a simple history and physical examination leading to a specific treatment (Rousseau, 1996b). The

| TABLE 19-1 | |
|---|---|
| *Causes of Cough in End-Stage Illness* | |
| **Category** | **Cause** |
| Cardiopulmonary | COPD, CHF, asthma, infections, tumors, pleural or peri-cardial effusion, pneumonia, sinus or postnasal drainage, paralysis of the vocal cords |
| Medications | Angiotensin-converting enzyme (ACE) inhibitors, ipra-tropium bromide, inhalation of nebulized water for hiccoughs or dry mouth |
| Esophageal | Gastroesophageal reflux |
| Aspiration | Motor neuron disease (e.g., amyotrophic lateral sclerosis [ALS]), multiple sclerosis (MS), stroke, gastroesoph-ageal reflux |

From Ahemdzai, S. (1998). Palliation of respiratory symptoms. In D. Doyle, G. W. C. Hanks, & N. MacDonald (Eds.), *Oxford textbook of palliative medicine* (2nd ed.) (pp. 583-616). New York: Oxford University Press; Kaye, P. (1994). *Notes on symptom control in hospice and palliative care.* Essex, CT: Hospice Education Institute; Rousseau, P. (1996a). Nonpain symptoms management in terminal care. *Clinics in Geriatric Medicine, 12,* 313-327; Rousseau, P. (1996b). Cough in the terminally ill: A brief synopsis. *American Journal of Hospice and Palliative Care, 13*(6), 45-46.

characteristics of cough can also serve to delineate the etiology. This important information can be gathered either through observation; the report of the patient or caregivers, including family members; or the directed history and physical examination. The characteristics of cough are summarized in Table 19-2.

## ■ HISTORY AND PHYSICAL EXAMINATION

In addition to the specific cough assessment as identified in Table 19-2, a complete history (unless already available) may provide clues regarding the possible cause. The history and physical examination will include reviewing patients' medical and nursing diagnoses and making a targeted systems assessment. The history includes the following important aspects:

- History and nature of any allergies, chronic sinusitis, asthma, chronic obstructive pulmonary disease (COPD), or other cardiopulmonary diseases
- History of the primary disease, including the association of disease progression and causes of cough
- History and nature of any gastroesophageal reflux disease or stroke and a thorough medication history, including over-the-counter medications and herbal or natural products
- Assessment of the cough, including frequency, duration, aggravating and alleviating factors, and sputum production, including color, amount, and frequency
- Identification of patient or caregiver perceptions of cause

## TABLE 19-2

### Common Causes of Cough

| Cough Characteristics | Possible Cause |
| --- | --- |
| Cough and dyspnea | Frequent association of cough and dyspnea (refer to the dyspnea clinical practice guideline) |
| Cough and choking | Aspiration, associated with a variety of conditions, including obstruction and fistula |
| Cough and choking; patient is also weak, has had significant weight loss, has a respiratory infection | Inability to clear sputum, causing sputum to be retained |
| Cough and hoarseness | Vocal cord paralysis, common in primary or secondary tumors of the chest |
| Cough and history or symptoms of cardiac disease, in particular CHF accompanied by anemia | Congestive heart failure |
| Cough with fever, upper respiratory infection (i.e., common cold) | Upper respiratory infection |
| Cough with history of COPD or other respiratory disease; cough that seems associated with environmental factors such as dry air or cigarette smoke | Preexisting condition or environmental factor |

From Cowcher, K., & Hanks, G. W. (1990). Long-term management of respiratory symptoms in advanced cancer. *Journal of Pain and Symptom Management, 5,* 320-330; Fanta, C. H. (1993). Respiratory complications. In J. F. Holland, E. Fei, R. C. Bast, D. W. Kufe, D. L. Morton, & R. W. Weischselbaum (Eds.), *Cancer medicine* (3rd ed.) (2349-2358). Philadelphia: Lea & Febiger; Hagen, N. A. (1991). An approach to cough in cancer patients. *Journal of Pain and Symptom Management, 6,* 257-262; Kemp, C. (1997). Palliative care for the respiratory problems in terminal illness. *The American Journal of Hospice and Palliative Care, 14*(1), 26-30.

- Evaluation of the distress caused by the cough, on a 0 to 10 scale
- Identification of the degree of relief that would allow the patient to rest and participate in valued activities
- Assessment of associated/accompanying symptoms, such as anxiety, pain, or dyspnea

In the target physical assessment:

- Assess breath sounds beginning auscultation at the base of the lungs rather than the apex, then returning to the base; allows atelectasis that clears with deep breathing to be detected.
- Assess for pleural and cardiac effusion.
- Note quality and recent changes in voice.
- Inspect the nose and mouth for drainage.
- Observe for signs and symptoms of heart failure.
- Note the patient's overall strength, activity, and functional ability.

# ■ DIAGNOSTICS

Evaluation of cough depends on several factors, including the prognosis/life expectancy of the patient and the risk/benefit evaluation of diagnostic measures, some of which may be invasive. Treatment, even for a suspected infection, is empiric. Diagnostic studies are generally not indicated unless the patient is undergoing anticancer treatment or if congestive heart failure (CHF) or COPD is suspected, but not yet ruled out (Rousseau, 1996b).

# ■ INTERVENTION AND TREATMENT

The pharmacologic treatment of cough is directed at the underlying cause. These interventions, with some additional nonpharmacologic measures, are summarized in Table 19-3. Note, however, that expectorants and mucolytics are of little value and generally not recommended, as they tend to cause nausea and vomiting and do not treat the underlying cough (Rousseau, 1996b). Although there is no agreement on the best choice of opioid for cough, all except meperidine have antitussive activity. Codeine, 15-30 mg PO q4h as needed, or morphine, 2.5 mg PO q4h as needed, is baseline. If the patient is already taking an opioid, the dose should be gradually increased until the cough is suppressed or side effects become intolerable (Rousseau, 1996a; Rousseau, 1996b). Some sources recommend giving opioids with an antihistamine to reduce the opioid-induced histamine release (Kemp, 1997). Although oral preparations are preferred, opioids for cough suppression can also be administered rectally, subcutaneously, or intravenously. Inhaled or nebulized opioids have no proven benefit in cough (Rousseau, 1996b). Over-the-counter products with dextromethorphan may also be an option in treating cough in end-stage illness (Ahemdzai, 1998).

If the cough is refractory to the treatment discussed in Table 19-3, consider the use of a nebulized anesthetic, which is thought to block the receptor responsible for bronchial irritation, although its use is controversial (Rousseau, 1996a). Bupivacaine 0.25% is recommended at a dose of 5 ml every 4 to 6 hours. Because of local anesthetic effects, the patient should be instructed not to eat or drink for 30 minutes after taking it to prevent aspiration and thus worsening of the cough (Ahemdzai, 1998; Rousseau, 1996a). Nebulized lidocaine, however, is not recommended as it is reported to precipitate bronchospasm and cause vasoconstriction and has a short duration of action (Horn, 1992; Rousseau, 1996a).

Inhaled local anesthetics are also beneficial for cough due to pooled saliva in those patients who have swallowing difficulties, most often persons with motor neuron disease or multiple sclerosis. Especially at night, this pooled saliva overflows into the trachea, resulting in prolonged bouts of coughing. A single dose of nebulized bupivacaine can lessen the pharyngeal and tracheal sensation, allowing better sleep. However, this treatment may increase the risk of saliva aspirations, and the risks and benefits must be discussed with the patient and family and considered in the context of disease stage and goals of treatment.

## TABLE 19-3

### Reversable Causes of Cough

| Causes | Treatment* |
|---|---|
| Cigarettes | Advise the patient to stop or reduce smoking; request family and visitors to smoke away from the patient. An air cleaner may also be helpful. |
| Postnasal drip | Prescribe antihistamine. |
| | Prescribe antibiotic (if purulent sputum). |
| Respiratory infection | Perform chest physiotherapy unless contraindicated by patient condition. |
| | Administer nebulized saline solution (especially helpful when followed by chest physiotherapy). |
| COPD/asthma | Prescribe bronchodilator and/or corticosteroid. |
| Cardiac failure | Administer diuretic. |
| Drug-induced | Administer ACE inhibitor and/or digoxin. |
| | Reduce dose or stop drug, then prescribe a drug other than an ACE inhibitor. |
| Esophageal reflux | Advise patient to sleep in a semiupright position. |
| | Stop or reduce dose of drug, causing a reduction of low esophageal sphincter tone.[†] |
| | Prescribe metoclopramide to increase lower esophageal sphincter tone. |
| | Use proton pump inhibitor to reduce acid content and volume of gastric secretion. |
| Aspiration of saliva | Use anticholinergic to reduce saliva. |
| Pleural effusion | Perform thoracentesis. |
| | Position the patient on the same side as the pleural effusion (positioning thought to reduce mediastinal shift that causes the cough). |
| Irritation of the pharynx | Prescribe local anesthetic lozenges. |
| Malignant obstruction | Prescribe corticosteroids (dexamethasone 4-8 mg PO qd or prednisone 20-60 mg PO qd). Evaluate for palliative radiation therapy or palliative chemotherapy. |

*Specific drug dosages for most suggested treatment are not listed; usual drug dosages for treatment of the underlying cause are advised.
†Medications that decrease the competence of the cardiac sphincter: nicotine, anticholinergics, benzodiazepines, calcium-channel blockers, nitrates and nitrites, estrogens, meperidine, theophylline.
Adapted from Twycross, R. (1997). *Symptom management in advanced cancer.* Oxon, UK: Radcliffe Medical Press.

## ■ OTHER COMPLEMENTARY TREATMENTS

In addition to the methods of treatment listed in Table 19-3, the following interventions may provide additional comfort:
- Stressing a side-lying position when one lung is completely obstructed
- Providing warm and humidified air
- Teaching coughing and deep breathing exercises
- Teaching effective coughing technique: it is impossible to cough effectively while lying supine

# ■ PATIENT AND FAMILY EDUCATION

To treat cough effectively, the following information is taught to patients and their family caregivers:

- Encourage monitoring for patterns and frequency of coughing episodes.
- Instruct them to notify their health care provider if:
  - The planned intervention is not effective.
  - The cough becomes worse or the patient is febrile and/or develops a productive cough.
- Instruct the patient and family about a treatment plan, including pharmacologic and complementary interventions.

As with all treatments for advanced illness, interventions for any symptom is driven by the patient-focused goals of care. The consequences of no treatment should be part of the overall goal-setting discussion with the patient and family.

# ■ EVALUATION AND PLAN FOR FOLLOW-UP

Success of the treatment of cough is determined by evaluating mutually established goals with the patient and family.

---

✔ **CASE STUDY**    Mr. Jones is a 65-year-old gentleman with end-stage lung cancer whose unremitting cough caused him to consult his physician, who made the eventual diagnosis. Cough remained a troublesome symptom until after his response to the initial chemotherapy and radiation therapy. He was admitted to home care after learning that his cancer had recurred, causing a left pleural effusion and a large mass in the mediastinum. His cough has returned; he is unable to rest, eat, or even interact with his family and friends. Most importantly, the cough serves as a constant reminder of his disease.

Mr. Jones has a history of COPD but denies any symptoms of CHF; the physical examination finding is negative as well. Although he is advised to stop smoking, he chooses to continue, citing it as one of the only things he still enjoys. A trial of codeine 15 mg q4-6, is ineffective in relieving his cough. The pleural effusion is drained by his health care provider, giving some relief of the cough. Because of suspicion of a malignant obstruction a radiation therapy consultation is ordered, and dexamethasone, 4 to 8 mg qd, is added, producing nearly complete relief. Mr. Jones is able to attend his daughter's wedding and enjoy the reception without his cough—and the ever-present reminder of his illness. He is fearful, however, of the cough's returning and robbing him of his quality of life in his final days and weeks. He is assured that his concern about cough and his desire to be free of this troublesome symptom will be priorities in his continued care plan.

Mr. Jones dies a month later, at home, still enjoying an occasional cigarette, with his cough controlled by nebulized bupivacaine.

## References

AHEMDZAI, S. (1998). Palliation of respiratory symptoms. In D. Doyle, G. W. C. Hanks, & N. MacDonald (Eds.), *Oxford textbook of palliative medicine* (2nd ed.) (pp. 583-616). New York: Oxford University Press.

COWCHER, K., & Hanks, G. W. (1990). Long-term management of respiratory symptoms in advanced cancer. *Journal of Pain and Symptom Management, 5,* 320-330.

FANTA, C. H. (1993). Respiratory complications. In J. F. Holland, E. Fei, R. C. Bast, D. W. Kufe, D. L. Morton, & R. W. Weischselbaum (Eds.), *Cancer medicine* (3rd ed.) (pp. 2349-2358). Philadelphia: Lea & Febiger.

HAGEN, N. A. (1991). An approach to cough in cancer patients. *Journal of Pain and Symptom Management, 6,* 257-262.

HORN, L. W. (1992). Terminal dyspnea: A hospice approach. *American Journal of Hospice and Palliative Care, 9,* 24.

KAYE, P. (1994). *Notes on symptom control in hospice and palliative care.* Essex, CT: Hospice Education Institute.

KEMP, C. (1997). Palliative care for the respiratory problems in terminal illness. *The American Journal of Hospice and Palliative Care, 14*(1), 26-30.

ROUSSEAU, P. (1996a). Nonpain symptoms management in terminal care. *Clinics in Geriatric Medicine, 12,* 313-327.

ROUSSEAU, P. (1996b). Cough in the terminally ill: A brief synopsis. *American Journal of Hospice and Palliative Care, 13*(6), 45-46.

STEGMAN, M. B. (1999). Evaluation and management of gastrointestinal symptoms. In R. S. Schonwetter, W. Hawke, & C. F. Knight (Eds.), *Hospice and palliative medicine: Core curriculum and review syllabus* (pp. 77-84). Dubuque, IA: Kendall/Hunt.

TWYCROSS R. (1997). *Symptom management in advanced cancer* (2nd ed.). Oxon, UK: Radcliffe Medical Press.

# *Dehydration*

KIM K. KUEBLER, SANDY MCKINNON

## ■ DEFINITION AND INCIDENCE

*Dehydration* is defined as the overall reduction of water content in the body. Dehydration may be isotonic, hypertonic/hypernatremic, or hypotonic/hyponatremic. Dehydration is a common condition in the dying patient population, resulting from decreased intake of fluids or from an abnormal loss of fluids. It is well known that dehydration in individuals who are not terminally ill precipitates fluid and electrolyte imbalances that lead to symptoms of headache, confusion, nausea, vomiting, muscle cramps, thirst, and dry mouth (xerostomia) (Bruera, Belzile, Watanabe, & Fainsinger, 1996; Dunphy, 1995; Fainsinger & Bruera, 1994). It is not clear that these same symptoms universally occur in the terminally ill despite a decrease in total body water content.

The dehydration that results from a decreased desire to take in fluids at the end of life is sometimes called the "natural dehydration of the dying" or "terminal dehydration." Many believe that terminal dehydration does not adversely affect well-being (Billings, 1985; McCann, Hall, & Groth-Juncker, 1994; Printz, 1992; Zerwekh, 1997). There may even be beneficial effects of dehydration at the end of life. The following have been identified as potential benefits of terminal dehydration: (1) decrease in incontinence or need for catheterization due to decreased urine output; (2) decrease in cough and congestion due to reduction in pulmonary secretions; (3) decrease in nausea and vomiting due to decreased gastric fluids; (4) decrease in pain due to less edema around tumors and a potential for a natural anesthetic effect from dehydration (Zerwekh, 1997).

Optimal palliative care of persons who have a decrease in body fluids relies on assessment and management of reversible causes, identification and management of actual or potential uncomfortable symptoms or toxicities associated with dehydration, evaluation of potential benefits associated with dehydration, and evaluation of the benefits and burdens of hydration.

## ■ ETIOLOGY AND PATHOPHYSIOLOGY

Dehydration may be isotonic, hypertonic, or hypotonic. Because serum sodium and its associated anions account for more than 90% of the solute in extracellular fluid, the plasma sodium concentration is a good indicator of plasma osmolarity (Guyton & Hall, 1996a). In isotonic dehydration there is a depletion of both sodium and water. The serum sodium level is within normal limits (135 to 148 mEq/liter) despite a fluid volume deficit. In hypertonic dehydration serum sodium is concentrated (>150 mEq/liter) as a result of lower fluid volume. Hypotonic dehydration occurs with excessive loss of sodium along with some fluid volume loss, leading to a serum sodium level <130 mEq/liter.

As death approaches and patients lose their ability or desire to drink fluids, the lack of fluid intake may lead to an isotonic depletion of water and sodium or, possibly, a tendency toward hypertonic dehydration with slight hypernatremia. In studies of persons experiencing dehydration at the end of life over half had normal or near-normal serum sodium concentrations (Burge, 1993; Ellershaw, Sutcliffe, & Saunders, 1995; Waller, Hershkowitz, & Adunsky, 1994). It must be noted, however, that the results of these studies cannot be generalized because of small sample sizes, potentially biased selection criteria, and missing data (Viola, Wells, & Peterson, 1997). It is also important to note that although over half had normal serum sodium concentration, a significant number had elevations in sodium concentration.

Persons with isotonic dehydration may demonstrate low blood pressure with dizziness and syncope, decreased skin turgor, dry mucous membranes, low-grade fever, decreased urine output, and weight loss. A complaint of thirst is common, although not universal. Because the serum is more concentrated, laboratory data may show elevated hemoglobin, hematocrit, and blood urea nitrogen (BUN) level.

Many of the patients in the studies noted who did not have an isotonic dehydration did appear to have a hypertonic/hypernatremic dehydration. Hypernatremia is possible with a prolonged decrease in fluid intake, as may be seen in the terminally ill; it also occurs in the presence of excessive diaphoresis and with diabetes insipidus. The signs and symptoms are the same as those of isotonic dehydration, except that thirst is almost universal because even slight increases in sodium concentration (as little as 2 mEq/liter above normal) activate the thirst mechanism (Guyton & Hall, 1996b). As the sodium level increases, anxiety and restlessness may also be present.

Fluid and electrolyte losses occurring with vomiting or diarrhea may lead to isotonic dehydration if the fluid and electrolyte loss is balanced. However, excessive sodium is often lost with prolonged gastrointestinal fluid losses leading to a hypotonic dehydration. This type of dehydration is also possible with excessive use of diuretics or with the diuretic effect associated with hypercalcemia. Persons with hypotonic dehydration may appear to have a normal urinary output, but, if intake and output records are kept, the clinician will note excessive output compared to intake. Like other types of dehydration the patient may have low blood pressure, poor skin turgor, dry mucous membranes, and weight loss. In addition fatigue and confusion are associated with hyponatremic dehydration.

The sensation of thirst is important to fluid balance. In dehydration patients experience thirst, due to either dry mucous membranes or increased serum sodium level, and are stimulated to drink to replace the fluid loss. It is important to note, however, that the presence of thirst does not necessarily indicate dehydration. Many medications, such as opioids, phenothiazines, antihistamines, antidepressants, and anticholinergics, can cause the sensation of thirst despite adequate hydration. Thus thirst alone is not a good indicator of a patient's hydration status.

The elderly are at an increased risk for dehydration, in part because a decrease in the sense of thirst accompanies the normal aging process. A lack of thirst may also be the result of a coexistent inability to respond physiologically to thirst from disease or disability (West, 1993). In addition the elderly are susceptible to the development of dehydration or hypovolemia as a result of chronic use of medications such as diuretic therapy, which can be responsible for significant water and vital electrolyte depletion.

Confusion, agitation, and restlessness are often associated with dehydration and may result from one of several of the following mechanisms. Dehydration directly affects the body's blood volume and circulatory reserve and can cause confusion and restlessness in non–terminally ill patients as well as those with an advanced illness (Fainsinger & Bruera, 1994; Fainsinger et al., 1994; Pereira & Bruera, 1997). In addition the decreased circulatory volume may lead to decreased renal perfusion and eventual renal failure. In persons receiving opioids, poor renal perfusion may cause accumulation of opioid metabolites, leading to confusion, myoclonus, and nausea (Bruera, Franco, Maltoni, Wantanabe, & Suarez-Almazor, 1995). Constipation, pyrexia, and electrolyte imbalance result from dehydration and can further contribute to disorientation, agitation, and neuromuscular irritability (Fainsinger & Bruera, 1994; Steiner & Bruera, 1998).

Providing fluids to persons who are dehydrated may alleviate many of the symptoms of dehydration and assist in flushing waste products and medication metabolites from the circulation. Providing fluids to persons whose kidneys cannot eliminate the additional fluid may lead to discomfort from fluid overload, with symptoms of edema, ascites, pulmonary congestion, and nausea and vomiting.

## ■ ASSESSMENT AND MEASUREMENT

The determination of a patient's hydration status is difficult in patients who have multiple problems associated with advanced diseases. Steiner and Bruera (1998) suggest the following factors as the most reliable when discerning dehydration:

- Severely restricted oral intake
- Decreased urine output in patients who do not have preexisting renal failure

- Poor skin turgor, dry mouth, and postural hypotension, noting that dehydration is not the only cause of these symptoms
- Changes in laboratory findings such as elevated urea, creatinine, hematocrit, sodium, and plasma proteins levels
  Other signs and symptoms of dehydration include the following:
- Confusion
- Restlessness
- Delirium
- Myoclonus
- Seizures
- Constipation
- Nausea/vomiting
- Decreased glomerular filtration rate (may also be the result of renal failure)
- Presence of bed sores
- Higher than normal systolic blood pressure
- Tachycardia
- Thready pulse

Adequate renal function is necessary for the elimination of medication metabolites. In the absence of adequate hydration, medications such as opioids must be adjusted. As renal failure occurs, consider decreasing opioid doses or changing to "prn" dosing to minimize opioid toxicities (Fainsinger & Bruera, 1994; Regional Palliative Care Program Capital Health Authority, 1998; West, 1993).

It is important to note that the presence of edema is not a good indicator of the patient's hydration status. Edema in the advanced cancer population is often the result of low serum albumin level or tumor blockage of the venous or lymphatic systems. Patients taking corticosteroids may also experience edema. Despite excessive fluid in the interstitial spaces, there may be inadequate intravascular fluid.

# ■ DIAGNOSTICS

The following should be evaluated (Fainsinger & Bruera, 1994; Twycross, 1997; Twycross & Lichter, 1998):
- Blood pressure
- Hematocrit
- Sodium
- BUN
- Serum creatinine level
- Calcium levels (to rule out hypercalcemia)

# ■ INTERVENTION AND TREATMENT

Providing hydration to persons with advanced illness remains controversial for some clinicians and further research is required in this area. Studies in the 1990s indicated that maintaining artificial hydration in dying patients alleviates some symptoms that interfere with their quality of life. In addition, providing hydration may relieve the emotional distress experienced by some patients and their families who have concerns about dehydration (Fainsinger & Bruera, 1991; Fainsinger & Bruera, 1994; Fainsinger et al., 1994; Parkash & Burge, 1997; Twycross, 1997). It is interesting to note, however, that some families view hydration as burdensome and inappropriate (Parkash & Burge, 1997). Thus patient and family views regarding dehydration and artificial hydration provide important information for clinical decision making.

There seems to be an ongoing debate about the benefits of hydration. The ethical basis of most clinical decision making is the assessment of the benefits, risks, and burdens conferred by any particular intervention. In the terminal phase of advanced diseases attention is directed at attempts to maintain or improve the quality of life; symptom control and patient comfort are the primary goals for both medical and nursing care. Optimal palliative care necessitates remedial intervention for all treatable conditions causing discomfort (Dunphy, 1995). Hydration is being used in the terminal setting to provide symptom relief for many patients (Kuebler, 1999). Until a general consensus is reached, the decision to administer fluids to an individual patient must be based on a thorough physical assessment, review of the therapeutic benefits and adverse effects of hydration, and open discussion with patients and families regarding their fears and concerns (Steiner & Bruera, 1998).

One argument against parenteral hydration relates to the potential discomfort, cost, and complexity of maintaining this intervention. The utilization of hypodermoclysis can provide an inexpensive, comfortable method of replacing fluids (Fainsinger & Bruera, 1991; Pereira & Bruera, 1997; Regional Palliative Care Program Capital Health Authority, 1998).

## Hypodermoclysis

Hypodermoclysis (HDC) offers many advantages to symptomatic dehydrated patients who would have difficulty reversing their dehydration by the oral route. It is believed that HDC offers far more benefits of fluid replacement than the traditional intravenous route because (Fainsinger & Bruera, 1991; Fainsinger et al., 1994):

- There is no need for venous access.
- It is easy to teach family members how to use HDC in the home with a subcutaneous injection.
- HDC can be stopped and started without concern of a thrombus development.
- HDC can be administered in the home with no need for hospitalization.
- Subcutaneous sites can last for several days.

In the absence of large volume losses, 1 liter of fluid per 24 hours is usually sufficient to maintain renal function in the advanced cancer population and prevent potential problems related to overhydration.

**Method for initiating hypodermoclysis.**    The APN should:

- Select an insertion site. Preferred sites include the upper chest (avoid breast tissue), upper back, abdomen, back of upper arms, and upper thighs.
- Cleanse the skin over the selected site with alcohol or chlorhexidine.
- Gently pinch a well-defined amount of tissue and insert a small needle (25- or 23-gauge butterfly) at a 45-degree angle into the subcutaneous space.
- Dress the site with a transparent dressing.
- Select an electrolyte-containing solution such as 2/3, 1/3, or plain normal saline solution.
- Begin infusions slowly (50-75 ml/hr) to determine tolerance. Most people tolerate 50 to 100 ml/h without requiring hyaluronidase.
- Hyaluronidase is an enzyme that breaks down hyaluronic acid and aids in the rapid diffusion and absorption of injected fluids; although not always necessary, it can be used to improve absorption in patients experiencing difficulties in this area (Fainsinger & Bruera, 1994; Pereira & Bruera, 1997).
- The recommended amount of hyaluronidase in 1 liter of fluid varies from 150 to 750 units. The most common dose suggested is 150 units per liter of subcutaneous fluid (Fainsinger & Bruera, 1994).

A summary of hydration in palliative care, in particular when hypodermoclysis or an intravenous infusion is indicated, is found in Box 20-1.

---

| **BOX 20-1** | *Indications and Contraindications to Hydration in Palliative Care* |
|---|---|

**INDICATIONS**

Generally all the following criteria should be met:

- The patient is experiencing symptoms (e.g., thirst, malaise, delirium) for which dehydration seems the most likely cause.
- Increased oral intake is not feasible.
- There is anticipation that parenteral hydration will relieve the symptoms (e.g., in patients with severe dysphagia, vomiting, or diarrhea).
- The patient's underlying physical condition is relatively good (e.g., some patients with head and neck cancer).
- The patient is willing to have parenteral hydration.
- The patient and relatives understand that the purpose is to relieve symptoms and not to cure.

It is advisable initially to give a provisional time limit for parenteral hydration (e.g., 2-3 days), after which it will be discontinued if not helpful.

**CONTRAINDICATIONS**

- The patient requests to not have an invasive procedure.
- The sum of the burdens of parenteral hydration outweighs the likely benefits.
- The patient is moribund for reasons other than dehydration.

If it is not in the patient's best interests, parenteral hydration should not be introduced simply to satisfy relatives who insist that something must be done.

From Twycross, R. (1997). *Symptom management in advanced cancer.* Oxon, UK: Radcliffe Medical Press.

# ■ PATIENT AND FAMILY EDUCATION

Listening to the fears of family members about their loved one's dehydrated state is a valuable opportunity for the advanced practice nurse (APN) to discuss the normal signs and symptoms of the dying process. Terminally ill patients often lose interest in eating and drinking as they physically deteriorate (Twycross, 1997). Inform the family that this condition is often referred to as "natural dehydration" and there is reason to believe that this dehydration does not cause any discomfort. The one symptom persons with natural dehydration often experience is dry mouth. This can generally be relieved by providing good oral care and encouraging the patient to take sips of water or ice chips when appropriate.

Patients who experience acute dehydration as a result of vomiting, diarrhea, or polyuria often experience distressing thirst and would benefit from rehydration. However, patients and families who prefer to avoid exogenous hydration for whatever reason should be respected for their informed decisions. The aim of hydration in the palliative care setting is comfort, not the return to a normal fluid and electrolyte balance (Twycross, 1997). Patients and their families should be helped to understand that hydration is a temporary intervention to help relieve distressing symptoms that interfere with the quality of life.

# ■ EVALUATION AND PLAN FOR FOLLOW-UP

Ongoing assessment is essential to patients receiving hydration in order to discern their level of comfort. If symptoms improve with hydration and the patients' quality of living is improved, the intervention is maintained. If symptoms do not improve, or patients show signs and symptoms of fluid overload, hydration is discontinued.

---

✔ **CASE STUDY**

Mrs. Smith has advanced colon cancer with extensive metastases to bones, liver, and peritoneal lymph nodes. She has considerable edema of the lower extremities and abdominal ascites. Mostly confined to bed at home, Mrs. Smith has tremendous family support and is hoping to see her first grandchild's birth, expected within 2 weeks. Mrs. Smith has not been eating or drinking much and her urine output has decreased in spite of daily doses of furosemide. Her cognitive status has been excellent with a Mini–Mental State Examination (MMSE) score of 30/24 until 2 days ago. Today she is restless and disoriented with an MMSE score of 18/29. Blood drawn this morning shows elevated urea, creatinine, hematocrit, and sodium levels. Her serum albumin level is low. Current medications include furosemide, 20 mg every morning, and immediate-release morphine 50 mg q4h PO, with 20 mg q1h for breakthrough as needed. Mrs. Smith's family is very distressed by the rapid deterioration and concerned that

*Continued*

seeing her new grandchild may not be possible. The following plan of care is initiated by the APN:

- Discontinue the furosemide. The ascites is probably due to third spacing (low albumin level) and blockages of lymphatic circulation. Furosemide will only lead to further dehydration.
- Initiate hypodermoclysis of normal saline at 50 to 100 ml/h, depending on tolerance.
- Explore other possible causes of agitated delirium such as opioid toxicity and infection.

After a day of hypodermoclysis with plain normal saline solution Mrs. Smith scores a 30/29 on the MMSE and is communicating with her family about the plans for her grandchild's birth. She eventually becomes cognitively impaired and dies comfortably 2 weeks after seeing her first grandchild.

## References

BILLINGS, A. (1985). Comfort measures for the terminally ill: Is dehydration painful? *American Geriatric Society, 33,* 808-810.

BRUERA, E., Belzile, M., Watanabe, S., & Fainsinger, R. (1996). Volume of hydration in terminal cancer patients. *Support Care Cancer, 4,* 147-150.

BRUERA, E., Franco, J., Maltoni, M., Wantanabe, S., & Suarez-Almazor, M. (1995). Changing patterns of agitated impaired mental status in patients with advanced cancer: Association with cognitive monitoring, hydration and opioid rotation. *The Journal of Pain and Symptom Management, 10*(4), 287-291.

BURGE, F. I. (1993). Dehydration symptoms of palliative care cancer patients. *The Journal of Pain and Symptom Management, 8*(7), 454-464.

DUNPHY, K. (1995). Rehydration in palliative and terminal care: If not—why not? *Palliative Medicine, 9,* 221-228.

ELLERSHAW, J. I., Sutcliffe, J. M., & Saunders, C. M. (1995). Dehydration and the dying patient. *Journal of Pain and Symptom Management, 10,* 192-197.

FAINSINGER, R., & Bruera, E. (1991). Hypodermoclysis (HDC) for symptom control vs. the Edmonton injector (EI). *Journal of Palliative Care, 7*(4), 5-8.

FAINSINGER, R., & Bruera, E. (1994). The management of dehydration in terminally ill patients. *Journal of Palliative Care, 10*(3), 55-59.

FAINSINGER, R., MacEachern, T., Miller, M., Bruera, E., Spachynski, K., Kuehn, N., & Hanson, J. (1994). The use of hypodermoclysis for rehydration in terminally ill cancer patients. *Journal of Pain and Symptom Management, 9*(5), 298-302.

GUYTON, A. C., & Hall, J. E. (1996a). Body fluid compartments: Extracellular and intracellular fluids—interstitial fluid and edema. In *Textbook of medical physiology* (pp. 297-313), Philadelphia: W. B. Saunders.

GUYTON, A. C., & Hall, J. E. (1996b). Regulation of extracellular fluid osmolarity and sodium concentration. *Textbook of medical physiology* (pp. 349-365), Philadelphia: W. B. Saunders.

KUEBLER, K. (1999). Nurses have a responsibility to learn more about end-of-life care. *Oncology Nursing Forum, 26*(1), 17.

McCANN, R. M., Hall, W. J., & Groth-Juncker, A. (1994). Comfort care for terminally ill patients: The appropriate use of nutrition and hydration. *Journal of the American Medical Association, 272,* 1263-1266.

PARKASH, R., & Burge, F. (1997). The family's perspective on issues of hydration in terminal care. *Journal of Palliative Care, 13*(4), 23-27.

PEREIRA, J., & Bruera, E. (1997). *The Edmonton aid to palliative care* (pp. 58-60). Edmonton: Division of Palliative Care, University of Alberta, Edmonton.

PRINTZ, L. A. (1992). Terminal dehydration, a compassionate treatment (Commentary). *Archives of Internal Medicine, 152,* 697-700.

REGIONAL Palliative Care Program Capital Health Authority. (1998). *99 Common questions (and answers) about palliative care: A nurse's handbook* (pp. 40-53). Edmonton: Regional Palliative Care Program Capital Health Authority.

STEINER, N., & Bruera, E. (1998). Methods of hydration in palliative care patients. *Journal of Palliative Care, 14*(12), 6-13.

TWYCROSS, R. (1997). Dehydration. In *Symptom management in advanced cancer* (pp. 170-172). Oxon, UK: Radcliffe Medical Press.

TWYCROSS, R., & Lichter I. (1998). The terminal phase. In D. Doyle, G. Hanks, & N. MacDonald (Eds.), *Oxford textbook of palliative medicine* (2nd ed.) (pp. 979-981). New York: Oxford University Press.

VIOLA, R. A., Wells, G. A., & Peterson, J. (1997). The effects of fluid status and fluid therapy on the dying: A systematic review. *Journal of Palliative Care 13*(4), 41-52.

WALLER, A., Hershkowitz, M., & Adunsky, A. (1994). The effect of intravenous fluid infusion on blood and urine parameters of hydration and on state of consciousness in terminal cancer patients. *American Journal of Hospice and Palliative Care, 11*(6), 22-27.

WEST, C. (1993). Ischemia. In V. Carrieri-Kohlman, A. Lindsey, & C. West (Eds.), *Pathophysiological phenomena in nursing* (pp. 1-45). Philadelphia: W. B. Saunders.

ZERWEKH, J. V. (1997). Do dying patients really need IV fluids? *American Journal of Nursing, 97*(3), 26-30.

# CHAPTER 21

# Delirium/Acute Confusion

KIM K. KUEBLER, DEBRA E. HEIDRICH

## ■ DEFINITION AND INCIDENCE

Although reports of confusion in persons with advanced disease are common, the term *confusion,* lacks specificity. A patient described as confused could be feeling disoriented, exhibiting inappropriate behavior, or experiencing hallucinations or could have a medical diagnosis of delirium or dementia. To prevent miscommunication among health care professions, the advanced practice nurse (APN) must always qualify the term *confusion* by describing the type of cognitive or behavioral change the patient is experiencing.

Frequently the new onset of behavior labeled as "confusion" is indicative of the acute syndrome of delirium. Delirium is a serious complication in the management of persons with advanced diseases (Breitbart & Cohen, 1998). Significantly, delirium, unlike dementia, is potentially reversible and requires prompt recognition and management.

*Delirium* is defined as "an etiologically non-specific, global, cerebral dysfunction characterized by concurrent disturbances of the level of consciousness, attention, thinking, perception, memory, psychomotor behavior, emotion, and the sleep-wake cycle" (Breitbart, Chochinov, & Passik, 1998, p. 945). The *DSM-IV* criteria for delirium (American Psychiatric Association, 1994) and a brief discussion of each are as follows:

- Disturbance of consciousness with reduced ability to focus, sustain, or shift attention
- A change in cognition (such as memory deficit, disorientation, language disturbance) or the development of a perceptual disturbance that is not better accounted for by preexisting, established, or evolving dementia
- Disturbance that develops over a short period (usually hours to days) and tends to fluctuate over the course of the day
- Evidence from history, physical examination, or laboratory findings that indicates the disturbance is caused by a general medical condition

*Disturbed consciousness* means a reduced clarity or awareness of the environment that does not reach the level of stupor or coma. Altered attention is a critical feature of a disturbance in consciousness (Milisen, Foreman, Godderis, Abraham, & Broos, 1998). This altered attention may appear as a change in level of consciousness, slowed or inadequate reactions to stimuli or the environment, or easy distractibility. Persons with altered attention may be unable to follow conversations or complete simple tasks (Ingham & Caraceni, 1998; Trzepacz, Breitbart, & Franklin, 1999).

*Changes in cognition* include a variety of memory deficits, of which short-term memory deficits are the most common. These may result from inattention or easy distractibility (Milisen et al., 1998; Trzepacz et al., 1999). The short-term memory deficit may include disorientation to person, place, or time, but disorientation is not universal. Time orientation is the first to be affected, followed by disorientation to place. Progression of disorientation includes disorientation to other persons, and finally to the self. However, disorientation to self is quite rare (Trzepacz et al., 1999). Language disturbances may also be exhibited as a form of cognitive change. These include a lack of fluency and spontaneity in conversations, leading to long pauses, use of repetitive phrases, or difficulty in finding the correct word. The ability to write may actually be affected earlier than spoken language in the person with delirium (Chedru & Geschwind, 1972).

*Perceptual disturbances* are other signs of cognitive changes and can include illusions and hallucinations. Illusions are misinterpretations of real external stimuli (e.g., seeing spiders instead of the pattern on the wallpaper); hallucinations are subjective perceptions that occur in the absence of any relevant external stimuli (Luckmann, 1997). Perceptual disturbances are most commonly visual, but auditory, tactile, gustatory, and olfactory misperceptions can occur. When these illusions or hallucinations are believed to be real, persons often exhibit emotions and behavior consistent with the misconceptions (Trzepacz et al., 1999).

The features of *development over a short period* and *fluctuation over the course of the day* are important defining criteria for delirium. Noting the onset of the disturbances in consciousness or cognition assists in differentiating delirium from other syndromes that cause mental status changes, such as dementia.

The fourth criterion for the diagnosis of delirium is *evidence that the changes are due to an underlying medical condition.* In end-of-life care it may be difficult to identify the exact cause of delirium. An individual may have several potential causes at any one time (see "Etiology and Pathophysiology"). The challenge for the APN is to identify which of the potential causes is the most likely and then determine the appropriate approach to this problem.

Additional features commonly seen with delirium are sleep pattern disturbances, emotional disturbances, daytime sleepiness, nighttime agitation, and disturbances in sleep (Trzepacz et al., 1999). The predominant emotional symptom observed with delirium is anxiety. Fear, depression, irritability, anger, euphoria, and apathy are also relatively common. The delirious patient may show labile emotions, shifting rapidly and unpredictably from one emotional state to another (Ingham & Caraceni, 1998; Trzepacz et al., 1999).

There are two variants of delirium, hyperalert/hyperactive and hypoalert/hypoactive. The hyperalert/hyperactive variant of delirium is most commonly recognized (Milisen et al., 1998; Inouye, 1994). Characteristics of hyperactive-hyperalert delirium include agitation, increased alertness to stimuli, hallucinations, and mood lability. Hypoactive-hypoalert delirium is characterized by withdrawal from people and usual activities, sleepiness, and decreased responsiveness to stimuli (Breitbart & Cohen, 1998; Milisen et al., 1998). The hypoactive-hypoalert variant of delirium is often overlooked, and its symptoms are attributed to dementia, depression, or senescence (Chan & Brennan, 1999; Csokasy, 1999; Fainsinger, Tapper, & Bruera, 1993; Inouye, 1994; Pereira, Hanson, & Bruera, 1997; Stiefel, Fainsinger, & Bruera, 1992).

Terminal restlessness is sometimes described as a specific form of delirium seen in the last days or hours of life (Burke, 1997). The Hospice and Palliative Nurses Association has proposed the following definition: "a common observable syndrome occurring in patients with varying diagnoses and appearing during their last days of life" (Kuebler et al., 1997, p. 2). The observable indicators of terminal restlessness are identified as (1) frequent, nonpurposeful motor activity; (2) inability to concentrate or relax; (3) disturbances in sleep/rest patterns; (4) fluctuating levels of consciousness, cognitive failure, or anxiety; and (5) potential progression to agitation (Kuebler et al., 1997; Kuebler, English, & Heidrich, 2001). These indicators are congruent with many of the signs of delirium. In addition, the cause and management of terminal restlessness are similar to those for delirium.

Delirium is the most commonly encountered mental disorder in hospital settings (Lipowski, 1989; Breitbart & Cohen, 1998) and is very common in persons with advanced illness. More than 75% of terminally ill persons with cancer (Bruera et al., 1992; Ingham & Caraceni, 1998; Massie, Holland, & Glass, 1983) and 57% of those in the terminal stage of acquired immunodeficiency syndrome (AIDS) (Breitbart, Chochinov, & Passik, 1998) may experience delirium. Restlessness and agitation at the end of life, a possible description for terminal restlessness, are reported to occur in up to 42% of patients during the last 48 hours of life (Lichter & Hunt, 1990). Some 25% to 35% of these delirium episodes are reversible (Kuebler, English, & Heidrich, 2001; Fainsinger et al., 1993; Bruera, Franco, Maltoni, Wantanabe, & Suarez-Almazor, 1995). Thus prompt diagnosis and treatment are essential for improving outcomes in persons with advanced illness.

# ■ ETIOLOGY AND PATHOPHYSIOLOGY

Delirium has many potential causes in persons with advanced illness (Box 21-1), necessitating a thorough physical assessment of the patient and review of medications. It is important to consider the contribution of multiple medications to the development of delirium, especially in elderly patients. In

| BOX 21-1 | *Common Causes of Delirium in End-of-Life Care* |
|---|---|

**DISEASE**

Central nervous system tumors (primary or metastatic)

Dementia (e.g., human immunodeficiency virus [HIV], Alzheimer's disease, senile dementia)

Organ system failure

**DISEASE SYMPTOM**

Hypoxia

Infection

**CHEMICAL IMBALANCE**

Hypercalcemia

Hyponatremia

Uremia

Hepatic failure

**PHYSICAL DISCOMFORT**

Constipation

Dyspnea

Pain

Sleep disturbance

Urinary retention

**PSYCHOLOGIC**

Depression

Past or current substance abuse

Sensory overload or sensory deprivation

**EMOTIONAL/SPIRITUAL**

Anxiety

Fear

Guilt

Spiritual distress

Unfinished business

**MEDICATIONS**

Anticholinergics

Benzodiazepines

Chemotherapeutic agents

$H_2$ blockers

Opioids

Phenothiazines

Steroids

**MEDICATION/ SUBSTANCE WITHDRAWAL**

Alcohol

Benzodiazepines

Nicotine

Opioids

Steroids

From Breitbart, W., & Cohen, K. R. (1998). Delirium. In J. C. Holland (Ed.). *Psychooncology* (pp. 564-575). New York: Oxford University Press; Hanks, G., Portenoy, R. K., MacDonald, N., & Forbes, K. (1998). Difficult pain problems. In D. Doyle, G.W.C. Hanks, & N. MacDonald (Eds.). *Oxford textbook of palliative medicine* (2nd ed.) (pp. 454-477). New York: Oxford University Press; Kuebler, K. K. (Ed.). (1997). *Hospice and palliative care clinical practice protocol: Terminal restlessness.* Pittsburgh, PA: Hospice and Palliative Nurses Association.

addition, in individuals with impaired renal or hepatic function, medication toxicity related to slow elimination of the medication or accumulation of drug metabolites may develop.

Very little is known about the underlying pathophysiologic mechanisms of delirium, but it is believed to be a dysfunction of multiple regions of the brain (Breitbart & Cohen, 1998; Kuebler et al., 2001; Fainsinger et al., 1993; de Stoutz, Tapper, & Fainsinger, 1995). A disturbance of neurotransmitters is the probable mechanism leading to delirium. There may actually be a group of different disorders, involving different neurotransmitters, separately or simultaneously, that lead to delirium symptoms (Breitbart & Cohen, 1998). Some proposed mechanisms and examples of potential causes of each are identified in Table 21-1.

## TABLE 21-1

### Neurotransmitter System Changes Associated with Delirium

| Mechanism | Cause | Type |
|---|---|---|
| Suppression of cholinergic systems | Anticholinergics | Hyperactive |
| Antagonism of the serotonin system | Lysergic acid diethylamide (LSD) | Hyperactive |
| Blocking N-methyl-D-aspartate (NMDA) receptors | Phencyclidine (PCP) | Hyperactive |
| Overstimulation of the gamma-aminobutyric acid (GABA) systems | Hepatic encephalopathy, benzodiazepine intoxication | Hyperactive |
| Acute understimulation of the GABA systems | Benzodiazepine withdrawal, alcohol withdrawal | Hypoactive |
| Overactivation of the dopaminergic mesocortical system | Anticholinergics | Hyperactive |
| Alterations in multiple neurotransmitter systems | Infection, hypoxia, Alzheimer's disease | May be mixed |

From Ross, C. A. (1991). CNS arousal systems: Possible role in delirium. *International Psychogeriatrics, 3*, 353-371; Breitbart, W., & Cohen, K. R. (1998). Delirium. In J. C. Holland (Ed.). *Psychooncology* (pp. 564-575). New York: Oxford University Press.

## ■ ASSESSMENT AND MEASUREMENT

The prognosis for the patient experiencing delirium is often poor, yet this should not deter the clinician from looking for the underlying cause because a significant number of cases are reversible (Fainsinger et al., 1993; de Stoutz et al., 1995). Reversing delirium at the end of life makes a major difference to both the patient's and family's quality of life.

Many delirium assessment scales have been developed, some intended for clinical practice and others for research (APA, 1999). The review article by Smith, Breitbart, and Platt (1995) provides a comprehensive evaluation of the variety of instruments available for detecting, diagnosing, and rating delirium. The following section discusses those tools most often used in clinical practice.

### Screening Instruments

Screening instruments identify delirium symptoms but are not diagnostic. They are very helpful for identifying those patients who require follow-up evaluation in more depth. These scales may also be useful for monitoring improvement or deterioration in the patient with delirium (Chan & Brennan, 1999):

- Mini–Mental State Examination (MMSE): This is one of the most frequently used tools for the clinical evaluation of cognitive changes. It assesses orientation, instantaneous recall, short-term memory, serial subtraction or reverse spelling, constructional capacities, and use of language.

Although it is not designed to measure severity, some do use scores to indicate severity: 24 to 30 = no impairment; 18 to 23 = mild impairment; 0 to 17 = severe impairment (Tombaugh & McIntyre, 1992).

- NEECHAM Confusion Scale: This scale was designed for rapid and unobtrusive assessment and monitoring of acute confusion by the bedside nurse (Neelon, Champagne, Carlson, & Funk, 1996). It can detect changes in mental status as well as physiologic and behavioral manifestations of delirium, including those indicative of hypoactive/hypoalert delirium. Repeated measures can be used to monitor changes in mental status (Milisen et al., 1998; Coskasy, 1999). The validity on the physiologic control subscale of this tool has been criticized as a measurement for delirium by Smith and colleagues, who do not find it helpful in screening or as an indication of the severity of delirium (Smith et al., 1995).

## Diagnostic Instruments

Diagnostic instruments are used along with the clinical evaluation to make a formal diagnosis of delirium:

- Confusion Assessment Method (CAM): This valid and reliable tool was designed for efficient and effective detection of delirium (Inouye, van Dyck, Alessi, Siegal, & Horwitz, 1990). The four core *DSM-IV* criteria for delirium can be assessed by nonpsychiatric clinicians in less than 5 minutes. Milisen and coworkers (1998) recommend using the CAM to confirm delirium in persons who score less than 25 on the NEECHAM Confusion Scale.
- Delirium Symptom Interview (DSI): This is a valid and reliable tool for diagnosing delirium, assessing for the presence or absence of various symptoms. It was designed for ease of administration, but its administration has been noted often to require more than the proposed 15 minutes (Smith et al., 1995). A disadvantage of this instrument is that it requires substantial training for appropriate use (Inouye, 1994).
- Delirium Rating Scale (DRS): The scale is a delirium-specific tool based on the *DSM-III* criteria. Clinician ratings are obtained for 10 different domains. It is helpful for confirming the diagnosis of delirium, but not the severity (Breitbart & Cohen, 1998).

## Delirium Symptom Severity Rating Scales

Delirium symptom severity rating scales are designed to rate the severity of this syndrome, making them useful for monitoring the effect of interventions. Although not designed to do so, these scales are sometimes used for making the diagnosis of delirium (APA, 1999).

- Memorial Delirium Assessment Scale (MDAS): This scale was designed to quantify the severity of delirium symptoms for use in clinical intervention studies. It assesses disturbances in arousal, level of consciousness, cognitive functioning, and psychomotor activity. Completing requires about 10 minutes. Another tool, such as the CAM, should be used in conjunction with the MDAS for diagnostic purposes (Breitbart et al., 1997).

- As noted, both the MMSE and the NEECHAM Confusion Scale have been used to measure delerium severity. The NEECHAM Confusion Scale was designed for both screening and monitoring; the MMSE has been used for monitoring but was not designed for this purpose.

## Laboratory Evaluation

Laboratory evaluation is the fourth category of formal measures used to investigate the underlying cause of delirium. Slowing and disorganization of the electroencephalogram (EEG) is often associated with a clouded sensorium and frequently is often associated with hypoactive delirium. Individuals with hyperactive delirium may show low voltage fast activity on the EEG. These EEG changes are important diagnostic signs of delirium; however, the absence of abnormalities does not rule out delirium (Smith et al., 1995). Given that clinical evaluation is more reliable and EEG administration involves time, discomfort, and expense, there is a limited role for the use of an EEG in end-of-life care.

## ■ HISTORY AND PHYSICAL EXAMINATION

### History

- Review the recent history of the patient's mental status changes, including both patient and caregiver observations:
  - Note reported changes in arousal, level of consciousness, orientation, and cognition.
  - Note onset of changes and any fluctuation over the course of a day, asking specifically about changes at night.
- Review the medical history:
  - Note the terminal diagnosis as well as coexisting medical conditions.
  - Note diseases that directly affect the central nervous system and those associated with organ system failure.
- Review medications for risk of delirium (see Box 21-1):
  - Note medications directly associated with delirium.
  - Note medications with a potential for toxicity if given in high doses or in the presence of renal or hepatic dysfunction.
  - Note any recently discontinued/refused medications with a potential for a withdrawal response.
- Assess for a history of substance abuse.
- Assess for a history of psychiatric disorders, including depression.
- Assess sleeping patterns and signs of sleep deprivation.

### Physical Examination

The APN should use one of the screening tools discussed to identify persons with mental status or cognitive changes and a diagnostic tool to confirm the diagnosis of delirium. In addition, a targeted physical examination is essential for identifying the potential cause(s) of the delirium. The following aspects of the physical assessment assist in identifying the most common physical causes of delirium in persons with advanced illness:

- General survey:
  - Vital signs, especially fever and hyperpnea
  - Skin color, especially pallor, cyanosis, jaundice
  - Skin turgor
  - Pruritus
- Respiratory system:
  - Dyspnea or hypoxia
  - Cough or congestion
- Gastrointestinal system:
  - Pain or discomfort
  - Bowel patterns, including signs of constipation or obstruction
  - Nausea and vomiting
- Genitourinary system:
  - Pain or discomfort
  - Urinary output
  - Signs of retention or obstruction
- Musculoskeletal system:
  - Pain or discomfort
  - Weakness or agitation

### Environmental/Psychoemotional Assessment

The following assessment variables are best evaluated by an interdisciplinary team approach involving the APN, social worker, and spiritual counselor. The family's observations are very important while assessing the cause of delirium and should be included in a complete assessment of these variables:

- Signs of anxiety, fear, or guilt
- Potential of "unfinished business"—interpersonal, financial, or spiritual
- Depression (see Chapter 22)
- Signs of spiritual distress
- Potential for sensory overload or sensory deprivation

## ■ DIAGNOSTICS

The following diagnostic tests assist in confirming a diagnosis of an underlying medical cause of delirium. These tests are appropriate only when they directly influence the treatment plan. For example, laboratory work to confirm hypercalcemia is necessary only if the patient's quality of living will be enhanced by treating the hypercalcemia and if the diagnosis cannot be made on the basis of the underlying medical diagnosis and associated symptoms. Tests include:

- Blood glucose level
- Electrolyte (i.e., sodium, potassium, chloride, calcium) levels
- Urea and creatinine levels

- Liver function: aspartate aminotransferase (AST), alanine aminotransferase (ALT), lactate dehydrogenase (LDH)
- Oxygen saturation
- Blood, urine, or other cultures for infection

## ■ INTERVENTION AND TREATMENT

It may be possible to reverse delirium even in advanced illness, with the exception of possibly the last 24 to 48 hours of life (Breitbart & Cohen, 1998). When the cause of delirium is identified and the interdisciplinary team is in agreement that treatment of the underlying cause will improve quality of living, the focus of intervention is on reversal of the delirium. When the cause of delirium cannot be identified or cannot be reversed, the focus of care is on comfort.

### Manage Underlying Causes of Delirium

- Manage increased intracranial pressure: dexamethasone, 16 to 36 mg PO qd, in the morning (Waller & Caroline, 2000).
- Treat hypoxia: oxygen therapy.
- Treat infection: appropriate antiinfective agents.
- Correct metabolic abnormalities, as appropriate:
  - Hypercalcemia:
    - Mild: hydrate by using oral, parenteral, or hypodermoclysis fluids.
    - Moderate or severe: consider administering a bisphosphate (e.g., pamidronate disodium) if it will improve the quality of living.
  - Hyponatremia due to syndrome of inappropriate antidiuretic hormone (SIADH):
    - Mild: encourage moderate alcohol intake (e.g., glass of sherry before meals) and dietary sodium intake (Waller & Caroline, 2000).
    - Moderate: demeclocycline, 300 mg PO bid (Twycross, 1997; Waller & Caroline, 2000); fluid restriction is often not an issue in palliative care, but consider restricting to <1 liter/day.
    - Severe: Infusion of intravenous (IV) hypertonic saline solution is not without risk and is considered inappropriate in palliative care (Twycross, 1997).
- Treat physical discomforts (see Chapters 18, 24, 28, and 30 for constipation, dyspnea, pain, and pruritus).
- Treat psychoemotional discomforts (see Chapters 7, 16, and 22 for psychosocial care, anxiety, and depression):
  - Be aware that persons with major depression are at greater risk of suicide when experiencing delirium.
- Treat dehydration (see Chapter 20).
- Discontinue or decrease the dosage of the offending medication, as possible:
  - If accumulation of opioid metabolites is suspected, consider opioid rotation.
  - Be careful not to stop benzodiazepines abruptly.

- Taper corticosteroids to lowest effective dose (do not discontinue abruptly).
- Treat withdrawal syndrome: resume the responsible drug and then taper slowly.

## Encourage a Supportive Environment

- Provide orientation clues:
  - Orient frequently to time and place.
  - Encourage familiar persons to be present and keep familiar objects close by.
  - Keep a calendar and clock visible; open shades during the day and darken the room at night but use a night-light.
  - If the patient is experiencing illusions or hallucinations, gently correct misconceptions while reassuring the patient that he or she is safe.
- Ensure a calm environment by minimizing stimulation.
- Keep the patient safe by adequate supervision without the use of restraints.

## Manage Agitation Associated with Delirium

- The butyrophenone class of neuroleptics is considered first-line treatment for agitation, except for delirium associated with alcohol or benzodiazepine withdrawal (APA, 1999; Ingham & Caraceni, 1998). Benzodiazepines may worsen restlessness and cognitive impairment (Waller & Caroline, 2000):
  - Haloperidol is the drug of choice for hallucinations and agitation in the medically ill (Breitbart & Cohen, 1998; Ingham & Caraceni, 1998):
    - Mild agitation: 0.5 to 3 mg PO tid.
    - Moderate to severe agitation: 2 to 5 mg IV/SC; repeat every 20 to 60 minutes until symptoms are controlled, using the more frequent interval for most severe agitation. When calmed, the patient can be maintained with oral or subcutaneous doses similar to that required for mild agitation (Waller & Caroline, 2000). Doses generally do not exceed 20 mg/24 hrs, but some patients may require higher doses (Breitbart & Cohen, 1998).
  - To prevent extrapyramidal side effects of haloperidol the APN should also start diphenhydramine, 25 mg PO tid (Ingham & Carcaceni, 1998; Waller & Caroline, 2000).
  - When haloperidol alone does not control the delirium, a benzodiazepine, preferably lorazepam, may be added (Ingham & Caraceni, 1998). However, the practitioner is cautioned to observe for worsening delirium with the use of benzodiazepines.
- For delirium tremens:
  - Benzodiazepines are the medications of choice (Ingham & Caraceni, 1998): lorazepam, 1 to 2 mg PO bid-qid.
  - Transdermal clonidine, 0.1 to 0.2 mg/day for autonomic symptoms, such as anxiety and tachycardia (Waller & Caroline, 2000).
- Sedation may be required for agitation unresponsive to the preceding interventions. In one study of 39 cancer patients with delirium, 26% required sedation (Stiefel et al., 1992).

- Chlorpromazine suppository, 25 to 100 mg q6h is an alternative. This phenothiazine neuroleptic may assist in clearing the sensorium but is very sedating. It does have more anticholinergic and cardio-vascular side effects than haloperidol (Twycross, 1997). One advantage of chlorpromazine is its ease of administration in the home care environment.
- Midazolam, 1 to 2 mg/hr SC, by continuous infusion is recommended when agitation and restlessness are pronounced (Waller & Caroline, 2000) or when tremors and twitching are predominant and interfere with quality of life (Kuebler et al., 1997; Kuebler et al., 2001):
  - For severe agitation the APN can administer midazolam, 1 mg SC every 10 minutes, until symptoms are controlled by sedation. The hourly maintenance dose is then 25% to 33% of the dose required for induction (Kuebler et al., 1997).
  - This medication is primarily sedating and does not clear sensorium nor improve cognition (Breitbart & Cohen, 1998).
- Droperidol, 1.25 mg IV/IM q2-4h is considered if the phenobarbital suppository is not effective (Twycross, 1997). This is a butyrophenone and has the potential of clearing the sensorium as well as causing sedation.
- Phenobarbital can be administered by suppository (15 to 90 mg) or IV (100 to 200 mg), titrating to effect (Twycross, Wilcock, & Thorp, 1998). Phenobarbital is recommended for severe terminal illness on rare occasions when all other medications have been ineffective (Twycross, 1997). This barbiturate has sedative and anxiolytic properties. Barbiturates should be administered cautiously, at the lowest effective dose. Phenobarbital should be used only by skilled clinicians due to its CNS depressant effects. One advantage of phenobarbital is its ease of administration in the home care environment.

## ■ PATIENT AND FAMILY EDUCATION

The experience of delirium is frightening to both the patient and the family. Both need reassurance that the patient is not going crazy, that the delirium may be reversible, and that the symptoms can be managed:
- Explain the causes of delirium and the interventions being initiated to reverse it.
- Teach the family the following interventions:
  - Report changes in the patient's mental status or complaints of feeling confused or unable to concentrate.
  - Gently correct patient illusions or hallucinations and reassure that environment is safe (e.g., there are no spiders on walls).
  - Provide orientation clues:
    - Refer to the time of day often (e.g., "It looks like we're going to have a lovely fall day").
    - Keep the environment familiar. If the patient is unable to be at home, take familiar objects to the inpatient facility.

- Have familiar persons at the bedside.
- Have a visible clock and calendar and mark off days on the calendar.
- Keep a calm, yet pleasantly stimulating environment:
  - Provide calm music that is pleasing to the patient.
  - Use soft lighting.
  - Minimize disturbances.
  - Encourage people to talk with the patient.
- Teach appropriate administration of all medications (e.g., neuroleptics, benzodiazepines, or barbiturates for delirium symptoms).
- Teach the importance of maintaining the pain regimen even if the patient is not able to ask for medications or communicate pain.

If sedation is required to manage the patient's agitation, discuss the pros and cons of this intervention with the family. In the presence of terminal agitation the time before sedation may be the last time the family sees the patient awake. Encourage the family to say their good-byes and address unfinished business while there is a potential the patient can respond. Reinforce with the family that the patient can likely hear even when sedated and that it is important to continue to share supportive thoughts and feelings and share good-byes although the patient cannot respond.

## ■ EVALUATION AND PLAN FOR FOLLOW-UP

Patient status is monitored for improvement or decline in the symptoms of delirium. One of the delirium severity rating scales will be helpful for assessing and documenting these changes. When delirium cannot be reversed, the goal is comfort. The patient is monitored to assure that distressing symptoms, such as illusions, hallucinations, restlessness, and agitation, are optimally managed.

After the treatment of delirium related to medication side effects, the APN needs to use caution in the selection of medications for control of other symptoms that may emerge over time. The offending class of medication should not be used in the future, if possible. If that class of medication is required for comfort, the medication should be started at a low dose and the patient monitored frequently for early signs of delirium.

✔ **CASE STUDY** Mr. Allen is a 78-year-old gentleman with metastatic prostate cancer being cared for by his wife of 52 years. His medications for symptom management include sustained-release morphine, 60 mg PO bid, for pain; immediate-release morphine, 20 mg PO q1h prn, for breakthrough pain (which he uses approximately once daily); ibuprofen, 400 mg PO qid, for pain; Senokot-S, 3 tablets bid, for constipation; and lorazepam, 0.5 mg PO q4-6h prn, for anxiety. He has been taking the lorazepam two or three times a day for the past 2 weeks. His condition has been declining over the past month. The hospice interdisciplinary team is involved in his care and is providing assistance with personal care, symptom management, and psychosocial support. He is essentially bedbound at this time. He has been awake during the days, participating in conversations and watching TV, but dozing frequently.

Mrs. Allen calls the APN and reports that Mr. Allen had a terrible night. He is confused and keeps trying to get up out of bed. She reports that during the night she gave him two extra doses of lorazepam, which "only seemed to make him worse." She is very distraught and states, "He was talking nonsense all night and I don't think he knows who I am."

When the APN arrives at the home, Mrs. Allen reports that the patient is not as confused as he was during the night, but that he's still "not thinking right." He is lethargic, responding to voices, but dozing easily. Mr. Allen's score on the MMSE is 19/28, indicating some impairment. Using the CAM, the APN determines that Mr. Allen likely is experiencing delirium as the changes are acute in onset and fluctuate during the day, he is having difficulty focusing attention, he has had periods of being incoherent, and he is restless. In addition, the report that the patient's symptoms worsened on the lorazepam fits the diagnosis of delirium. Mrs. Allen reports that his urine output seems about normal; he is complaining of being thirsty but is not drinking all that is offered because of nausea. She also reports that Mr. Allen has not had a bowel movement in 3 days. Significant findings on physical examination include cachexia with poor skin turgor. He has slowed but audible bowel sounds. There is a large amount of soft stool in the rectal vault. The patient has been able to take all of his pills by mouth.

The APN identifies the following potential causes of Mr. Allen's delirium: hypercalcemia, pain/discomfort associated with constipation, dehydration, and accumulation of morphine metabolites. The APN explains that the confusion Mr. Allen experienced is likely due to one of these medical problems. The nurse administers a bisacodyl suppository now and instructs the family to follow up with a sodium biphosphate enema if there are no results. The lorazepam is discontinued. The nurse calls in a prescription for haloperidol, 0.5 mg tid, and tells Mrs. Allen that if Mr. Allen becomes agitated and restless during the night, she can give him an extra dose every 2 hours, but to call if he requires more than two extra doses. The APN also tells her that the haloperidol may help with the patient's nausea. Given that fluids can decrease the symptoms of hypercalcemia and dehydration, as well as the potential for morphine metabolite accumulation, the APN discusses the options of pushing oral fluids or hypodermoclysis for hydration. Mr. Allen and his wife ask to try oral fluids first to see whether he can take in enough. He is encouraged to sip fluids throughout the day and try to take in at least 8 to 10 8-oz. glasses; Mrs. Allen is instructed to call if he cannot. As the dose of morphine is relatively low and Mr. Allen appears to have adequate renal function, no change is made in the pain management regimen at this time.   (Had

*Continued*

the dose been higher or renal status impaired, opioid rotation might have been considered.)

The following day, Mr. Allen continues to be somewhat lethargic, but when awakened, he is oriented and able to answer questions coherently. His MMSE score is 25/28. His wife reports that he slept quietly throughout the night.

## References

AMERICAN Psychiatric Association. (1994). *Diagnostic and statistical manual of mental disorders* (4th ed.). Washington, DC: Author.

AMERICAN Psychiatric Association. (1999). Practice guideline for the treatment of patients with delirium. *American Journal of Psychiatry, 156* (suppl. 5), 1-20.

BREITBART, W., Chochinov, H. M., & Passik, S. (1998). Psychiatric aspects of palliative care. In D. Doyle, G.W.C. Hanks, & N. MacDonald (Eds.). *Oxford textbook of palliative medicine* (2nd ed.) (pp. 933-954). New York: Oxford University Press.

BREITBART, W., & Cohen, K. R. (1998). Delirium. In J. C. Holland (Ed.). *Psychooncology* (pp. 564-575). New York: Oxford University Press.

BREITBART, W., Rosenfeld, B., Roth, A., Smith, M. J., Cohen, K., & Passik, S. (1997). The Memorial Delirium Assessment Scale. *Journal of Pain and Symptom Management, 13,* 128-137.

BRUERA, E., Franco, J., Maltoni, M., Wantanabe, S., & Suarez-Almazor, M. (1995). Changing patterns of agitated impaired mental status in patients with advanced cancer: Association with cognitive monitoring, hydration, and opioid rotation. *Journal of Pain and Symptom Management, 9*(3), 4-8.

BRUERA, E., Miller, L., McCallion, J., Macmillan, K., Krefting, L., & Hanson, J. (1992). Cognitive failure in patients with terminal cancer: A prospective study. *Journal of Pain and Symptom Management, 7,* 192-195.

BURKE, A. L. (1997). Palliative care: An update on "terminal restlessness." *Medical Journal of Australia, 166*(1), 39-42.

CHAN, D., & Brennan, N. J. (1999). Delirium: Making the diagnosis, improving the prognosis. *Geriatrics, 54*(3), 28-42.

CHEDRU, F., & Geschwind, N. (1972). Writing disturbances in acute confusional state. *Neuropsychologia, 10,* 343-353.

CSOKASY, J. (1999). Assessment of acute confusion: Use of the NEECHAM Confusion Scale. *Applied Nursing Research, 12,* 51-55.

DE STOUTZ, N. D., Tapper, M., & Fainsinger, R. L. (1995). Reversible delirium in terminally ill patients. *Journal of Pain and Symptom Management, 10,* 249-253.

FAINSINGER, R. L., Tapper, M., & Bruera, E. (1993). A perspective on the management of delirium in terminally ill patients on a palliative care unit. *Journal of Palliative Care, 9*(3), 4-8.

HANKS, G., Portenoy, R. K., MacDonald, N., & Forbes, K. (1998). Difficult pain problems. In D. Doyle, G.W.C. Hanks, & N. MacDonald (Eds.). *Oxford textbook of palliative medicine* (2nd ed.) (pp. 454-477). New York: Oxford University Press.

INGHAM, J. M., & Caraceni, A. T. (1998). Delirium. In A. M. Berger, R. K. Portenoy, & D. E. Weissman (Eds.). *Principles and practice of supportive oncology* (pp. 477-495). Philadelphia: Lippincott-Raven.

INOUYE, S. K. (1994). The dilemma of delirium: Clinical and research controversies regarding diagnosis and evaluation of delirium in hospitalized elderly medical patients. *American Journal of Medicine, 97,* 278-288.

INOUYE, S. K., van Dyck, D. H., Alessi, C. A., Siegal, A. P., & Horwitz, R. I. (1990). Clarifying confusion: The confusion assessment method (a new method for detection of delirium). *Annals of Internal Medicine, 113,* 941-948.

KUEBLER, K., Boistelmann, L., Heidrich, D., Deshotels, J., Powers, D., Gores, F., Hunt, J., Jaskar, D., & Kimber, G. (1997). *Hospice and palliative care clinical practice protocol: Terminal restlessness.* Pittsburgh, PA: Hospice and Palliative Nurses Association.

KUEBLER, K., English, N., & Heidrich, D. (2001). Delirium, confusion, agitation and restlessness. In B. Ferrell and N. Coyle (Eds.). *Textbook of palliative nursing* (pp. 290-308). New York: Oxford University Press.

LICHTER, I., & Hunt, E. (1990). The last 48 hours of life. *Journal of Palliative Care, 6*(4), 7-15.

LIPOWSKI, Z. J. (1989). Delirium in the elderly. *New England Journal of Medicine, 320,* 578-582.

LUCKMANN, J. (1997). Caring for people with mental disorders. In J. Luckmann (Ed.). *Saunders manual of nursing care* (pp. 1899-1930). Philadelphia: W. B. Saunders.

MASSIE, M. J., Holland, J., & Glass, E. (1983). Delirium in terminally ill cancer patients. *American Journal of Psychiatry, 140,* 1048-1050.

MILISEN, K., Foreman, M. D., Godderis, J., Abraham, I. L., & Broos, P.L.O. (1998). Delirium in the hospitalized elderly: Nursing assessment and management. *Nursing Clinics of North America, 33,* 417-439.

NEELON, V. J., Champagne, M. T., Carlson, J. R., & Funk, S. G. (1996). The NEECHAM Confusion Scale: Construction, validation, and clinical testing. *Nursing Research, 45,* 324-330.

PEREIRA, J., Hanson, J., & Bruera, E. (1997). The frequency and clinical course of cognitive impairment in patients with terminal cancer. *Cancer, 79,* 835-842.

ROSS, C. A. (1991). CNS arousal systems: Possible role in delirium. *International Psychogeriatrics, 3,* 353-371.

SMITH, M. J., Breitbart, W. S., & Platt, M. M. (1995). A critique of instruments and methods to detect, diagnose, and rate delirium. *Journal of Pain and Symptom Management, 10,* 35-77.

STIEFEL, F., Fainsinger, R., & Bruera, E. (1992). Acute confusional states in patients with advanced cancer. *Journal of Pain and Symptom Management, 7,* 94-98.

TOMBAUGH, T. N., & McIntyre, N. J. (1992). The Mini–Mental State Examination: A comprehensive review. *Journal of the American Geriatric Society, 40,* 922-935.

TRZEPACZ, P., Breitbart, W., & Franklin, J. (1999). American psychiatric association practice guidelines: Practice guidelines for the treatment of patients with delirium. *American Journal of Psychiatry, 156* (Suppl. 5), 1-20.

TWYCROSS, R. (1997). *Symptom management in advanced cancer* (2nd ed.). Oxon, UK: Radcliffe Medical Press.

TWYCROSS, R., Wilcock, A., & Thorp, S. (1998). *Palliative care formulary.* Oxon, UK: Radcliffe Medical Press.

WALLER, A., & Caroline, N. L. (2000). *Handbook of palliative care in cancer* (2nd ed.). Boston: Butterworth-Heinemann.

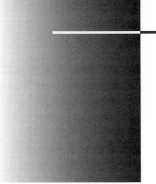

CHAPTER **22**

# *Depression*

KIM K. KUEBLER

## ■ DEFINITION AND INCIDENCE

The term *depression* can be used to describe (1) an emotional effect that is a subjective feeling of short duration, (2) a mood that is a state sustained over a longer period of time, (3) an emotion that comprises subjective feelings along with objective observations, or (4) a disorder that has characteristic symptom clusters and complexes of signs and symptoms (Zung, 1973). Depression is often described as a feeling of gloom, emptiness, numbness, or despair, which can occur in the physically healthy, the psychiatrically ill, and often those living with a chronic illness (Much & Barsevick, 1999). Persons who are depressed often experience feelings of helplessness, changes in appetite and sleep patterns, lethargy, and lack of concentration (Howland, Shelton, & Trivedi, 2000; Much & Barsevick, 1999).

Reactive, or situational, depression is a common and expected response to a life-threatening disease. Reactive depression is generally self-limiting and resolves as the individual uses education, support, and other coping resources to face the threat against well-being.

A depressed mood becomes a problem for patients when it is prolonged or severe and interferes with daily functioning. Depressed mood related to an identifiable psychosocial stressor that exceeds what would be normally expected or that impairs social or occupational functioning may fit the *Diagnostic and Statistical Manual of Mental Disorders, Fourth Edition (DSM-IV)* criteria for an Adjustment Disorder with Depressed Mood (Strain, 1998). Although less specific than the criteria for Major Depressive Disorder, this diagnosis does allow for identification of early or temporary depressed states and can assist in obtaining appropriate treatment.

Major Depressive Disorder is a serious medical condition that disrupts an individual's mood, behavior, thought processes, and physical health (American Psychiatric Association, 2000a). The *DSM-IV* criteria for this diagnosis are listed in Box 22-1.

Many studies document the prevalence of depression in various populations. However, these studies are somewhat difficult to compare as the researchers do not always differentiate among reactive depression, adjustment disorders, and major depressive disorders. The incidence of depressive symptoms in cancer patients ranges from 10% to 47% and may

| BOX 22-1 | *Criteria for Major Depressive Episode* |

At least five of the following symptoms have been present most of the day, or almost every day, for at least 2 weeks. At least one of the symptoms must be item 1 or 2.
1. Depressed mood (feeling sad or empty; appears tearful).
2. Markedly decreased interest or pleasure in all, or almost all, activities.
3. Significant weight loss.
4. Insomnia or hypersomnia.
5. Psychomotor agitation or retardation.
6. Fatigue or loss of energy.
7. Feelings of worthlessness, or excessive or inappropriate guilt.
8. Diminished ability to think or concentrate, or indecisiveness.
9. Recurrent thoughts of death (not just fear of dying), recurrent suicidal ideation, or suicide attempt.

From American Psychiatric Association (2000a). *Major depressive disorder: A patient and family guide.* Washington, DC: Author; American Psychiatric Association (2000b). *Practice guidelines for the treatment of patients with major depression* (2nd ed.). Washington, DC: Author.

increase with higher levels of functional loss, advancing illness, and unmanaged symptoms such as pain (Breitbart, Chochinov, & Passik, 1998; Massie & Popkin, 1998; Twycross, 1997). Depression is also associated with many medical illnesses and may be more prevalent in neurologic diseases than others (Massie & Popkin, 1998). The data on incidence of major depressive episodes in persons with advanced cancer show less variability than do the preceding studies, probably because the criteria for major depression are well defined. Approximately 5% to 10% of patients with advanced cancer have a major depressive disorder (Derogatis, Morrow, & Fetting, 1983; Twycross, 1997).

## ■ ETIOLOGY AND PATHOPHYSIOLOGY

A history of depression appears to have a direct correlation with abnormal amounts of serotonin (5-hydroxytryptamine [5-HT]) and norepinephrine in the central nervous system (Much & Barsevick, 1999; Sterling, 1999). Other neurotransmitters such as gamma-aminobutyric acid (GABA) have also been closely linked to unconditioned anxiety in persons with depressive symptoms (Sterling, 1999). It is not clear whether depression causes these changes or whether these neurochemical changes cause depression. Current studies suggest that depression is caused by a dysregulation of the limbic-hypothalamic-pituitary-adrenal (LHPA) axis (Much & Barsevick, 1999). Clearly more research is required in this area.

There are a number of risk factors associated with a diagnosis of depression. Again it is not clear whether these factors directly cause disturbances in neurotransmission or have an indirect effect via stress or mood alterations. The following have been linked to an increased incidence of depression (Breitbart et al.,1998; Massie & Popkin, 1998; Much & Barsevick, 1999; Twycross, 1997):

- Older age
- Diagnosis with a chronic or life-threatening illness
- Unmanaged symptoms, especially pain
- Self-concept disturbance, due to changes in body image or ability to carry out roles
- History of substance use
- Personal or family history of depression
- Difficulty in expressing emotions
- Spiritual distress
- Use of medications with depressive side effects, including antihypertensives, benzodiazepines, corticosteroids, neuroleptics, amphotericin B, and certain chemotherapy agents
- Disease-related metabolic changes, nutritional deficiencies, or systemic infections, hypercalcemia, the syndrome of inappropriate antidiuretic hormone (SIADH), hypo- or hyperthyroidism, and adrenal insufficiency

## ■ ASSESSMENT AND MEASUREMENT

As individuals face the end of life the emotions that accompany the dying process can be overwhelming. The terminally ill experience multiple losses and naturally grieve these losses. Although reactive depression is normal, it is nonetheless distressing and should be not be ignored. It is extremely important that the advanced practice nurse (APN) assess for signs of a depressed mood and determine the severity of the patient's depression—from mood change to adjustment disorder to major depression—and to provide for the appropriate management for all levels of depression.

### Assessment of Depression

The problem often cited when assessing major depression in persons with advanced diseases is that many of the somatic symptoms of depression (e.g., weight loss, fatigue, sleeping alterations) overlap with the symptoms of the disease process itself. Thus the APN must focus on the psychologic symptoms of depressed mood, decreased interest in activities, inability to concentrate, feelings of worthlessness or excessive guilt, and recurrent death wishes as potential signs of depression (Breitbart et al., 1998; Massie & Popkin, 1998; Twycross, 1997). In a major depression these symptoms are present every day or almost every day for at least 2 weeks.

Major depression may be classified as mild, moderate, or severe on the basis of the severity of the symptoms. Mild depressive episodes have minimal symptoms and minor functional impairment. Moderate depression is characterized by symptoms that exceed the minimum and a greater degree of functional impairment. Severe episodes of depression involve the presence of several symptoms in excess of the minimum, and these symptoms markedly interfere with social or occupational functioning (American Psychiatric Association, 2000b).

It is often helpful to use a screening tool to assist in identifying the presence and to some degree the severity of depressed mood states. Information from one of the following assessment tools assists the APN in identifying those persons who require a more detailed evaluation of their depressed mood. The APN and collaborative physician should select one that best fits their practice setting:

- Beck Depression Inventory: The patient is asked a series of 21 questions that are scored to determine depression (Beck & Steer, 1987; Much & Barsevick, 1999). This tool is based on the *DSM* criteria for depression.
- Hospital Anxiety and Depression (HAD) Scale: This 14-item self-report tool excludes most of the somatic symptoms of depression that are often symptoms of advanced disease. Completing it takes about 5 to 7 minutes (Zabora, 1998). This tool cannot distinguish between depression and sadness (Carroll, Callies, & Noyes, 1993; Twycross, 1997).
- Geriatric Depression Scale: This tool is designed specifically for assessing depression in the elderly. It is a 30-item subjective questionnaire that excludes somatic complaints, focusing on the psychosocial symptoms of depression (Koenig, Meador, & Cohen, 1988).
- Brief Symptom Inventory: Although this self-report tool has 53 items, completing it requires only 5 to 7 minutes. This tool screens for general psychologic distress and includes a depression subscale (Zabora, 1998). It is helpful in identifying those at risk for other psychologic symptoms in addition to depression.

## Assessment of Suicide Risk

Although suicide is relatively uncommon among cancer patients, this population has a risk of committing suicide twice that of the general population (Massie & Popkin, 1998). Essentially all persons in palliative care programs have one of the risk factors for suicide: advanced disease and poor prognosis. Thus a suicide assessment is essential for all persons with depressed mood states.

The APN must assess for additional factors associated with a higher risk for suicide (Breitbart et al., 1998; Lucas, 1999; Massie & Popkin, 1998):

- Uncontrolled symptoms, including pain, fatigue, and emotional suffering
- Feelings of hopelessness and despair
- Delirium
- History of substance abuse, psychiatric disorder, or suicide attempt

- Familial history of suicide
- Social isolation
- Recent death of a loved one

It is essential that the APN assess the seriousness of suicidal intent by asking patients whether they have ever considered taking their own lives. Further questioning is then necessary to determine whether the individual has a plan for self-harm, to establish the specificity of the plan, and to determine whether the patient has the means to carry it out. Mental health experts emphasize that any patient who has devised a plan and a means to commit suicide should be immediately referred for a thorough psychiatric evaluation. The assessment for suicide risk is ongoing. It is especially important to reevaluate the severely depressed patient who is frequently undergoing treatment for depression. A patient without the energy to follow through on a suicidal act while severely depressed may indeed have the energy as the depression lessens.

## ■ HISTORY AND PHYSICAL EXAMINATION

The patient's feelings of hopelessness or worthlessness or suicidal ideation must be fully explored along with a thorough physical assessment of the somatic responses to depression (Breitbart et al., 1998). Changes in heart rate and respiratory rate may indicate anxiety, which often accompanies depression.

The APN must identify other potential causes for the patient's somatic complaints, as well as disease-, symptom-, or medication-related causes of the depressive symptoms. A thorough assessment includes identification of uncontrolled symptoms, metabolic abnormalities, endocrine abnormalities, and medications associated with depressive symptoms.

## ■ INTERVENTION AND TREATMENT

The APN must utilize the entire team when caring for persons with depressive symptoms. The supportive care of the nurse, social worker, spiritual counselor, and primary care physician may be sufficient to address the distress associated with a depressed mood. However a clinical psychiatrist should be consulted when caring for the individual with major depression (American Psychiatric Association, 2000b).

Optimal therapy for major depression is often a combination of supportive psychotherapy, cognitive-behavioral techniques, and pharmaceutic management (Breitbart et al., 1998; Breitbart, Jaramillo, & Chochinov, 1998; Massie & Popkin, 1998: Zabora, 1998). For mild major depression psychotherapy alone, antidepressant medication alone, or a combination of the two may be used. Moderate and severe major depressions often require the combination of psychotherapy and antidepressant medications. Electroconvulsive therapy may be a consideration for major depression with a high degree of symptom severity and impaired functioning (American Psychiatric Association, 2000b); however this therapy is rarely used in the palliative care setting.

Short-term psychotherapy for depression uses a crisis intervention model. Interventions include listening actively, offering verbal support, providing information to assist the individual in coping with the situation, identifying past strengths, and supporting previously successful ways of coping (Massie & Popkin, 1998). For the individual at risk for suicide it is essential to consult a skilled psychiatrist, maintain a supportive relationship, and focus on improved quality of living (Massie & Popkin, 1998).

For individuals with a high risk of suicide the APN must take steps to assure safety. Supervision, either in the patient's residence or in a facility, may be required 24 hours a day. Objects or medications that may be used for self-harm must also be removed from the environment.

Antidepressant medications are effective in the treatment of depression. There are several different classes of antidepressant medications, whose effectiveness is comparable among and within classes. Medication selection is based on anticipated side effects, patient preference, quantity and quality of clinical trial data, and medication costs. Based on these considerations, the following medications can be considered: selective serotonin reuptake inhibitors (SSRIs), desipramine, nortriptyline, bupropion, and venlafaxine (American Psychiatric Association, 2000b). The elderly are particularly prone to the orthostatic hypotensive and anticholinergic side effects of tricyclic antidepressants and tend to have fewer side effects if one of the antidepressants listed is used (Breitbart et al., 1998). The axiom "Start low and go slow" is certainly appropriate when titrating antidepressants in the elderly. Table 22-1 lists some of the more frequently used antidepressants by class and indicates the prevalence of various side effects.

Psychostimulants are another class of medications used for the treatment of depression in the terminally ill. These medications enhance mood, decrease fatigue, and stimulate appetite, leading to an overall improved sense of well-being (Woods, Tesar, Murray, & Cassem, 1986). Unlike the antidepressants, which tend to require several days to weeks to achieve therapeutic effect, the psychostimulants generally have a more immediate effect. Potential adverse side effects include tremor, tachycardia, insomnia, nightmares, and psychosis (Massie & Popkin, 1998; Waller & Caroline, 2000). These medications are generally started at low doses and titrated up for desired effect or until untoward side effects occur. Dextroamphetamine is usually started at 2.5 to 5 mg PO qd. The starting dose for methylphenidate is 5 mg PO in the morning and 2.5 mg PO at noon.

Anxiety often accompanies depression. Cognitive-behavioral interventions, active listening, and psychosocial support, alone or in combination with administration of benzodiazepines, are helpful in managing this symptom. See Chapter 16 for a more detailed discussion.

# TABLE 22-1

## Antidepressents

| Drug | Dose | Effect* Anticholin-ergic Effects | Sedation | Orthostatic Effects | Sexual Effects | GI Upset | Agitation/ Insomnia | Comments |
|---|---|---|---|---|---|---|---|---|
| **TRICYCLICS†** | | | | | | | | |
| Amitriptyline (Elavil) | 100-300 mg/day | ++++ | ++++ | ++++ | +++ | + | None | Used for neuropathic pain/hypnotic |
| Desipramine (Norpramin) | 100-300 mg/day | ++ | ++ | ++ | +++ | + | + | |
| Doxepin (Sinequan) | 100-300 mg/day | ++++ | ++++ | ++++ | +++ | + | None | |
| Imipramine (Tofranil) | 100-300 mg/day | ++++ | +++ | ++++ | +++ | + | None | |
| Nortriptyline (Pamelor) | 50-200 mg/day | ++ | ++ | ++ | +++ | + | None | "Therapeutic window" plasma level; must be within 50-150 ng/ml for efficacy |
| **SELECTIVE SEROTONIN REUPTAKE INHIBITORS§** | | | | | | | | |
| Citalopram hydrobromide (Celexa) | 20-60 mg/day | None | + | None | ++++ | +++ | + | Used for neuropathic pain/hypnotic |
| Fluoxetine (Prozac) | 10-80 mg/day | None | None | None | ++++ | +++ | ++++ | |
| Paroxetine (Paxil) | 20-60 mg/day | + | + | None | ++++ | +++ | + | |
| Sertraline HCl (Zoloft) | 50-200 mg/day | None | + | None | ++++ | ++++ | ++ | |

Continued

## TABLE 22-1

*Antidepressants—cont'd*

| Drug | Dose | Effect* | | | | | | Comments |
|------|------|---------|---|---|---|---|---|----------|
| | | Anticholinergic Effects | Sedation | Orthostatic Effects | Sexual Effects | GI Upset | Agitation/ Insomnia | |
| **SEROTONIN/NOREPINEPHRINE REUPTAKE INHIBITORS[s]** | | | | | | | | |
| Venlafaxine HCl (Effexor) | 37.5-375 mg/day | None | + | + | +++ | ++++ | ++ | "Therapeutic window" plasma level; must be within 50-150 ng/ml for efficacy[s] |
| **NOREPINEPHRINE/DOPAMINE REUPTAKE INHIBITORS[‖]** | | | | | | | | |
| Bupropion HCl (Wellbutrin) | 150-450 mg/day | None | None | None | None | ++ | ++++ | |
| **OTHER ANTIDEPRESSANTS[¶]** | | | | | | | | |
| Maprotiline HCl (Ludiomil) | 150-225 mg/day | ++ | ++ | ++ | ++ | + | None | |
| Mirtazapine (Remeron) | 15-45 mg/day | None | +++ | None | None | + | None | |
| Nefazodone HCl (Serzone) | 300-600 mg/day | None | +++ | + | None | ++ | + | |
| Trazodone HCl (Desyrel) | 200-600 mg/day | + | ++++ | ++++ | None | ++ | None | |

\* Prevalence: +++, very high; +++, high; ++, moderate; +, low.

[†] All tricyclics cause slowed cardiac conduction; have the propensity to lower seizure threshold; 2000 mg can be a fatal overdose in adults; some tricyclics have established therapeutic plasma levels; moderately priced.

[‡] The lower dosages are most appropriate for depressed symptoms; no need to titrate as in the tricyclics; caution warranted when coprescribed with other medications that undergo extensive hepatic metabolism, especially in the elderly; costly.

[s] Side effects similar to those of the SSRIs; daily dosing for extended-release capsules, twice-daily and thrice-daily dosing for tablets; should be considered when a trial of SSRIs has been ineffective; costly.

[‖] Sustained-release form given twice daily, tablets thrice daily; avoid use in patients with a history of seizure disorders; most activating antidepressant available; costly.

[¶] Moderate to costly medications; often good for depression mixed with insomnia.

Complementary interventions also play a role in the treatment of depression. These interventions can improve mood and outlook, decrease feelings of hopelessness and helplessness, and decrease anxiety. Chapter 6 addresses the use and benefits of complementary therapies in end-of-life care. The APN should consider the following for patients who have depressed mood states:

- Pet therapy
- Color therapy
- Music therapy
- Guided imagery
- Aromatherapy

## ■ PATIENT AND FAMILY EDUCATION

Depression, like many psychiatric illnesses, is often perceived as an embarrassment or disgrace. Patients and families need support and education about the diagnosis of depression, with emphasis that it is not a sign of weakness or a character flaw. Some persons find written information helpful, such as the *Major depressive disorder: A patient and family guide* (American Psychiatric Association, 2000a).

The following information must be included in the teaching plan for the patient and family:

- Take medications as prescribed, noting that antidepressants may not produce the full therapeutic benefit for a few weeks.
- Report any untoward side effects of the medications so that they can be addressed.
- Report any worsening of symptoms.
- Keep a record of the depressive symptoms to assist in evaluating the effectiveness of interventions.
- Use the interdisciplinary team for support and information.

## ■ EVALUATION AND PLAN FOR FOLLOW-UP

Early detection and ongoing assessment of depression are important considerations for the APN caring for patients at the end of life. Timely interventions are not always possible, and therefore thoughtful consideration should be given to the appropriate medications that can be used to improve patient outcomes.

✔ **CASE STUDY**    Louise is an 88-year-old active woman whose diagnosis of congestive heart failure was made several years ago. Louise lives alone with her dog and spends the majority of her time worrying about dying. She often wakes in the middle of the night experiencing "paniclike" attacks and often lies in bed worrying about her health. Reporting shortness of breath, chest pressure, and difficulty with concentration, Louise has undergone extensive diagnostic tests to investigate her complaints (i.e., magnetic resonance imaging [MRI] of the brain, echocardiogram, and angiogram) all of which yielded negative findings and indicated no further disease progression.

Louise's daughter lives out of town but is concerned about her mother and asks the APN to make a home evaluation. The APN finds Louise sitting in her darkened apartment and later learns that she spends most of her days in this manner. With further investigation the APN learns that Louise has experienced several losses within the last year. Her grandson was killed in an auto accident 6 months ago, her son was killed in an accident several years ago, and her husband recently died after 68 years of marriage. Louise begins to open up to the APN and describes her life as limited and worthless; she believes that there is no reason for her to live any longer and she is ready to join her husband.

Further assessment reveals that Louise is not eating or drinking, sleeps most of the time, and does not engage in any of her previous social activities. Louise tells the APN that if it weren't for her dog she would have taken her own life.

On the basis of the assessment the APN initiates the following plan:

- Admit the patient to the local hospital for evaluation.
- Investigate physical symptoms and medication compliance.
- Schedule an electrocardiogram (ECG) to evaluate chest pain.
- Schedule a chest radiograph to evaluate dyspnea.
- Consult a cardiologist.
- Consult the psychiatrist or clinical psychologist regarding suicidal ideologies.
- Initiate Paroxetine, 10 mg qd for depression. (Because of the patient's age the initial dose is low; SSRIs are less likely to lead to untoward side effects than the tricyclic antidepressants in the elderly).
- Initiate buspirone, 5 mg tid, for her anxiety.
- Facilitate the patient's support system (identify other family members, friends, or a religious or social group available to the patient for support).
- Utilize home care referrals to others on the palliative care team: the social worker, chaplain, and volunteers.

After 2 weeks Louise returns home and tells the APN how much better she is feeling. She denies feeling hopeless and has asked her sister to move into her two-bedroom apartment with her. The APN continues to visit Louise, monitors her well-being and helps facilitate her ongoing visits to the clinical psychologist and cardiologist.

# References

American Psychiatric Association (2000a). *Major depressive disorder: A patient and family guide.* Washington, DC: Author.

American Psychiatric Association (2000b). *Practice guidelines for the treatment of patients with major depression* (2nd ed.). Washington, DC: Author.

BECK, A., & Steer, R. (1987). *Beck depression inventory (BDI) manual.* San Antonio, TX: The Psychological Corporation, Harcourt Brace Jovanovich.

BREITBART, W., Chochinov, H. M., & Passik, S. (1998). Psychiatric aspects of palliative care. In D. Doyle, G.W.C. Hanks, & N. MacDonald (Eds.). *Oxford textbook of palliative medicine* (2nd ed.) (pp. 933-954). New York: Oxford University Press.

BREITBART, W., Jaramillo, J. R., & Chochinov, H. M. (1998). Palliative and terminal care. In J. C. Holland (Ed.), *Psycho-oncology* (pp. 437-449). New York: Oxford University Press.

CARROLL, B., Callies, A., & Noyes, R. (1993). Screening for depression and anxiety in cancer patients using the hospital anxiety and depression scale. *General Hospital Psychiatry, 15,* 69-74.

DEROGATIS, L. R., Morrow, G. R., & Fetting, J. (1983). The prevalence of psychiatric disorders among cancer patients. *Journal of the American Medical Association, 249,* 751-757.

HOWLAND, R., Shelton, R., & Trivedi, H. (2000). Chronic depression: Now a treatable condition. *Patient Care for the Nurse Practitioner, 3*(1), 54-71.

KOENIG, H., Meador, K., & Cohen, H. (1988). Self-rated depression scales and screening for major depression in the older hospitalized patient with medical illness. *Journal of the American Geriatric Society, 36,* 699-706.

LUCAS, B. (1999). Coping with psychiatric emergencies in the office. *Patient Care for the Nurse Practitioner, 2*(2), 31-42.

MASSIE, M. J., & Popkin, M. K. (1998). Depressive disorders. In J. C. Holland (Ed.), *Psycho-oncology* (pp. 518-540). New York: Oxford University Press.

MUCH, J., & Barsevick, A. (1999). Depression. In C. Yarbro, M. Frogge, & M. Goodman (Eds.), *Cancer symptom management* (2nd ed.) (pp. 594-607). Sudbury, MA: Jones & Bartlett.

STERLING, L. (1999, March). Pharmacological review of SSRIs in panic disorder. In *Therapeutic spotlight: Psychiatric illness in primary care: A supplement to clinician reviews,* 10-13.

STRAIN, J. J. (1998). Adjustment disorders. In J. C. Holland (Ed.), *Psycho-oncology* (pp. 509-517). New York: Oxford University Press.

TWYCROSS, R. (1997). *Symptom management in advanced cancer* (2nd ed.). Oxon, UK: Radcliffe Medical Press.

WALLER, A., & Caroline, N. L. (2000). *Handbook of palliative care in cancer* (2nd ed.). Boston: Butterworth-Heinemann.

WOODS, S. W., Tesar, G. E., Murray, G. B., & Cassem, N. H. (1986). Psychostimulant treatment of depressive disorders secondary to medical illness. *Journal of Clinical Psychiatry, 47,* 12-15.

ZABORA, J. R. (1998). Screening procedures for psychosocial distress. In J. C. Holland (Ed.), *Psycho-oncology* (pp. 653-661). New York: Oxford University Press.

ZUNG, W. (1973). The diagnosis and treatment of depression. *Archives of General Psychiatry, 29,* 328-337.

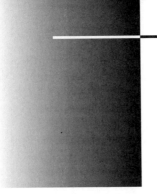

CHAPTER 23

# *Diarrhea*

DEBRA E. HEIDRICH

## ■ DEFINITION AND INCIDENCE

*Diarrhea* is defined as an increase in stool volume and liquidity, resulting in the passage of three or more loose or unformed stools per day (Carpenito, 2000; Sykes, 1998). However this symptom is somewhat subjective: Whereas some may report three soft stools in a day as diarrhea, others may report only stools that are liquid and occur in large volume. Diarrhea is often associated with abdominal cramping and rectal urgency (Carpenito, 2000; Levy, 1991). Uncontrolled diarrhea can lead to fluid and electrolyte imbalances, resulting in lethargy, weakness, and orthostatic hypotension. In addition, persistent diarrhea may lead to malnutrition, impaired skin integrity, altered sleeping patterns, social isolation, anxiety, and self-concept disturbances.

Approximately 5% to 10% of persons with advanced cancer report diarrhea (Levy, 1991; Sykes, 1998; Waller & Caroline, 2000), and as many as 27% to 50% or more of those with human immunodeficiency virus (HIV) disease may experience this symptom (Simon, 1998; Sykes, 1998). The number of acquired immunodeficiency virus (AIDS) patients admitted to the hospital for uncontrolled diarrhea may be decreasing with the use of highly active antiretroviral therapy. A review of data from the state of New York in 1998 revealed that of the 15,000 persons with AIDS admitted to hospitals 2.8% had a diarrheal diagnosis (Anastasi & Capili, 2000). This study does not indicate the number of persons with AIDS who experience diarrhea that is not severe enough to warrant hospitalization. It is important to recognize that even mild to moderate diarrhea can have a debilitating effect.

Most diarrhea is acute, lasting only a few days, and is generally due to infection. Diarrhea that lasts more than 3 weeks is considered chronic and is usually due to organic disease (Sykes, 1998).

## ■ ETIOLOGY AND PATHOPHYSIOLOGY

The three most common causes of diarrhea in persons with advanced cancer are laxative overdose, fecal impaction with overflow diarrhea, and partial bowel obstruction (Levy, 1991; Twycross, 1997). Other common causes are radiation enteritis, medications, and steatorrhea. In persons with AIDS infection is often the cause, although the pathogen is not always identifiable.

Any condition that increases secretion within the gastrointestinal (GI) tract, interferes with reabsorption from the GI tract, increases the motility of the GI tract, or causes excretion of mucus, fluids, or blood can cause diarrhea. These correspond with the general mechanisms of diarrhea: secretory, osmotic, hypermotile, and exudative. Diarrhea in the terminally ill often involves more than one mechanism (Levy, 1991; Luckmann, 1997). The pathophysiologic characteristics of these mechanisms are discussed later. Table 23-1 includes many of the conditions that lead to diarrhea in the palliative care setting, the pathophysiologic mechanism(s), descriptors that may be helpful in determining the type and cause of this symptom, and suggested interventions.

## Pathophysiologic Characteristics of Secretory Diarrhea

The lining of the walls of the small intestine includes small pits, called the *crypts of Lieberkühn,* that lie between the intestinal villi. The villi and crypts are covered with epithelium composed of either mucus-producing goblet cells or enterocytes. The mucus of the goblet cells lubricates and protects the surfaces of the bowel lumen. The enterocytes of the crypts secrete large quantities of water and electrolytes, and those of the villi reabsorb water and electrolytes along with the products of metabolism (Guyton & Hall, 1996a). Active secretion that overwhelms the absorptive processes of the GI tract leads to diarrhea that generally persists with fasting (Mercadante, 1998). Substances that increase bowel secretions (secretagogues) include vasoactive intestinal polypeptide (VIP), calcitonin, serotonin, bradykinin, substance P, prostaglandins, and gastrin (Guyton & Hall, 1996a; Levy, 1991; Mercadante, 1998). Conditions that lead to the production of one or more of these secretagogues include the following:

- Inflammation in the bowel wall causes the release through the cyclooxygenase pathway of prostaglandins, which stimulate bowel secretions. In addition, the inflammation interferes with the absorption process, further contributing to diarrhea (Mercadante, 1998). This is the likely mechanism for the diarrhea associated with acute radiation enteritis, chemotherapy, and infection.

- Two infections that lead to significant fluid and electrolytes losses from secretory diarrhea are cryptosporidiosis and pseudomembranous colitis. *Crytosporidium* sp., a common cause of diarrhea in the AIDS population, impairs absorption and enhances secretion within the intestinal tract (Clark, 1999). The diarrhea of cryptosporidiosis is profuse and watery and is associated with abdominal cramping, fever, and vomiting (Welsby, Richardson, & Brettle, 1998). Pseudomembranous colitis is caused by colonization with *Clostridium difficile* after antibiotic therapy. *C. difficile* produces toxins that damage the mucosa, leading to a secretory diarrhea (Twycross, 1997). Symptoms begin within 1 week to 1 month of starting antibiotic therapy.

*Text continued on p. 288*

## TABLE 23-1

### Causes, Character, and Treatment of Diarrhea

| Cause | Mechanism(s) | Descriptors | Treatment |
|---|---|---|---|
| **CANCER-RELATED DIARRHEA** | | | |
| Endocrine-producing tumor | Secretory via production or stimulation of secretagogues | High volume, watery Associated with abdominal cramping | Encourage/replace fluids, as needed Control diarrhea: antidiarrheals Inhibit intestinal secretion (if severe): octreotide, clonidine Treat pain: anticholinergics |
| Obstruction | Exudative and hypermotility | Alternating constipation and diarrhea, often with mucus and blood; colicky pain | Reduce inflammation: steroids Treat pain: anticholinergics Control diarrhea: cautious use of antidiarrheals |
| Biliary or pancreatic obstruction | Osmotic due to fat malabsorption | Steatorrhea: large volume, pale, foul odor; feces floats in toilet | Decrease dietary fat Treat fat malabsorption: pancreatic enzymes, famotidine |

From Bickley, L. S., & Hoekelman, R. A. (1999b). An approach to symptoms. In L. S. Bickley & R. A. Hoekelman (Eds.), *Bates' guide to physical examination and history taking* (7th ed.) (pp. 43-105). Philadelphia: Lippincott-Raven; Mercadante, S. (1998). Diarrhea, malabsorption, and constipation. In A. Berger, R. K. Portenoy, & D. E. Weissman (Eds.), *Principles and practice of supportive oncology* (pp. 191-205). Philadelphia: Lippincott-Raven; Levy, M. H. (1991). Constipation and diarrhea in cancer patients. *The Cancer Bulletin, 43*, 412-422; Luckmann, J. (1997). Caring for people with gastrointestinal disorders. In J. Luckmann (Ed.), *Saunders' manual of nursing care* (pp. 1241-1299). Philadelphia: W. B. Saunders; Sykes, N. P. (1998). Constipation and diarrhea. In D. Doyle, G. W. C. Hanks, & N. MacDonald (Eds.), *Oxford textbook of palliative medicine* (2nd ed.) (pp. 513-526). New York: Oxford University Press; Welsby, P. D., Richardson, A., & Brettle, R. P. (1998). AIDS: Aspects in adults. In D. Doyle, G. W. C. Hanks, & N. MacDonald (Eds.), *Oxford textbook of palliative medicine* (2nd ed.) (pp. 1121-1148). New York: Oxford University Press.

Continued

## TABLE 23-1

### Causes, Character, and Treatment of Diarrhea—cont'd

| Cause | Mechanism(s) | Descriptors | Treatment |
|---|---|---|---|
| **CANCER TREATMENT-RELATED DIARRHEA** | | | |
| *Chemotherapy* | Secretory due to damage to villi, inhibiting absorption; hypermotility due to irritation | High volume, watery; may be explosive<br>Associated with colicky pain | Encourage/replace fluids, as needed<br>Slow motility: antidiarrheals<br>Inhibit intestinal secretion (if severe): octreotide, clonidine<br>Treat pain: anticholinergics |
| *Radiation therapy*<br>• Acute | Secretory (due to inflammation and bile salt malabsorption), osmotic, and hypermotility due to effects of bile salts | High volume, watery, explosive<br>Associated with: abdominal cramping<br>Usually self-limiting | Encourage/replace fluids, as needed<br>Treat inflammation: nonsteroidal antiinflammatory drugs (NSAIDs)<br>Absorb bile salts: cholestyramine<br>Slow motility: antidiarrheals |
| • Chronic (may occur 5-15 years after treatment) | Ischemic enteritis, ulcerations, or impaired cellular functioning; may be secretory and/or osmotic | Depends on mechanism; generally high volume and watery | Encourage/replace fluids, as needed<br>Control diarrhea: antidiarrheals<br>Absorb bile salts: cholestyramine |

*Surgery*

| | Mechanism | Characteristics | Management |
|---|---|---|---|
| • Gastrectomy | Secretory, osmotic, and hypermotility due to "dumping syndrome" and potential for bile salt malabsorption | High volume with undigested food. Associated with nausea, vomiting, flatulence, and colicky pain | Frequent, small meals. Control diarrhea: antidiarrheals. Bile salt malabsorption: cholestyramine. Treat pain: simethicone for gas pain; anticholinergics for colicky pain |
| • Ileal resection | Secretory, osmotic, and hypermotility due to poor reabsorption of bile salts | High volume with undigested food | Frequent, small meals. Control diarrhea: antidiarrheals. Bile salt malabsorption: cholestyramine. Treat pain: simethicone for gas pain; anticholinergics for colicky pain |
| • Short bowel syndrome | Osmotic due to decreased fluid absorption | Depends on length of bowel resected: loose to watery | Increase bulk of stool: bulk-forming laxatives. Slow motility: antidiarrheals |

From Bickley, L. S., & Hoekelman, R. A. (1999b). An approach to symptoms. In L. S. Bickley & R. A. Hoekelman (Eds.), *Bates' guide to physical examination and history taking* (7th ed.) (pp. 43–105). Philadelphia: Lippincott-Raven; Mercadante, S. (1998). Diarrhea, malabsorption, and constipation. In A. Berger, R. K. Portenoy, & D. E. Weissman (Eds.), *Principles and practice of supportive oncology* (pp. 191–205). Philadelphia: Lippincott-Raven; Levy, M. H. (1991). Constipation and diarrhea in cancer patients. *The Cancer Bulletin, 43,* 412–422; Luckmann, J. (1997). Caring for people with gastrointestinal disorders. In J. Luckmann (Ed.), *Saunders' manual of nursing care* (pp. 1241–1299). Philadelphia: W. B. Saunders; Sykes, N. P. (1998). Constipation and diarrhea. In D. Doyle, G. W. C. Hanks, & N. MacDonald (Eds.), *Oxford textbook of palliative medicine* (2nd ed.) (pp. 513–526). New York: Oxford University Press; Welsby, P. D., Richardson, A., & Brettle, R. P. (1998). AIDS: Aspects in adults. In D. Doyle, G. W. C. Hanks, & N. MacDonald (Eds.), *Oxford textbook of palliative medicine* (2nd ed.) (pp. 1121–1148). New York: Oxford University Press.

*Continued*

## TABLE 23-1

### Causes, Character, and Treatment of Diarrhea—cont'd

| Cause | Mechanism(s) | Descriptors | Treatment |
|---|---|---|---|
| **INFECTION-RELATED DIARRHEA** | | | |
| Noninflammatory infections (e.g., viruses, Escherichia coli, Staphylococcus aureus) | Secretory due to stimulation of secretagogues via endotoxins | Often self-limiting Watery, without pus or mucus Associated with periumbilical cramping, nausea, and vomiting Temperature normal or slightly elevated | If prolonged: Treat infection, when possible Encourage/replace fluids, as necessary Control diarrhea: antidiarrheals, using bismuth subsalicylate (Pepto-Bismol) as first choice, if required Treat pain: anticholinergics |
| Inflammatory infections (e.g., Shigella, Salmonella, Campylobacter spp., invasive E. coli) | Secretory | Loose to watery, often with blood, pus, or mucus Associated with lower abdominal cramping, rectal urgency, and fever | Treat infection, when possible Encourage/replace fluids, as necessary Control diarrhea: antidiarrheals Treat pain: anticholinergics |
| Cryptosporidiosis | Secretory | High volume, watery, explosive; associated with abdominal cramping, fever, and vomiting | Treat infection: metronidazole or vancomycin Encourage/replace fluids, as necessary Control diarrhea: antidiarrheals Treat pain: anticholinergics |
| **OTHER TREATMENT-RELATED DIARRHEA** | | | |
| Overuse of laxatives | Depends on type(s) of laxative; usually osmotic or hypermotility | Frequent, loose stools Rectal leakage with too much softener; cramping with too much stimulant | Discontinue or decrease dose of laxatives |
| Impaction | Exudative | Small amounts of dark, mucuslike liquid; rectal pressure | Perform disimpaction Begin/adjust laxative protocol |

**OTHER TREATMENT-RELATED DIARRHEA—CONT'D**

| | | |
|---|---|---|
| Enteral supplements/feedings | Osmotic due to hyperosmolality of supplement or due to lactose intolerance | Large volume and watery<br>Associated with abdominal cramping, distension, and flatulence<br>Low stool pH | Dilute supplement with water and gradually increase strength<br>Consider using bulk-forming agents<br>Evaluate need for lactose-free supplement |
| Celiac plexus block | Hypermotility due to suppression of sympathetic nervous system | Moderate to large volume, loose stool<br>May be self-limiting | Slow motility: antidiarrheals; anticholinergics |
| Anxiety | Hypermotility and secretory of lower GI tract via parasympathetic stimulation | Generally moderate to large volume; loose stool<br>Stool may contain mucus | Treat anxiety: address psychosocial concerns; teach relaxation techniques; evaluate need for anxiolytic |
| Medication | Often secretory | Secretory generally large volume; but diarrhea character may vary with offending medication | Stop offending medication, when possible |

From Bickley, L. S., & Hoekelman, R. A. (1999b). An approach to symptoms. In L. S. Bickley & R. A. Hoekelman (Eds.), *Bates' guide to physical examination and history taking* (7th ed.) (pp. 43-105). Philadelphia: Lippincott-Raven; Mercadante, S. (1998). Diarrhea, malabsorption, and constipation. In A. Berger, R. K. Portenoy, & D. E. Weissman (Eds.), *Principles and practice of supportive oncology* (pp. 191-205). Philadelphia: Lippincott-Raven; Levy, M. H. (1991). Constipation and diarrhea in cancer patients. *The Cancer Bulletin, 43,* 412-422; Luckmann, J. (1997). Caring for people with gastrointestinal disorders. In J. Luckmann (Ed.), *Saunders' manual of nursing care* (pp. 1241-1299). Philadelphia: W. B. Saunders; Sykes, N. P. (1998). Constipation and diarrhea. In D. Doyle, G. W. C. Hanks, & N. MacDonald (Eds.), *Oxford textbook of palliative medicine* (2nd ed.) (pp. 513-526). New York: Oxford University Press; Welsby, P. D., Richardson, A., & Brettle, R. P. (1998). AIDS: Aspects in adults. In D. Doyle, G. W. C. Hanks, & N. MacDonald (Eds.), *Oxford textbook of palliative medicine* (2nd ed.) (pp. 1121-1148). New York: Oxford University Press.

- Certain tumors, including small-cell lung cancer, ganglioneuroma, pheochromocytoma, carcinoma of thyroid, malignant carcinoids, and gastrinomas, produce one or more of these secretagogue substances (Levy, 1991; Mercadante, 1998).
- The inability to reabsorb bile acids from the small intestine leads to diarrhea via the secretory effect of these substances on the mucosa of the colon and their osmotic effect in the colon. The result is diarrhea that is watery and explosive (Mercadante, 1998; Sykes, 1998). Ileal resection, gastrectomy with vagotomy, and postradiation enteritis may interfere with bile acid reabsorption.
- Some medications can also cause secretory diarrheas (see Box 23-1) (Mercadante, 1998) via direct simulation of secretions or secondary to irritation of the epithelial cells.

## Pathophysiologic Characteristics of Osmotic Diarrhea

The small bowel is highly permeable to sodium and water transport, but not to solute. When large amounts of nonabsorbable sugar (e.g., lactulose and sorbitol) are ingested, the GI tract's ability to compensate may be overwhelmed, resulting in diarrhea from the osmosis of fluid into the lumen. The diarrhea due to carbohydrate malabsorption is chacterized by a low pH, high content of carbohydrates, high stool osmolality, and flatulence. Other substances that cause osmotic diarrhea are magnesium, sulfate, and poorly absorbed salts, including bile salts. The pH of diarrhea caused by one of these latter substances is usually normal (Mercadante, 1998).

Persons with lactose intolerance and those receiving high-carbohydrate supplements or enteral feedings are at risk for osmotic diarrhea. The sorbitol in sugar-free elixirs and enteral feedings is often overlooked as a cause of this symptom (Sykes, 1998). The overuse of osmotic laxatives is also a cause of diarrhea for some persons with advanced disease.

Malabsorption of fat is another cause of osmotic diarrhea. Most dietary intake of fat is absorbed in the small intestines and only small amounts of lipids enter the colon. The absorption of fat from the small intestines is dependent on pancreatic enzymes to break down the fats and bile salts to

| BOX 23-1 | *Medications Associated with Secretory Diarrhea* |
|---|---|

**DIURETICS**
Caffeine
Theophylline
Antacids
Antibiotics
Poorly absorbable osmotic laxatives

From Mercadante, S. (1998). Diarrhea, malabsorption, and constipation. In A. Berger, R. K. Portenoy, & D. E. Weissman (Eds.), *Principles and practice of supportive oncology* (pp. 191-205). Philadelphia: Lippincott-Raven.

make the fat particles soluble. Pancreatic cancer or resection of the pancreas may cause a deficiency of pancreatic enzymes, leading to malabsorption of fat and steatorrhea. Biliary tract obstruction, terminal ileal resection, and cholestatic liver disease cause a decrease in bile salt formation, again contributing to malabsorption of fat and steatorrhea (Mercadante, 1998). Steatorrhea is characterized by loose, pale, foul-smelling feces. The feces may be greasy in appearance and tend to float in the toilet, making them difficult to flush.

## Pathophysiologic Characteristics of Diarrhea Due to Hypermotility

When GI tract motility is abnormally stimulated, bowel contents are moved through the intestines too quickly to prevent adequate absorption, leading to diarrhea. Several factors may contribute to GI hypermotility.

Parasympathetic stimulation enhances GI motility and can lead to diarrhea. Both the small and the large intestine receive parasympathetic stimulation from the spinal cord via the pelvic nerves. The sigmoidal, rectal, and anal regions are more abundantly supplied with parasympathetic fibers than other intestinal areas (Guyton & Hall, 1996b). Stress can stimulate the parasympathetic system, leading to hypermotility and secretion of mucus in the large intestine. This condition is sometimes referred to as *psychogenic diarrhea* (Guyton & Hall, 1996c).

Stimulation of the sympathetic nervous system inhibits activity of the GI tract and generally acts to balance parasympathetic activity. Sympathetic innervation originates in the spinal cord between the fifth thoracic (T5) and second lubar (L2) vertebrae and innervates all portions of the GI tract. If sympathetic activity is blocked, leaving the parasympathetic activity unopposed, hypermotility and diarrhea may result (Guyton & Hall, 1996b). This is the likely mechanism for the diarrhea associated with celiac plexus block (Mercadante, 1998).

- Peristaltic activity of the small intestine is initiated by a combination of factors, including entry of partially digested food into the duodenum and mechanical and hormonal activation of the gastroenteric reflex. Peristaltic activity is generally weak. However in the presence of intense irritation powerful peristaltic contractions occur. The resultant "peristaltic rush" leads to elimination of the irritative bowel contents or excessive distension (Guyton & Hall, 1996d). Food poisoning and infections may cause this type of diarrhea. This is generally considered a protective mechanism to rid the body of the irritative substance.
- Movement of fecal material through the large intestine occurs via a modified type of peristalsis, called *mass movements*. Mass movements generally occur only one to three times each day. However irritation of the colon, as may be seen with ulcerative colitis or tumors, initiates intense mass movements (Guyton & Hall, 1996d).
- Medications that increase bowel motility, including stimulant laxatives and cholinergics (e.g., metoclopramide), may also lead to diarrhea.

## Pathophysiologic Characteristics of Exudative Diarrhea

The discharge of serum proteins, blood, or excessive amounts of mucus into the bowel leads to diarrhea. The large intestine has many crypts of Lieberkühn lined with epithelial cells. The primary purpose of these epithelial cells is to secrete mucus. The rate of secretion is regulated by direct, tactile stimulation of the mucous cells (Guyton & Hall, 1996a). Normally this mucus serves to lubricate the bowel lumen and soften the stool. In the presence of abnormal tactile stimulation excessive amounts of mucus may be secreted. Irritation to the bowel produced by tumors, partial or complete obstruction, or impaction may cause excessive mucus formation and contribute to diarrhea.

Obstruction, whether by tumor or stool, may lead to a blockage of venous blood flow in the intestinal circulation, increasing the intestinal capillary pressure. Fluid, along with serum proteins, leaks into the intestinal lumen (Guyton & Hall, 1996e). This increased fluid alone may lead to diarrhea. It is made worse however by the osmotic effect of the serum proteins in the bowel.

The disruption of the bowel wall caused by tumor or ulceration from inflammatory processes may lead to the discharge of blood into the bowel lumen. Like serum proteins, blood has an osmotic effect, pulling fluid into the bowel and leading to diarrhea.

### The Diarrhea of AIDS

Most diarrheas in AIDS patients are due to infection. Cryptosporidiosis is the most common causative organism, but other protozoal, viral, fungal, and bacterial infections are also seen in this population (Welsby et al., 1998). At times no pathogens can be identified (Holodniy et al., 1999).

## ■ ASSESSMENT AND MEASUREMENT

A thorough assessment and physical examination of the patient are required to identify the causes of diarrhea and guide appropriate intervention. Measurement of the severity of diarrhea is based on the number and quantity of loose stools per day and any associated symptoms. The National Cancer Institute (NCI) developed a grading tool for diarrhea severity related to cancer treatment on a 0 to 4 scale (see Table 23-2). This scale is useful in categorizing responses to treatment for research purposes and could be used in the clinical setting. However many patients and health care practitioners use the number of diarrhea stools per day as a "rating scale." The rating scale used must be clear to all persons as a 4 on the NCI scale is very different from 4 diarrhea stools in one day.

Assessment of the character and amount of diarrhea provides clues regarding the underlying cause.

- Disorders of the small intestine or proximal colon tend to cause large amounts of diarrhea that is light in color and watery or greasy. Undigested food may be present, but blood usually is not.

| TABLE 23-2 | | | | |
|---|---|---|---|---|
| **Common Toxicity Criteria for Diarrhea for Patients Without Colostomy** | | | | |
| Grade | 0 | 1 | 2 | 3 | 4 |

| Grade | 0 | 1 | 2 | 3 | 4 |
|---|---|---|---|---|---|
| Symptoms | None | Increase of <4 stools/ day over pretreat- ment | Increase of 4-6 stools/ day or nocturnal stools | Increase to ≥7 stools/ day or incon- tinence; need for parenteral support for dehydration | Physiologic conse- quences requiring intensive care; or hemody- namic collapse |

From National Cancer Institute. (1999). *Common toxicity criteria: Version 2.0.* Bethesda, MD: Author.

- Disorders of the left side of the colon or rectum tend to cause small amounts of diarrhea that is dark in color and contains mucus or blood. This diarrhea may also be accompanied by a sense of rectal urgency (Mercadante, 1998).
- Stools that are pale and fatty and have an offensive odor indicate steatorrhea and fat malabsorption.
- Diarrhea that follows several days of constipation suggests fecal impaction or partial obstruction (Mercadante, 1998; Sykes, 1998).
- Osmotic diarrheas tend to stop with fasting, whereas diarrhea that persists after a 2 or 3 day fast suggests a secretory process. Hypermotility disorders are suspected when osmotic and secretory diarrhea is ruled out (Levy, 1991).

  The history and physical examination includes the following:
- General history:
  - Terminal diagnosis and its potential effect on bowel functioning or risk of infection:
    - Bowel tumors
    - Immunosuppression
  - History of chronic bowel diseases (e.g., ulcerative colitis)
  - History of food intolerances or allergies, especially intolerance of milk or milk products due to lactase deficiency
  - Recent history of chemotherapy
  - Recent or past history of radiation therapy
  - Recent food and fluid intake, including alcohol consumption
  - Current medications:
    - Laxatives (excessive stimulative laxatives causes colic and urgency; excessive softening leads to fecal leakage) (Sykes, 1998)
    - Antibiotics
    - Any new medications, notably those listed in Box 23-1

- Diarrhea history:
  - Duration (how long diarrhea has been present)
  - Whether diarrhea was preceded by constipation
  - Frequency (number of diarrhea stools in 24 hours)
  - Timing (times of day when diarrhea is worse or absent):
    - Association with intake of food or fluids
    - Wakening of the patient from sleep
  - Quantity (size of diarrhea stools):
    - Consistency (e.g., semiformed, unformed, liquid)
    - Color (light or dark)
    - Other characteristics (e.g., foul odor, tendency to float in toilet)
    - Discomfort (e.g., location of associated pain—periumbilical colicky pain often indicates small intestinal origin, whereas left-sided lower abdominal pain may indicate lower colon or rectal origin)
- Physical examination:
  - Auscultation of bowel sounds:
    - Hyperactivity with most diarrheas
    - Intestinal obstruction indicated by high-pitched sounds accompanied by abdominal cramping (Bickley & Hoekelman, 1999a)
  - Palpation of abdomen for fecal or tumor mass
  - Noting of any ascites or abdominal distension
  - Examination of the rectum for tone, presence of feces in ampulla, or signs of rectal discharge
  - Assessment for the presence of fever, indicative of an infectious process
  - Noting of any signs of dehydration:
    - Postural hypotension
    - Poor skin turgor
    - Decreased urine output
  - Assessment of nutritional status (in advanced diseases, it may be difficult to determine whether the cause of poor nutritional status is related more to terminal illness or malabsorption of nutrients)

## ■ DIAGNOSTICS

Often a careful history and clinical examination identify the cause and further diagnostic evaluation is not necessary. If information is not sufficient, examination of the stool for pus, blood, fat, and ova and parasites as well as stool culture may be appropriate (Levy, 1991; Mercadante, 1998; Twycross, 1997). Guaiac-positive diarrhea indicates an exudative mechanism, such as chronic radiation colitis, cancerous tumor, or infectious diarrhea.

Bowel obstructions are often diagnosed on the basis of findings from the patient's history and physical examination. Abdominal radiography to confirm a bowel obstruction is generally not necessary in palliative care settings. If a surgical intervention for the bowel obstruction is a consideration, radiography is appropriate.

Calculating the stool anion gap (stool anion gap = stool osmolality − 2 [stool sodium + stool potassium]) can assist in determining whether the diarrhea is osmotic or secretory:

- If the anion gap is more than 50 mmol/liter, the diarrhea is osmotic.
- If the anion gap is less than 50 mmol/liter, diarrhea is secretory.

In addition to calculation of the anion gap, the presence of secretory agents in the serum, such as vasoactive protein, gastrin, and calcitonin, may indicate a secretory diarrhea (Levy, 1991).

Endoscopy, biopsy, or barium radiography may be necessary to determine the cause of inflammatory processes (Levy, 1991). The patient's physical status and ability to tolerate the procedure as well as the likelihood of identifying a treatable cause of the diarrhea are important considerations when determining the appropriateness of these invasive, uncomfortable procedures.

## INTERVENTION AND TREATMENT

Appropriate interventions are aimed at treating reversible causes of diarrhea, preventing complications, promoting comfort, and improving quality of living. All medication dosages are from *Mosby's 2001 Nursing Drug Reference* (Skidmore-Roth, 2001).

### General Measures

Discontinue any laxatives and begin a clear liquid diet to promote bowel rest. It is helpful to avoid very hot and very cold foods, as well as any milk products. Gradually, add semisolids such as bananas, rice, applesauce, and crackers or plain toast. The diet can be advanced as tolerated. Encourage a gluten-free diet to reduce abdominal cramping and avoid fatty foods, whole grain products, and fresh fruits and vegetables.

Monitor hydration status by tracking intake and output. Most diarrhea in palliative care other than HIV-associated diarrhea is rarely of sufficient amount or duration to require rehydration (Sykes, 1998). When rehydration is necessary, oral hydration is preferred. The rehydration solution should contain glucose, electrolytes, and water. Use commercial sports drinks (e.g., Gatorade) or dextrose and electrolyte solutions available at pharmacies (e.g., Resol, Rehydralyte, Pedialyte). Alternatively, make a solution of ½ teaspoon salt, ½ teaspoon baking soda, and 4 tablespoons sugar in 1 liter of water (Carpenito, 2000). The World Health Organization's recommended rehydration solution is 2 g salt plus 2 g sugar in 1 liter of water. This can be flavored with lemon juice if desired (Waller & Caroline, 2000). Homemade solutions should be used within 24 hours of preparation. Intravenous replacement may be required if the patient is unable to tolerate sufficient oral intake.

It is essential to provide good skin care. Keep the perianal area clean. Use of a squeeze bottle with warm, soapy water to cleanse the area is superior to use of toilet paper (Kemp, 1999). Sitz baths also help cleanse and promote comfort. After cleansing, apply a petroleum-based ointment to the intact skin and a protective powder (e.g. Stomahesive) to denuded skin followed with a petroleum-based ointment (Kemp, 1999). If the patient is experiencing massive amounts of diarrhea, consider the use of a fecal incontinence bag to protect skin, decrease caregiver burden, and help control odor.

## Treat Cause of Diarrhea

- If the diarrhea is related to medications, stop the offending agents(s) when possible.
- If the diarrhea is due to fecal impaction, perform a manual disimpaction. Premedicate patients for this procedure. Waller and Caroline (2000) suggest sedation with midazolam, 1 mg IV, titrated up by 0.5-mg increments as needed, plus morphine. An oral benzodiazepine and opioid is also effective if the patient is premedicated 1 to 1½ hours before the procedure. Provide local anesthesia by applying lidocaine jelly on the anus and then instilling 10 ml of 1% lidocaine jelly into the rectum. Wait 10 minutes before performing the digital removal of stool (Waller & Caroline, 2000). Then adjust laxatives to prevent future constipation.
- If the diarrhea is caused by infection, assess the potential of treating the infection. In acute, self-limited diarrhea, such as common viral-related diarrhea, no antiinfective treatment may be necessary. When pseudomembranous colitis is suspected, begin either metronidazole, 500 mg PO q8h × 10 days (inexpensive) or vancomycin, 125 mg PO q6h × 10 days (expensive) (Skidmore-Roth, 2001; Sykes, 1998; Twycross, 1997).
- For more prolonged infection-related diarrhea, which most often occurs in the AIDS population, the antiinfective is ideally selected based on the documented causative agent. Evaluation of the patient's physical status and preferences regarding treatment and the likelihood of disease response to treatment is essential in planning appropriate treatment. Consultation with an infectious disease specialist is recommended:
  - *Salmonellae* spp. are usually treated with standard antimicrobials.
  - *Isospora belli* sp. are effectively treated with trimethoprim-sulfamethoxazole (Verdier, Fitzgerald, Johnson, & Pape, 2000; Welsby et al., 1998).
  - Cytomegalovirus (CMV) often responds to treatment with ganciclovir or foscarnet.
  - A broad-spectrum antiinfective, such as ciprofloxacin or metronidazole, may be initiated if findings of studies are negative (Welsby et al., 1998). Antiviral agents should also be considered when culture results are negative.
  - AIDS patients with diarrhea respond better to antidiarrheal therapy and have fewer relapses of diarrhea when concurrently treated with antiretroviral therapy or protease inhibitors (Bini & Cohen, 1999; Maggi et al., 2000).
- If diarrhea is caused by fat malabsorption, consider administering pancreatic enzymes. The starting dose of pancreatin or pancrelipase is 2 capsules/tablets PO with meals and 1 capsule/tablet with snacks. The

dose can be increased to 3 capsules/tablets with meals, if needed. Famotidine, an $H_2$ histamine receptor antagonist, has also been noted to increase fat absorption (Waller & Caroline, 2000). The recommended dose is 20 mg PO bid.

- If the diarrhea is due to bile salt malabsorption, administer cholestyramine. This medication absorbs and combines with bile acids to form an insoluble complex that is then eliminated in the feces (Skidmore-Roth, 2001). Administer 4 to 12 g PO tid (Waller & Caroline, 2000).

## Treat Discomfort

Discomfort associated with diarrhea includes gas pain and colicky pain. Simethicone is helpful for gas-related discomfort. Anticholinergic medications treat most colicky pain effectively. Examples of anticholinergic medications include propantheline (Pro-Banthine), 15 mg PO tid; hyoscyamine (Anaspaz, Levsin), 0.125 to 0.25 mg PO tid to qid; and dicyclomine (Antispas, Bentyl), 10 to 20 mg PO tid to qid.

## Control Diarrhea

Because diarrhea can be protective by flushing out irritative substances, avoid antidiarrheals for acute diarrhea. Adsorbent agents, such as attapulgite (Kaopectate), work by taking up substances nonspecifically including bacteria, toxins, and water. They may be helpful for mild diarrhea in the healthy population. However, the large volumes required and their moderate effectiveness make them undesirable for palliative care (Sykes, 1998).

Mucosal prostaglandin inhibitors are helpful for acute diarrhea that requires an antidiarrheal for comfort and for those that involve an inflammatory process (e.g., radiation enteritis). Any nonsteroidal antiinflammatory drug (NSAID), except indomethacin, may be helpful (Sykes, 1998). Bismuth subsalicylate (Pepto-Bismol) is also a mucosal prostaglandin inhibitor. The recommended dosage is 30 ml or 2 tablets PO every 30 to 60 minutes, not to exceed 8 doses per day for more than 2 days (Skidmore-Roth, 2001). Another gastrointestinal antiinflammatory medication is mesalamine (Asacol). Administer 800 mg PO tid.

Opioids are the mainstay of general antidiarrheal treatment in palliative settings (Sykes, 1998). They work by decreasing intestinal motility, leading to increased fluid absorption. Loperamide is the preferred opioid for diarrhea as it does not cross the blood-brain barrier and therefore has the highest antidiarrheal/analgesic ratio of the opioid-like agents (Mercadante, 1998). Loperamide is also about three times more potent than diphenoxylate and 50 times more potent than codeine. It is also long-acting, requiring only twice-daily dosing when long-term management of diarrhea is required. Codeine is the least expensive of these three opioids but has a greater potential for systemic effect (Twycross, 1997). Tincture of opium (paragoric), which is sometimes used when diarrhea is refractory to loperamide, crosses the blood-brain barrier and thus causes systemic opioid effects. The bitter taste of tincture of opium may be nauseating to some persons. Dosages for all of these opioid antidiarrheals are as follows:

- Loperamide (Imodium): Initial dose of 4 mg, followed by 2 mg after each loose stool. The generally accepted maximal dose is 16 mg/day (Waller & Caroline, 2000); doses up to 32 mg/day can be used (Twycross, 1997).
- Diphenoxylate (in Lomotil): 2.5 to 5 mg PO qid, titrated to patient response; not to exceed 8 tablets in 24 hours (Skidmore-Roth, 2001).
- Codeine phosphate: 30 to 60 mg PO tid to qid (Twycross, 1997).
- Tincture of opium: 0.3 to 1 ml PO qid (Skidmore-Roth, 2001; Waller & Caroline, 2000).

Octreotide, an analog of the hormone somatostatin, inhibits GI motility, pancreatic secretion, and intestinal absorption. It has been demonstrated to be effective in the management of chemotherapy-induced diarrhea, diarrhea associated with dumping syndrome, and chronic diarrhea not responsive to specific antimicrobial therapy. It has also been shown to be helpful in controlling diarrhea due to secretory tumors and celiac plexus block (Cascinu, Fedeli, Fedeli, & Catalano, 1993; Dudl, Anderson, Forsythe, Ziegler, & O'Dorisio, 1987; Fried, 1999; Mercadante, 1995). Side effects include nausea, pain at the injection site, and headache. Because octreotide is expensive, this medication is generally reserved for those whose condition is refractory to other interventions. Dosages range from 150 to 600 μg SC/day, either in divided doses or by continuous infusion. Waller & Caroline (2000) suggest the following:

- For chemotherapy or radiation therapy–induced diarrhea, administer 100 μg SC bid.
- For postgastectomy dumping syndrome, administer 300 μg/d SC by continuous infusion.
- For carcinoid syndrome, administer 150 to 300 μg SC bid or 300 to 600 μg/day SC by continuous infusion.

Clonidine may be helpful for some secretory diarrheas. This medication probably acts on enterocytes to suppress the release of secretory substances. The side effects of hypotension and sedation may limit its usefulness in palliative care (Mercadante, 1998).

# ■ PATIENT AND FAMILY EDUCATION

Detailed information from the patient and family is required in order to assess the potential causes of diarrhea and plan appropriate interventions. The APN must teach the importance of prompt and detailed reporting of any changes in bowel patterns:

- Discuss the importance of reporting bowel functioning, include frequency, amount, color, and consistency of stools and any discomforts associated with bowel movements to the health care team.
- Encourage adequate oral fluid intake to replace fluid losses due to diarrhea:
  - Provide instruction on the purchase or preparation of fluids with sugar and electrolytes.

- If intravenous (IV) hydration is required at home, provide instruction on IV site care and maintenance of the IV fluids.
- Teach the following dietary modifications to lessen diarrhea, taking into consideration the patient's desire and ability to eat:
  - Eat/provide small, frequent meals.
  - Avoid excessively hot, cold, or spicy foods.
  - Avoid caffeine.
  - Avoid milk products, fat, whole grains, and fresh fruits and vegetables.
  - Broaden the diet as tolerated, beginning with white bread, pasta, potatoes, rice, and fruits. The old mnemonic "BRAT" may be helpful in remembering acceptable foods: **b**ananas, **r**ice or rice cereals, **a**pplesauce, **t**oast.
  - In persons with a lactase deficiency, teach the use of lactose-free dairy products.
- Teach appropriate use of all medications, including antidiarrheals, anticholinergics, and antiinfective agents:
  - Patients with prolonged diarrhea may require antidiarrheal medications on a schedule rather than as needed.
  - As appropriate to the patient's condition and goals, teach patients with AIDS the importance of maintaining antiretroviral therapy during and after treatment for diarrhea.
  - Instruction on giving subcutaneous injections or maintaining subcutaneous infusions is required for patients who are receiving octreotide.
- Discuss the importance of perianal care:
  - Teach the patient and family good, gentle cleansing techniques using a squeeze bottle of warm water.
  - Teach how to monitor for skin breakdown.
  - Teach appropriate use of petroleum-based ointments and other protective agents (e.g., Stomahesive).

## EVALUATION AND PLAN FOR FOLLOW-UP

The APN frequently monitors the patient's bowel status, hydration status, and level of comfort. If diarrhea continues after instituting a treatment, appropriate changes must occur in the treatment plan. Determine if the cause was not correctly diagnosed or if a different treatment might be more effective. Encourage patients whose diarrhea continues for several days to keep intake and output records. This will assist in evaluating the need for oral or parenteral fluids.

At all times, the patient is evaluated for comfort, including abdominal pain due to gas or gastrointestinal spasm and discomfort associated with skin excoriation. Encourage the patient to describe the type of abdominal discomfort so that appropriate interventions are prescribed. Teach good skin care to prevent skin excoriation and instruct the patient and caregivers to report skin discomfort or any changes in the condition of the skin.

✔ **CASE**

**STUDY**
The daughter of Mrs. Anderson, an 82-year-old patient with advanced ovarian cancer, calls to report that her mother has had several bouts of diarrhea over the last 2 days. The daughter states that she gave her mother a few doses of loperamide (Imodium) both yesterday and today, but the diarrhea continues. She also reports that her mother is complaining of abdominal pain and cramping with the diarrhea. Mrs. Anderson's medications include the following:

- Sustained-release oxycodone, 40 mg PO bid, with a rescue of oxycodone, 10 mg PO q1-2h prn for pain
- Docusate sodium, 100 mg, plus casanthranol, 2 30 mg capsules PO hs for constipation
- Lorazepam, 1 mg PO q6h prn for anxiety
- Spironolactone, 200 mg PO qd, and furosemide, 40 mg PO, for ascites and peripheral edema
- Digoxin, 0.125 mg PO qd for heart failure (well-controlled)

The APN's questions elicit the following information. The diarrhea is dark and has the consistency of mucus. It occurs in small amounts, "maybe a quarter of a cup or so," five or six times during the day and night. There is no pattern related to food intake. Mrs. Anderson is complaining of intermittent cramping pains in her lower abdomen and a sensation of rectal fullness: "like her bowels are still full even after the diarrhea." The patient's last regular bowel movement was 5 days ago. Mrs. Anderson's ascites is markedly improved since adding the furosemide to the spironolactone 7 days ago.

The APN suspects a fecal impaction with overflow diarrhea and instructs the family to give no additional loperamide and to give Mrs. Anderson a dose of her immediate-release oxycodone for the discomfort. The APN schedules a home visit for later in the afternoon. Upon arrival the APN notes that the patient's mucous membranes are dry and that she has poor skin turgor. The physical assessment reveals a distended abdomen, with mild ascites. Bowel sounds are intermittent, high-pitched, and tinkling. There is dark liquid stool around the rectum, and a digital rectal examination reveals a large mass of hard, dry stool in the rectum.

The APN tells the patient and family that the diarrhea is caused by a blockage of the bowel with hard stool. She explains the need for removal of the impaction, gives the patient an oil retention enema, and instructs the daughter to give Mrs. Anderson her lorazepam and immediate-release oxycodone.

While waiting for the stool to soften as much as possible with the enema and for the medications to begin to work, the APN explains that the combination of the pain medication, decreased fluid intake, and medications for the ascites contributed to the patient's impaction. The APN discusses the following instructions with the patient and family:

- Withhold the furosemide.
- Increase the docusate sodium, 100 mg plus casanthranol 30 mg to 2 capsules bid.

- Monitor bowel movements:
  - If no bowel movement occurs in 2 days, give a 10-mg bisacodyl suppository. If there are no results, call the APN.
  - If diarrhea occurs, call the APN.
- Increase fluid intake by mouth, as tolerated:
  - Mix a solution of ½ teaspoon salt, ½ teaspoon baking soda, and 4 tablespoons sugar in 1 liter of water. Mrs. Anderson should sip the drink during the day, aiming to drink 1 liter of the fluid each day.
  - If the patient is unable to drink at least 1 liter a day, contact the APN.

The APN also writes these instructions because the patient's discomfort and medications may interfere with her understanding at the present time.

After providing local anesthesia of the anus and rectum with lidocaine jelly, the APN digitally removes the impaction and gives a cleansing enema. The nurse cleans the rectal area with a squeeze bottle of warm water and applies petroleum jelly to the reddened but intact skin. She reinforces the instructions and plans a follow-up phone call in the morning.

## References

Anastasi, J. K., & Capili, B. (2000). HIV and diarrhea in the era of HAART: 1998 New York State hospitalizations. *American Journal of Infection Control, 28,* 262-266.

Bini, E. J., & Cohen, J. (1999). Impact of protease inhibitors on the outcome of human immunodeficiency virus–infected patients with chronic diarrhea. *American Journal of Gastroenterology, 94,* 3553-3559.

Bickley, L. S., & Hoekelman, R. A. (1999a). The abdomen. In L. S. Bickley & R. A. Hoekelman (Eds.), *Bates' guide to physical examination and history taking* (7th ed.) (pp. 355-386). Philadelphia: Lippincott.

Bickley, L. S., & Hoekelman, R. A. (1999b). An approach to symptoms. In L. S. Bickley & R. A. Hoekelman (Eds.), *Bates' guide to physical examination and history taking* (7th ed.) (pp. 43-105). Philadelphia: Lippincott.

Carpenito, L. J. (2000). *Nursing diagnosis: Application to clinical practice* (8th ed.). Philadelphia: Lippincott.

Cascinu, S., Fedeli, A., Fedeli, S. L., & Catalano, G. (1993). Octreotide versus loperamide in the treatment of fluorouracil-induced diarrhea: A randomized trial. *Journal of Clinical Oncology, 11,* 148-151.

Clark, D. P. (1999). New insights into human cryptosporidiosis. *Clinical Microbiology Review, 12,* 554-563.

Dudl, R., Anderson, D., Forsythe, A., Ziegler, M., & O'Dorisio, T. (1987). Treatment of diabetic diarrhea and orthostatic hypotension with somatostatin analogue SMS 201-995. *American Journal of Medicine, 83,* 584-588.

Fried, M. (1999). Octreotide in the treatment of refractory diarrhea. *Digestion, 60* (suppl. 2), 42-46.

Guyton. A. C., & Hall, J. E. (1996a). Secretory functions of the alimentary tract. In A. C. Guyton & J. E. Hall (Eds.), *Textbook of medical physiology* (9th ed.) (pp. 815-832). Philadelphia: W. B. Saunders.

Guyton. A. C., & Hall, J. E. (1996b). Principles of gastrointestinal function—motility, nervous control, and blood circulation. In A. C. Guyton & J. E. Hall (Eds.), *Textbook of medical physiology* (9th ed.) (pp. 793-803). Philadelphia: W. B. Saunders.

GUYTON. A. C., & Hall, J. E. (1996c). Physiology of gastrointestinal disorders. In A. C. Guyton & J. E. Hall (Eds.), *Textbook of medical physiology* (9th ed.) (pp. 845-851). Philadelphia: W. B. Saunders.

GUYTON. A. C., & Hall, J. E. (1996d). Transport and mixing of food in the alimentary tract. In A. C. Guyton & J. E. Hall (Eds.), *Textbook of medical physiology* (9th ed.) (pp. 803-813). Philadelphia: W. B. Saunders.

GUYTON. A. C., & Hall, J. E. (1996e). Circulatory shock and physiology of its treatment. In A. C. Guyton & J. E. Hall (Eds.), *Textbook of medical physiology* (9th ed.) (pp. 285-294). Philadelphia: W. B. Saunders.

HOLODNIY, M., Koch, J., Mistal, M., Schmidt, J. M., Khandwala, A., Pennington, J. E., & Porter, S. B. (1999). A double-blind, randomized, placebo-controlled phase II study to assess the safety and efficacy of orally administered SP-303 for the symptomatic treatment of diarrhea in patients with AIDS. *American Journal of Gastroenterology, 94,* 3267-3273.

KEMP, C. (1999). *Terminal illness: A guide to nursing care* (2nd ed.). Philadelphia: Lippincott.

LEVY, M. H. (1991). Constipation and diarrhea in cancer patients. *The Cancer Bulletin, 43,* 412-422.

LUCKMANN, J. (1997). Caring for people with gastrointestinal disorders. In J. Luckmann (Ed.), *Saunders' manual of nursing care* (pp. 1241-1299). Philadelphia: W. B. Saunders.

MAGGI, P., Larocca, A. M., Quarto, M., Serio, G., Brandonisio, O., Angarano, G., & Pastore, G. (2000). Effect of antiretroviral therapy on cryptosporidiosis and microsporidiosis in patients infected with human immunodeficiency virus type 1. *European Journal of Clinical Microbiology and Infectious Disease, 19,* 213-217.

MERCADANTE, S. (1995). Octreotide in the treatment of diarrhea induced by celiac plexus block. *Pain, 61,* 345-346.

MERCADANTE, S. (1998). Diarrhea, malabsorption, and constipation. In A. Berger, R. K. Portenoy, & D. E. Weissman (Eds.), *Principles and practice of supportive oncology* (pp. 191-205). Philadelphia: Lippincott-Raven.

NATIONAL Cancer Institute. (1999). *Common toxicity criteria: Version 2.0.* Bethesda, MD: Author.

SIMON, D. (1998). Evaluation of diarrhea in HIV-infected patients. *Gastrointestinal Endoscopy Clinics of North America, 8,* 857-867.

SKIDMORE-ROTH, L. (2001). *Mosby's 2001 nursing drug reference.* St. Louis: Mosby.

SYKES, N. P. (1998). Constipation and diarrhea. In D. Doyle, G.W.C. Hanks, & N. MacDonald (Eds.). *Oxford textbook of palliative medicine* (2nd ed.) (pp. 513-526). New York: Oxford University Press.

TWYCROSS, R. (1997). *Symptom management in advanced cancer* (2nd ed.). Oxon, UK: Radcliffe Medical Press.

VERDIER, R., Fitzgerald, D., Johnson, W., & Pape, J. (2000). Trimethoprim-sulfamethoxazole compared with ciprofloxacin for treatment and prophylaxis of *Isospora belli* and *Cyclospora cayetanensis* infection in HIV-infected patients: A randomized controlled trial. *Annals of Internal Medicine, 132,* 885-888.

WALLER, A., & Caroline, N. L. (2000). *Handbook of palliative care in cancer* (2nd ed.). Boston: Butterworth-Heinemann.

WELSBY, P. D., Richardson, A., & Brettle, R. P. (1998). AIDS: Aspects in adults. In D. Doyle, G. W. C. Hanks, & N. MacDonald (Eds.), *Oxford textbook of palliative medicine* (2nd ed.) (pp. 1121-1148). New York: Oxford University Press.

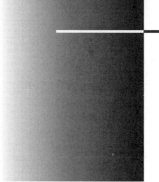

# Dyspnea

KIM K. KUEBLER

## ■ DEFINITION AND INCIDENCE

At the end of life, 50% to 75% of persons are affected by dyspnea, cited as one of the most prevalent symptoms in advanced disease (Ahmedzai, 1990; Ahmedzai, 1993; Bruera, MacEachern, Ripamonti, & Hanson, 1993; Dudgeon, 1997; Twycross, 1997). Dyspnea is a subjective symptom, and is most often defined or described as "difficult breathing" or "an uncomfortable awareness of breathing" (Bruera, Macmillan, Pither, & MacDonald, 1990; Cohen, Johnson-Anderson, Krasnow & Wadleigh, 1992). Patients with dyspnea further describe their breathing as "labored" or as a "severe shortness of breath" or as a sensation of "suffocation." Recognizing the multidimensional nature of dyspnea, the American Thoracic Society (ATS) broadened its definition to include the interplay among physiologic, psychologic, social, and environmental factors, characterizing dyspnea as "a subjective experience of breathing discomfort that consists of qualitatively distinct sensations that vary in intensity. The physiologic factors of dyspnea may also induce secondary physiological and behavioral responses" (American Thoracic Society, 1999, pg. 322).

Dyspnea accounts for much of affected persons' inability to carry out activities of daily living, gravely affecting their quality of life (American Thoracic Society, 1999; Cohen et al., 1992; Cowcher & Hanks, 1990; Dudgeon & Rosenthal, 1996; Gift & Pugh, 1993; Twycross, 1997). Regardless of cause, the continuous exhaustion accompanying breathlessness is described as one of the most devastating symptoms for both patient and the observing family (Bruera et al, 1990; Kuebler et al., 1996).

## ■ ETIOLOGY AND PATHOPHYSIOLOGY

Dyspnea should be viewed as a warning of a potential underlying medical condition (Ahmedzai, 1998; Twycross, 1997). Identification of these causative mechanisms is critical to the appropriate management of dyspnea. In the palliative care setting although the underlying medical condition may not be treatable, the symptom almost always responds to intervention or treatment. A patient may have more than one specific cause of breathlessness, leading to greater distress, and in addition to the physiologic mechanism, the patient's psychologic and emotional state may also produce or exacerbate the symptom of dyspnea.

## Normal Control of Breathing

In order to understand the many processes leading to dyspnea, it is helpful to review the normal physiologic characteristics of breathing. The respiratory center in the medulla oblongata responds to stimuli from four primary sources (American Thoracic Society, 1999; Guyton & Hall, 1996):

- Chemoreceptors in the aorta, carotid arteries, and medulla sense changes in $Po_2$, $Pco_2$, and pH and transmit signals back to the respiratory center to adjust breathing. The peripheral chemoreceptors (i.e., those in the aortic arch and carotid arteries) are most sensitive to changes in $Po_2$. When $Po_2$ decreases, ventilation increases. However, hypoxia must be fairly profound before this change in respiratory pattern is seen. The central chemoreceptors of the medulla are very sensitive to changes in pH. Changes in pH are closely related to $Pco_2$. Hypercapnia leads to a decrease in pH, which then stimulates ventilation.
- Mechanoreceptors in the diaphragm and chest wall sense changes in the work of breathing. When an increased work load is sensed, the respiratory center stimulates the diaphragm and respiratory muscles and attempts to expand the lungs.
- Vagal receptors in the airways and lungs also influence breathing. Afferent impulses are generated when (1) stretch receptors in the lungs are stimulated as the lungs expand, (2) irritant receptors in the bronchial walls are stimulated, or (3) C fibers in the interstitium of the lungs respond to increases in pulmonary interstitial or capillary pressure.
- Cortical areas of the brain affect breathing by allowing individuals to consciously increase or decrease their respiratory rate. It also appears that the chemoreceptors, mechanoreceptors, and respiratory center itself send messages to higher brain centers, leading to a cognitive awareness of the ventilatory demand.

## Mechanisms Leading to Dyspnea

Several factors lead to dyspnea, that is, "uncomfortable awareness of breathing." Blood-gas abnormalities are sensed by the chemoreceptors. As stated, the central chemoreceptors of the medulla are particularly sensitive to changes in pH. Any condition causing retention of $CO_2$, such as chronic obstructive pulmonary disease (COPD), leads to hypercapnia and a lowering of the pH. Even a slight lowering of the pH stimulates ventilation. Persons with hypercapnia experience dyspnea. It is not clear whether dyspnea is a direct effect of chemoreceptor stimulation to higher brain centers or the cognitive perception of the increased ventilatory demand. However, hypoxia must be fairly profound to stimulate the peripheral chemoreceptors, leading to increased ventilation. Hypoxia may cause the perception of dyspnea even in the absence of increased ventilatory demand (American Thoracic Society, 1999; Guyton & Hall, 1996).

Increased ventilatory demand, as occurs during exercise, certainly increases respiratory rate. When a healthy person performs strenuous exercise, for example, this increased demand is perceived as hyperpnea (increased depth) or tachypnea (increased rate), but not dyspnea (difficulty breathing). Some disease processes such as cardiovascular disease and lung parenchymal diseases increase the ventilatory demand to compensate for enlarged dead space. This increased demand is often perceived as dyspnea. In addition, persons with prolonged inactivity become deconditioned. In a deconditioned state even normal activities lead to an increased ventilatory demand via early lactic acid production by skeletal muscles. If hyperpnea results from routine or minimal activity, it is perceived as dyspnea (American Thoracic Society, 1999).

Respiratory muscle abnormalities lead to a mismatch between the central respiratory motor output and the achieved ventilation. Respiratory muscle weakness, whether caused by generalized weakness or a neuromuscular disorder, is perceived as dyspnea. Many persons with advanced diseases experience anorexia, cachexia, and generalized weakness and are at risk for experiencing dyspnea. In diseases that cause overinflation of the lung and overexpansion of the thorax the muscles of inspiration become weakened, leading to the sensation of dyspnea (American Thoracic Society, 1999; Guyton & Hall, 1996). This dyspnea may be mediated via mechanoreceptor messages to the cortex.

Abnormal ventilatory impedance (e.g., narrow airways or increased airway resistance) leads to stimulation of increased central respiratory motor output. When the effort expended to breathe is not matched by the level of ventilation, dyspnea is perceived (American Thoracic Society, 1999). This perception may result from vagal or mechanoreceptor stimulation of the cortex.

Cognitive factors also influence the perception of dyspnea (American Thoracic Society, 1999; Guyton & Hall, 1996; Kuebler et al., 1996; Twycross, 1997). Although many physiologic mechanisms lead to a perception of dyspnea, not all dyspnea is a direct result of pathologic structural characteristics. Psychologic states are interrelated to the dyspneic experience, which may be caused or exacerbated by anxiety, fear, hopelessness, and depression. Breathlessness that precipitates anxiety, leading to increased breathlessness and even more anxiety, is commonly called the "snowball effect." Shortness of breath is less frightening when individuals believe that it is treatable and that they have prompt access to treatment, and their level of perceived dyspnea decreases.

Dyspnea is predominantly experienced by persons with pulmonary, cardiac, and neuromuscular diseases (Ahmedzai, 1998; Carrieri-Kohlman & Janson-Bjerklie, 1993; Twycross, 1997). Table 24-1 summarizes many of the causes of dyspnea in the terminally ill. Note also that cognitive factors may contribute to all causes of dyspnea; thus they are not included. Although respiratory muscle abnormality due to weakness may be present in almost all advanced diseases, also listed in Table 24-1 are diseases in which weakness is most profound.

## ■ ASSESSMENT AND MEASUREMENT

The assessment of dyspnea in palliative care should be aimed at characterization of the symptom rather than understanding of the functional and gas-exchange abnormalities (Ripamonti & Bruera, 1997). This assessment of dyspnea includes the collection of both subjective and objective data; numerous assessment tools to this end have been identified (Ahmedzai, 1998; Bruera, Kuehn, Miller, Selmser, & Selmser, 1991; Gift, 1997; Gift & Narsavage, 1998; Ripamonti & Bruera, 1997), though not all are suited to the palliative care setting.

### Subjective Indicators

As stated by the ATS, the dyspneic experience is what the person describes it to be (American Thoracic Society, 1999). Thus it is important to elicit pa-

| TABLE 24-1 | | | | |
|---|---|---|---|---|
| **Causes of Dyspnea in Terminal Illness** | | | | |
| Disease Process | Blood-Gas Abnormalities | Increased Ventilatory Demand | Respiratory Muscle Abnormality | Ventilatory Impedance |
| **PULMONARY DISEASE** | | | | |
| COPD | X | X | X | X |
| Asthma | | X | | X |
| Cystic fibrosis | X | | X | X |
| Pneumonia | X | | | X |
| Pleural effusion | X | X | | X |
| Malignancy | X | X | X | X |
| Radiation pneumonitis | X | | | X |
| Pulmonary embolism | X | | | X |
| **CARDIOVASCULAR DISEASE** | | | | |
| Heart failure | | X | | X |
| Myopathies | X | X | | |
| Anemia | X | | X | |
| Superior vena cava syndrome | X | | | X |
| **NEUROMUSCULAR DISEASE** | | | | |
| Muscular dystrophy | | X | X | |
| Myasthenia gravis | | X | X | |
| Amyotrophic lateral sclerosis | | X | X | |
| Paralysis of diaphragm | | X | X | |

tients' subjective descriptions of their breathing. A visual analogue scale with "Not at all breathless" at the low end and "Severely breathless" at the high end of the scale may be most clinically useful to evaluate, document, and communicate the assessment (Kuebler et al., 1996). The descriptors patients use may be helpful in identifying the cause of dyspnea. Words such as *rapid* and *heavy* correlate with exercise, *tight* is associated with asthma, and persons with congestive heart failure often use the word *suffocation* (Simon, Schwartzstein & Weiss, 1990).

An assessment of patients' psychoemotional status, including anxiety, fear, depression, and powerlessness, and the perceived effect of dyspnea on quality of living must be included in the overall evaluation of this symptom.

## Objective Indicators

Observation of the patient's respiratory rate, depth, and effort is helpful to assessment. Note that tachypnea, hyperpnea, and hyperventilation, although they should be assessed and documented, should not be used to define dyspnea (Ahmedzai, 1998; Twycross, 1997).

The reductions in functional activities and the effect of dyspnea on the patient's perceived quality of life should be considered when assessing the multidimensional person (Ahmedzai, 1998; American Thoracic Society, 1999). Functional assessment requires further inquiry into the patient's activity or exercise tolerance. It is important for the clinician assessing the severity of dyspnea in the terminal setting to consider the patient's position on the continuum of the disease state. For example, assessing exercise tolerance is not appropriate for the bedridden patient. When documenting activity tolerance identify the degree of dyspnea caused by various activities such as walking, talking, eating, and self-care.

Observational data are essential for the management of the unresponsive dyspneic patient. Behavioral signs that indicate difficulty in breathing, such as increased respiratory rate, restlessness, diaphoresis, use of accessory muscles, or gasping, must be documented. Note that rapid and difficult respiration breathing indicates discomfort and requires further assessment to determine whether the discomfort is due to dyspnea or some other physical or emotional discomfort (Kuebler & Ogle, 1998).

## ■ HISTORY AND PHYSICAL EXAMINATION

The entire respiratory system, including the nose, mouth, pharynx, larynx, lungs, airways, bony and muscular thoracic cage, and peripheral and central centers involving respiratory drive, should be evaluated in the physical examination (Ahmedzai, 1998). Aging and gender affect airflow and chest wall dynamics and should be considered. A positive history of smoking and the effects of chronic illness are also significant contributors to the subjective dyspneic experience (Ahmedzai, 1998; Shepherd & Geraci, 1999).

## History

- Medical diagnosis, including pulmonary, cardiovascular, and neuromuscular disorders
- Treatment history, including surgery, radiation therapy, and chemotherapy
- Smoking history
- Allergies

## Physical Examination

- Cardiovascular
- Heart assessment (heart and vessels)
- Distant heart sounds (severe heart failure, pericardial effusions, and pulmonary hyperinflation)
- Second prominent pulmonic sound (pulmonary hypertension of any cause, pulmonary embolism)
- Third heart sound (systolic heart failure)
- Fourth heart sound (diastolic ventricular dysfunction, ischemic heart disease, cardiomyopathy)
- Murmurs (stenosis, insufficiency, septal defects, congenital heart disease, pericardial rubs)
- Jugular venous distension (pulmonary hypertension)
- Lung/ventilatory mechanics (upper and lower airways, lungs, pleura, and thoracic)
- Use of accessory muscles
- Percussion (subcutaneous crepitus)
- Rales, rhonchi, and wheezing (bronchial narrowing from edema or constriction)
- Friction rub (inflammation in pleura or pericardium)
- Popping, clicking, or crunching near the heart (mediastinal emphysema)
- Tracheal deviation (mediastinal mass, atelectasis, pneumothorax)
- Ability to finish a sentence without pausing
- Tissue oxygenation (skin, nails, mucous membranes, and mental status)
- Abdomen (ascites, organomegaly, obesity)
- Thyroid assessment
- Fever
- Nutrition and fluid status

## ■ DIAGNOSTICS

Although diagnostic procedures can be helpful in identifying the causes of dyspnea and monitoring the course of the illness, the practitioner must use sound judgment in evaluating the appropriateness of these diagnostic tests in palliative care. Diagnostic tests are appropriate when the information provided influences the course of treatment. When a diagnosis can reasonably be based on clinical presentation alone, the burdens and costs of diagnostic tests must be considered. For example a patient with COPD who is experiencing with moist rales, productive cough, and fever does not necessarily need chest radiography to identify pneumonia; radiography would certainly be appropriate, however, when verifying the presence and extent of pleural effusion before placement of a chest tube. With these precautions in mind the following diagnostic tests may provide helpful information in the dyspneic patient.

Ripamonti and Bruera (1997) point out that a chest radiograph, digital oximetry, and simple blood tests rule out significant causes of dyspnea. Pulmonary function tests can be useful when assessing obstructive and restrictive pulmonary diseases as well as neuromuscular weakness. These tests are easily performed at the bedside and can also help determine the response of bronchodilator therapies. Other diagnostics may include (Ahmedzai, 1998; Harwood, 1999; Kuebler et al., 1996; Shepherd & Geraci, 1999; Twycross; 1997) the following:

- Exercise tests (ergometer tests)
- Pulmonary function tests (proof of airflow obstruction and efficacy of specific interventions)
- Chest radiographs used to exclude conditions such as pleural effusion or heart failure (both treatable conditions)
- Ultrasound
- Ventilation perfusion scan
- Blood counts (hemoglobin and hematocrit, complete blood count [CBC], blood chemical tests)
- Skin oxygen saturation ($Spo_2$)

The following tests are rarely used in the palliative setting as a result of patient burden and cost considerations:

- Arterial blood gases
- Echocardiography
- Pulmonary angiography
- Computed tomography (CT)

## ■ INTERVENTION AND TREATMENT

The underlying cause of dyspnea should be treated, whenever possible, paying attention to prognosis, adverse effects, cost, and potential outcomes (Ahmedzai, 1998). All reasonable treatment options should be reviewed with the patient and family, including, possibly no treatment. The support of an interdisciplinary team of experts is essential in the management of dyspnea. The following discussion predominantly focuses on the pharmacologic management of dyspnea, remembering that all other dimensions of the human experience require ongoing assessment and intervention. Table 24-2 summarizes options for management of dyspnea based on its cause. The content of each intervention includes additional details of these interventions.

| TABLE 24-2 | |
| --- | --- |

### Correctable Causes of Dyspnea/Breathlessness

| Causes | Management |
| --- | --- |
| Respiratory infection | Antibiotics |
| | Expectorant |
| | Physiotherapy |
| COPD | Bronchodilators |
| Asthma | Corticosteroids |
| | Physiotherapy |
| Hypoxia | Trial of oxygen |
| Bronchial obstruction/lung collapse | Corticosteroids |
| Mediastinal obstruction | Radiotherapy |
| | LASER therapy |
| | Stint |
| Lymphangitis carcinomatosa | Corticosteroids |
| | Diuretics |
| | Bronchodilators |
| Pleural effusion | Paracentesis |
| | Pleurodesis |
| Ascites | Diuretics |
| | Paracentesis |
| Pericardial effusion | Paracentesis |
| | Corticosteroids |
| Anemia | Blood transfusion |
| | Erythropoietin |
| Cardiac failure | Diuretics |
| | Digoxin |
| | ACE inhibitors |
| Pulmonary embolism | Anticoagulants (if appropriate) |

From Twycross, R. (1999). Correctable causes of breathlessness. In *Introducing palliative care* (p. 123). Oxon, UK: Radcliffe Medical Press.

## Pharmacologic Interventions

**Opioids.**  Morphine, the most widely used pharmaceutical in the relief of dyspnea, is the basis of treatment (Ahmedzai, 1998; Dudgeon, 1997; Kuebler et al., 1996; Twycross, 1997). However, as Ahmedzai points out, this does not mean the use of opioids for dyspnea is properly understood; nor does it ensure proper opioid utilization for treatment (Ahmedzai, 1998).

Opioids may alleviate dyspnea by blunting the perceptual response to the symptom (American Thoracic Society, 1999). Twycross (1997) relates that morphine reduces the respiratory drive and can be used to relieve the symptom of breathlessness. Data from several clinical studies reveal that 80% to 95% of terminal cancer patients found significant relief through the utilization of morphine (Harwood, 1999; Mahler, 1990). The required dose of morphine for relief of dyspnea is influenced by the patient's current opioid regimen. The opioid naive patient may begin with 5 to 6 mg of morphine q4h as a starting dose. If the patient is on morphine for pain and remains dyspneic increasing the dose by 50% is recommended (Twycross, 1997).

Nebulized morphine is used for the treatment of dyspnea but has received mixed reviews. Opioid receptors are present on the sensory nerves within the respiratory tract (American Thoracic Society, 1999; Harwood, 1999). Ahmedzai (1998) postulates that morphine given via a nebulizer has a direct pulmonary effect. Despite the anecdotal evidence of many studies supporting the use of nebulized morphine, more recent controlled studies have yielded either inconclusive or negative results of this route of administration (Davis et al., 1994; Leung, Hill & Burdon, 1996; Masoud, Reed, & Thomas, 1995). Davis (1996) demonstrated nebulized morphine has no effect on dyspnea better than or different from that of nebulized saline solution. The usual starting dose for nebulized morphine is 2 to 2.5 mg preservative-free morphine in 3 cc of sterile saline solution. The dose may be titrated up to 10 to 20 mg morphine.

**Anxiolytics.**    Both benzodiazepines and phenothiazines have been shown to be effective in the management of dyspnea. Each has the potential to depress hypoxic and ventilator responses and can alter the emotional responses to dyspnea (Ahmedzai, 1998; Leung et al., 1996). Findings of controlled studies assessing the efficacy of benzodiazepines used for the treatment of dyspnea have proved inconsistent, and these medications are poorly tolerated in long-term therapy (Ahmedzai, 1998; American Thoracic Society, 1999; Dudgeon, 1997). There have been both beneficial and negative therapeutic results associated with diazepam and alprazolam (Dudgeon, 1997). Benzodiazepines are metabolized by the liver to long-acting metabolites.

Phenothiazines such as chlorpromazine and promethazine have been found useful in patients experiencing anxiety associated with the dyspneic experience (Dudgeon, 1997; McIver, Walsh, & Nelson, 1994; Woodcook, Gross, & Geddes, 1981). Combining morphine with chlorpromazine or promethazine was effective, unlike using a combination of morphine and prochlorperazine. Chlorpromazine and promethazine alone without morphine have been found to be effective in reducing symptoms of breathlessness in healthy persons and those with COPD (Dudgeon, 1997). Phenothiazines have anticholinergic properties that can also be used for respiratory secretions and are also useful as antiemetics. The following anxiolytics have been used to treat dyspnea:

- Lorazepam, 0.5 mg q4-6h titrated to effect
- Diazepam, 5 to 10 mg stat in the very anxious patient; 2 to 5 mg in the elderly
- Chlorpromazine (titrated to effect), 10 mg q4-6h and prn
- Promethazine (titrated to effect), 12.5 mg q4-6h and prn

Given the prevalence of anxiety associated with the experience of breathlessness it is considered good palliative care to institute anxiolytic therapy on an individual basis, paying attention to pathophysiology, metabolism, symptomatic response, and the presence of adverse effects.

**Corticosteroids.** Corticosteroids are frequently used in palliative care for the treatment of dyspnea. The mechanism of action is not clear; it is believed that the reduction in perceived dyspnea is due to the decrease in inflammation and increase in bronchodilatation (Carrieri-Kohlman & Janson-Bjerklie, 1993). Initiation of corticosteroid therapy is usually indicated when bronchodilators prove ineffective in relieving airflow obstruction. Ahmedzai (1998) believes that it is justifiable to administer steroids to almost all patients with problematic chronic airway disease. He recommends that the dose of steroid be high enough to work efficiently yet not cause gastric irritation or fluid retention (Ahmedzai, 1998).

The following is recommended for the treatment of dyspnea with corticosteroids (Pereira & Bruera, 1997):

- Prednisone, 30 to 60 mg/day
- Dexamethasone, 6 to 8 mg tid to qid

**Bronchodilators.** Bronchodilators help to decrease the effort of breathing, and several studies note their effect on breathlessness. The significant decrease in dyspnea produced by theophylline is believed to result from an improvement in the length-tension relationship of the diaphragm (Carrieri-Kohlman & Janson-Bjerklie, 1993).

Most bronchodilators fall under the category of medications termed *sympathomimetic drugs*. Most of these drugs are direct-acting agonists that stimulate the adrenergic receptors and range from being totally nonselective to being highly selective. Selective sympathomimetic medications stimulate only alpha and beta receptors. Table 24-3 highlights the most frequently used bronchodilators with attention to usefulness, dose, and route. Note that the most frequently used bronchodilators are the selective beta-2 agonists (Shlafer & Marieb, 1989).

An important consideration in choosing a specific bronchodilator for symptomatic treatment of bronchial asthma, emphysema, and other common respiratory disorders is understanding the effects of the medications. Patients with pulmonary disease who have an associated cardiac disorder can benefit from a nonselective agonist (Shlafer & Marieb, 1989). Excessive use of the beta-adrenergic agents may cause cardiac stimulation and may be particularly harmful in the elderly and those with cardiac disease (Ahmedzai, 1998; Carrieri-Kohlman & Janson-Bjerklie, 1993). Selective beta-2 agonists are widely used as bronchodilators for both chronic and acute pulmonary disorders such as asthma, bronchitis, and emphysema. Tolerance to bronchodilators does occur over time and requires ongoing evaluation (Shlafer & Marieb, 1989).

## Nonpharmacologic Interventions

**Oxygen therapy.** The literature does not support the utilization of oxygen therapy for the relief of dyspnea in and of itself. Therapeutic indications for oxygen use include hypoxemia or a tendency to development of pulmonary hypertension. If $O_2$ saturation is below 90% on room air the clinician may want to consider $O_2$ by nasal cannula at 1 to 3 liter/min, rechecking the

| TABLE 24-3 | | |
|---|---|---|

### Reversable Causes of Cough

| Prototype | Clinical Usefulness | Dose/Route |
|---|---|---|
| **NONSELECTIVE AGONISTS** | | |
| Epinephrine | Acute bronchoconstriction | SC: titrate 0.2-1 mg prn |
| | Sus-Phrine: longer-acting broncho-dilation, acute asthma, anaphylaxis | SC: titrate 0.5-1.5 mg q6h prn |
| | Epinephrine inhaler, Primatene, Vapo-nefrin: wheezing, bronchoconstriction, asthma | Inhaler: 1 puff (200 $\mu$g) q3-4h prn |
| **NONSELECTIVE BETA AGONISTS** | | |
| Isoproterenol | Isuprel: intraoperative bronchospasm | IV push: 0.2 mg (1 ml) in 10 ml NaCl or 5% dextrose; titrate 0.01-0.02 mg (0.5-1 ml) prn |
| | Isuprel: chronic bron-choconstriction, asthma | SL: titrate 10-15 mg tablet prn |
| | Isuprel inhaler: bron-choconstriction in asthma, COPD | Inhaler: 1-2 puffs (130 $\mu$g each) up to five times/day prn Nebulizer: 5-15 deep inhalations of 10 mg/ml solution |
| Ethylnorepi-nephrine | Acute bronchospasm | SC, IM: 1-2 mg (0.5-1 ml) prn |
| **SELECTIVE BETA-2 AGONISTS** | | |
| Albuterol sulfate | Proventil/Ventolin: bronchodilation in asthma, COPD Alupent: bronchodila-tion for chronic pul-monary disease | Inhaler: 1-2 puffs (90 $\mu$g each) q4-6h PO: 2-4 mg q3-4h; maximum, 8 mg qid Inhaler: 3-4 puffs q3-4h prn; maxi-mum, 12 puffs/day Nebulizer: 10 deep inhalations of undiluted 5% solution q4h prn PO: 10- to 20-mg tablets tid/qid |

Twycross, R., Wilcock, A., & Thorp, S. (1998). *Palliative care formulary.* Oxon, UK: Radcliffe Medical Press.

patient's $O_2$ saturation in 20 to 30 minutes and titrating up to 6 liters/min if necessary by nasal cannula (Ahmedzai, 1998; Pereira & Bruera, 1997).

**Cancer treatments.**   Patients who have obstructive lung tumor or supe-rior vena cava syndrome may benefit from palliative use of chemotherapy or radiation therapy to shrink the tumor. The appropriateness of these interven-tions depends on the patient's overall performance status, previous exposure to the treatments, benefit-burden assessment, and patient/family preferences.

**Procedures.**   If dyspnea is caused by accumulation of fluid in the pleural or abdominal cavities, thoracentesis or paracentesis is indicated.

**Complementary therapies.**   The following nonpharmacologic interventions are very effective in modifying the perception of dyspnea and can assist in decreasing respiratory rate and managing anxiety:
- Pursed-lip breathing
- Breathing exercises
- Positioning
- Cool air (bedside fan)
- Cool compresses on face
- Coping techniques
- Calming presence
- Relaxation therapy
- Massage
- Visualization
- Acupuncture
- Hypnosis.

# ■ PATIENT AND FAMILY EDUCATION

The goal of palliative therapy is to lessen the effect of dyspnea on the patient's quality of life. Ongoing assessment and patient family education about contributory factors, and pharmacologic and nonpharmacologic management can help relieve the dyspneic experience.

# ■ EVALUATION AND PLAN FOR FOLLOW-UP

Severe changes in the patient's pattern and onset of dyspnea should be drawn to the attention of the advanced practice nurse (APN). Frequent and ongoing communication with the patient, family, and health care team is paramount to ensure a multidimensional approach in the care and quality of life for the dyspneic patient.

✔ **CASE STUDY**

Thomas, a 56-year-old white male, presents with a diagnosis of stage IV metastatic squamous cell carcinoma of the left lung. His initial computed tomography (CT) scan identifies tumor extension from the upper left lung into the posterior chest wall. Thomas experiences long-standing chest pain that he describes as anterior left-sided "sharp pain" accompanied by debilitating dyspnea and hemoptysis. Findings from a thorough cardiac assessment are negative.

Exploratory thoracotomy reveals an unresectable tumor of the left lung with possible metastatic nodules in the right lung. The tests of the liver yield negative findings for metastatic disease. Bone scanning shows scapular involvement. Thomas and his wife are offered chemotherapy and radiation. He has tremendous fear of these interventions, however, because he believes that his mother-in-law suffered needlessly as a result of aggressive therapies in her advanced malignancy. He refuses any therapy and enters into a local hospice program.

His initial medications include transdermal fentanyl, which does not manage either his pain or dyspnea. Tom rates his pain intensity at a 9 on a 0 to 10 scale and his dyspnea is "off the scale" as he struggles to complete a sentence. His respiratory rate is 32. He is frustrated by his inability to perform any functions of daily living. After a complete physical examination, the APN employs the following interventions:

- Discontinuation of the transdermal fentanyl and administration of equianalgesic sustained-release morphine and its equivalent breakthrough dose
- Addition of prednisone, 20 mg qd, for both somatic pain and the antiinflammatory effects of dyspnea
- Titration of chlorpromazine from the initial dose of 10 mg q6-8h to 50 mg tid for the relief of anxiety that frequently accompanied his breathlessness
- Consultation of the interdisciplinary team to support his recent diagnosis and functional limitation as well as his negative perception of his mother-in-law's terminal experience
- Instruction of Tom and his wife in the use of pursed-lip breathing, fans, and position changing and reporting of any changes in his symptoms

## References

AHMEDZAI, S. (1990). Palliative care in oncology: Making quality the endpoint. *Annals of Oncology, 1*(6), 396-398.

AHMEDZAI, S. (1993). Palliation of respiratory symptoms. In D. Doyle, G. W. C. Hanks, & N. MacDonald (Eds.), *Oxford textbook of palliative medicine* (pp. 354-373). New York: Oxford University Press.

AHMEDZAI, S. (1998). Palliation of respiratory symptoms. In D. Doyle, G. W. C. Hanks, & N. MacDonald (Eds.), *Oxford textbook of palliative medicine* (2nd ed). (pp. 583-616). New York: Oxford University Press.

AMERICAN Thoracic Society (1999). Dyspnea mechanisms, assessment and management: A consensus statement. *American Journal of Respiratory Critical Care Medicine, 159,* 321-340.

BRUERA, E., Kuehn, N., Miller, M., Selmser, P., & Selmser, P. (1991). The Edmonton Symptom Assessment System (ESAS): A simple method for the assessment of palliative care patients. *Journal of Palliative Care, 7*(2), 6-9.

BRUERA, E., MacEachern, T., Ripamonti, C., & Hanson, J. (1993). Subcutaneous morphine on the dyspnea of terminal cancer patients. *Annals of Internal Medicine, 119*(9), 906-907.

BRUERA, E., Macmillan, K., Pither, T., & MacDonald, R. (1990). Effects of morphine on the dyspnea of terminal cancer patients. *Journal of Pain and Symptom Management, 5*(6), 341-344.

CARRIERI-KOHLMAN, V., Janson-Bjerklie, S. (1993). Dyspnea. In Carrieri-Kohlman, V., Lindsey, M., & West, C. (Eds.), *Pathophysiological phenomena in nursing* (2nd ed.) (pp. 247-278). Philadelphia: W. B. Saunders.

COHEN, M., Johnson-Anderson, A., Krasnow, S., & Wadleigh, R. (1992). Treatment of intractable dyspnea: Clinical and ethical issues. *Cancer Investigation, 10*(4), 317-321.

COWCHER, K., & Hanks, G. (1990). Long-term management of respiratory symptoms in advanced cancer. *Journal of Pain and Symptom Management, 5*(5), 320-330.

DAVIS, C. (1996). Single-dose, randomized, controlled trial of nebulized morphine in patients with cancer-related breathlessness. *Palliative Medicine, 10,* 64-65.

DAVIS, C., Hodder, C., Love, S., Slevin, M., & Wedzicha, J. (1994). Effect of nebulized morphine and morphine 6-glucuronide on exercise endurance in patients with chronic obstructive airway disease. *Thorax, 49*(4), 393.

DUDGEON, D. (1997). Dyspnea clinical perspectives. In *Symptoms in terminal illness: A research workshop, treating symptoms at the end-of-life* (pp. 1-22). Rockville, MD: National Institutes of Health.

DUDGEON, D., & Rosenthal, S. (1996). Management of dyspnea and cough in patients with cancer. *Hematology/Oncology Clinics of North America, 10*(1), 151-171.

GIFT, A. (1997). Dyspnea methods perspective. In *Symptoms in terminal illness: A research workshop, treating symptoms at the end-of-life* (pp. 1-22). Rockville, MD: National Institutes of Health.

GIFT, A., & Narsavage, G. (1998). Validity of the numeric rating scale as a measure of dyspnea. *American Journal of Critical Care, 7*(3), 200-204.

GIFT, A., & Pugh, L. (1993). Dyspnea and fatigue. *Nursing Clinics of North America, 28*(2), 373-384.

GUYTON, A. C., & Hall, J. E. (1996). Respiratory insufficiency-pathophysiology, diagnosis, oxygen therapy. In *Textbook of medical physiology* (9th ed.) (pp. 537-545). Philadelphia: W. B. Saunders.

HARWOOD, K. (1999). Dyspnea. In C. Yarbro, M. Frogge, & M. Goodman, (Eds.), *Cancer symptom management* (pp. 45-55). Sudbury, MA: Jones & Bartlett.

KUEBLER, K., Dahlin, C., Heidrich, D., Ladd, L., Montonye, M., & Zeri, K. (1996). *Hospice and palliative care clinical practice protocol: Dyspnea monograph.* Pittsburgh: Hospice Nurses Association.

KUEBLER, K., & Ogle, K. (1998). Psychometric evaluation of an objective assessment instrument to measure pain, dyspnea and restlessness. *Journal of Palliative Care, 14*(3), 125.

LEUNG, R., Hill, P., & Burdon, J. (1996). Effect of inhaled morphine on the development of breathlessness during exercise in patients with chronic lung disease. *Thorax, 51,* 596-600.

MAHLER, D. (1990). Acute dyspnea. In D. Mahler (Ed.), *Dyspnea* (pp. 127-144). Mt. Kisco, NY: Futura.

MASOUD, A., Reed, J., & Thomas, S. (1995). Lack of effect of inhaled morphine on exercise-induced breathlessness in chronic obstructive pulmonary disease. *Thorax, 50,* 629-634.

McIver, B., Walsh, D., & Nelson, K. (1994). The use of chlorpromazine for symptom control in dying cancer patients. *Journal of Pain and Symptom Management, 9*(5), 341-345.

Pearson, L. (1998). *Nurse practitioner's drug handbook.* Springhouse, PA: Springhouse.

Pereira, J., & Bruera, E. (1997). Dyspnea. In *The Edmonton aid to palliative care* (pp. 62-63). Edmonton, Canada: Division of Palliative Care, University of Alberta.

Ripamonti, C., & Bruera, E. (1997). Dyspnea: Pathophysiology and assessment. *Journal of Pain and Symptom Management, 13*(4), 220-232.

Shepherd, S., & Geraci, S. (1999). The differential diagnosis of dyspnea: A pathophysiological approach. *Clinician Reviews, 9*(4), 52-71.

Shlafer, M., & Marieb, E. (1989). *The nurse, pharmacology, and drug therapy.* Redwood City, CA: Addison-Wesley.

Simon, P., Schwartzstein, R., & Weiss, J. (1990). Distinguishable types of dyspnea in patients with shortness of breath. *American Review of Respiratory Disease, 142,* 1909-1914.

Twycross, R. (1997). Respiratory symptoms. In R. Twycross (Ed.), *Symptom management in advanced cancer* (pp.143-148). Oxon, UK: Radcliffe Medical Press.

Twycross, R. (1999). Correctable causes of breathlessness. In *Introducing palliative care* (p. 123). Oxon, UK: Radcliffe Medical Press.

Twycross, R., Wilcock, A., & Thorp, S. (1998). *Palliative care formulary.* Oxon, UK: Radcliffe Medical Press.

Woodcock, A., Gross, E., & Geddes, D. (1981). Oxygen relieves breathlessness in "pink puffers." *Lancet, 1,* 907-909.

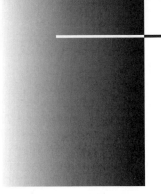

C H A P T E R **25**

# *Fatigue*

SANDY MCKINNON

## ■ DEFINITION AND INCIDENCE

The experience of fatigue is subjective and not unlike pain and anxiety is challenging to define. Although several authors offer definitions that highlight various aspects of the experience of extreme tiredness, there is as yet no universal or "gold standard" definition of fatigue in the context of health and disease (Glaus, 1998; Neuenschwander & Bruera, 1998; Portenoy & Miaskowski, 1998).

Growing interest in the treatment and study of fatigue is heightening the need for a common understanding of this symptom. Glaus (1998) notes that defining fatigue remains difficult in part because there are so many unanswered questions: It is not clear whether fatigue is a single entity or involves various related phenomena. Nor is it clear whether physiologic or psychologic processes take precedence. We do not yet understand what causes extreme tiredness in people with advanced illness. Although most practitioners are aware of a difference between fatigue that is normal and fatigue that is distressing, a clear definition including specific criteria such as severity, duration, and effect would help to increase the visibility of this problem and provide a focus for research (Portenoy & Miaskowski, 1998; Winningham et al., 1994).

Fatigue may include or overlap symptoms similar to malaise, weakness, asthenia, lassitude, loss of strength, and decreased energy (Tiesinga, Dassen, & Halfrens, 1996). Some authors use the terms fatigue and asthenia interchangeably (Neuenschwander & Bruera, 1998). Cella, Peterman, Passik, Jacobsen, and Breitbart (1998) conceptualize fatigue as a multidimensional phenomenon that includes physical, emotional, and cognitive components. Ferrell, Grant, Dean, Funk, and Ly (1996) note that fatigue has a significant effect on all dimensions of quality of life including physical, spiritual, psychologic, and social. Aaronson and colleagues (1999) define fatigue as the awareness of a decreased capacity for physical and/or mental activity due to an imbalance in the availability, utilization, and/or restoration of resources needed to perform activity.

Most researchers agree that fatigue is a multicausal, multidimensional symptom (Cella et al., 1998; Glaus, 1998; Neuenschwander & Bruera, 1998; Piper et al., 1998; Portenoy & Miaskowski, 1998, Winningham et al., 1994).

The lack of a clear definition has made it difficult to determine the incidence of fatigue in the terminally ill, though most reports place it between 60% and 90%. It is one of the most common symptoms reported by people with cancer and can clearly be both extremely distressing and debilitating (Clark & Lacasse, 1998; Glaus, 1998; Portenoy & Miaskowski, 1998). Fatigue is also a common symptom in many chronic diseases such as rheumatoid arthritis, diabetes, multiple sclerosis, and acquired immunodeficiency syndrome (AIDS), as well as the poorly understood chronic fatigue syndrome (Aaronson et al., 1999). Fatigue may precede a diagnosis of cancer and may be debilitating enough to lead people to refuse further anticancer treatment (Neuenschwander & Bruera, 1998).

Most research into cancer-related fatigue has focused on the period surrounding treatment, and there is much work to be done to further our understanding of fatigue in terminal illness. Several issues may contribute to the paucity of research in this area. Fatigue in cancer patients may be perceived as inevitable by care providers, family, and patients themselves (Neuenschwander & Bruera, 1998), and complaints may not be taken seriously (Clark & Lacasse, 1998). Fatigue-related problems often emerge after the more distressing symptoms such as pain or nausea have been relieved.

# ■ ETIOLOGY AND PATHOPHYSIOLOGY

Fatigue as a physiologic phenomenon may be a beneficial and protective symptom against overexertion during both prolonged physical and intellectual efforts (Neuenschwander & Bruera, 1996). The feeling of being tired after a good exercise session or a hard day's work can even be pleasant (Clark & Lacasse, 1998; Glaus, 1998). This phenomenon is to be distinguished from fatigue as a pathologic finding that is distressing and serves no beneficial function. Fatigue associated with cancer has been found to be more persistent and more emotionally overwhelming and lacks the normal circadian rhythm (Glaus, 1998). It is not relieved by a good sleep and paradoxically may contribute to sleep difficulties (Engstrom, Strohl, Rose, Lewandowski, & Stefanek, 1999).

Fatigue has been associated with most severe and chronic illnesses, including cancer, end-stage organ failure, neuromuscular disorders, and major depression. However the pathogenesis of fatigue is not yet well understood and is the subject of much speculation, conjecture, and research. Cella and associates (1998, p. 370) list several factors that may contribute to cancer-related fatigue:

- Preexisting conditions (e.g., congestive heart failure [CHF], fibromyalgia)
- Direct effects of cancer ("tumor burden")
- Cancer-treatment effects
- Surgery
- Chemotherapy
- Radiation therapy

- Biologic response modifiers
- Conditions related to cancer or its treatment:
  - Anemia
  - Dehydration
  - Malnutrition
  - Infection
  - Cytokine production
  - Altered muscle metabolism (e.g., decreased protein synthesis or accumulation of metabolites)
- Symptoms of cancer or its treatment (e.g., pain, nausea)
- Disruption of sleep/rest cycle
- Immobility
- Emotional demands of dealing with cancer
- Stress
- Anxiety
- Depression

Most often fatigue is the result of several factors, each requiring individual attention and treatment, if possible (Cella et al., 1998). Some of the potential causes listed are considered in more detail in the discussion that follows.

## Anemia

Anemia is one of the few conditions with a direct causal relationship to fatigue. However this does not mean that we can state with certainty that there is a threshold hemoglobin (Hb) level below which a person experiences fatigue (Portenoy & Miaskowski, 1998). Transfusions of packed red cells in people with low Hb level may or may not provide relief from distressing fatigue. It appears that persons with slowly decreasing Hb levels may have less severe symptoms than those whose Hb level drops rapidly. Thus, some persons with terminal illnesses may have significant anemia but few physical signs and symptoms.

## Medications

Many medications used to treat cancer cause drowsiness or fatigue, including opioids, hypnotics, benzodiazepines, tricyclic antidepressants, and dopamine antagonists. Many persons with terminal illnesses are taking one or more of these medications to treat other uncomfortable symptoms. Careful titration of medications to their lowest effective dose may assist in minimizing this effect.

## Cytokines

Cells within the body's immune system, and possibly within the tumor itself, produce proteins called cytokines (such as interleukins, interferons, and tumor necrosis factor). It is theorized that cytokines play a role in producing fatigue in illnesses such as cancer, infections, and chronic fatigue syndrome, but the exact mechanism is not yet known (Cella et al., 1998; Glaus, 1998).

## Malnutrition and Cachexia

The profound fatigue or asthenia associated with advanced cancer was once thought to be the result of malnutrition and cachexia (Neuenschwander & Bruera, 1998). It is now believed to be more complex than insufficient caloric intake. Cytokine production may be the underlying mechanism for the anorexia-cachexia syndrome and may also cause the symptom of fatigue. Similarly, cytokines may contribute to the fatigue associated with some infections (Walker, Schleinich, & Bruera, 1998). There is yet no explanation; for example, many breast cancer patients are extremely fatigued but do not experience weight loss (Walker et al., 1987).

## Neurologic Dysfunction

Autonomic dysfunction associated with malignancy may cause postural hypotension, occasional syncope, fixed heart rate, and nausea (Neuenschwander & Bruera, 1998).

## Metabolic and Endocrine Disorders

Preexisting illnesses and secondary conditions including diabetes mellitus; Addison's disease; electrolyte imbalances such as low sodium, potassium, and magnesium levels; and hypercalcemia may produce fatigue (Neuenschwander & Bruera, 1998; Portenoy & Miaskowski, 1998).

## Overexertion

Trying to keep up with a preillness lifestyle may contribute to exhaustion (Neuenschwander & Bruera, 1998). Having unrealistic expectations about physical capacities should trigger further emotional evaluation.

## Sleep Disruption

Lack of sleep may be related to several concerns including symptom distress (pain, dyspnea), waking for care needs (medication, repositioning), side effects of medication (steroids, methylphenidate, etc.), and daily inactivity (Engstrom et al., 1999). Rest and immobility may have the paradoxic effect of increasing fatigue and decreasing the efficiency of neuromuscular functioning (Cella et al., 1998; Portenoy & Miaskowski, 1998).

## Depression

Fatigue may be the physical expression of feelings of hopelessness and demoralization as the illness progresses. In addition depression may be masked. Treatments for major depression may involve medications that can exacerbate fatigue (Cella et al., 1998).

# ■ ASSESSMENT AND MEASUREMENT

Although researchers and clinicians agree that accurate assessment and measurement of fatigue are critical to advancing the knowledge and ability to treat effectively. However, there are few appropriate and valid tools in existence with which to assess and measure fatigue (Piper et al., 1998). Piper and coworkers (1998) suggest that a simple rating of fatigue intensity from 0 to 10 is reasonable in many circumstances. The authors add that patients should be asked the following as well:

- How has fatigue affected activities of daily living?
- Has the ability to concentrate or remember been affected?
- How has fatigue affected mood?

These screening questions are helpful in determining the need for further assessment, referrals, and the need for supportive therapies such as home care, occupational therapy, or assistive equipment (Piper et al., 1998). The symptoms of fatigue must be viewed in the context of the person's life, level of distress, and overall treatment goals, recognizing these goals may change over time (Portenoy & Miaskowski, 1998).

Initial assessment includes identifying temporal features, such as onset and daily patterns, determining any relationship between the fatigue and events such as chemotherapy, and assessing relieving and exacerbating factors. Screening lab tests may include complete blood count (CBC), electrolyte, serum calcium, creatinine, glucose, and transaminase levels, and possibly a thyrotropin (TSH) evaluation if hypothyroidism is suspected (Walker et al., 1998).

Fatigue is a multidimensional problem and more sophisticated assessment may be helpful in some cases (Piper et al., 1998; Portenoy & Miaskowski, 1998). Although most fatigue assessment instruments have been developed for research, they may be helpful in clinical practice if they are easy to use. Multidimensional tools such as the Piper Fatigue Self-Report Scale, which looks at severity, distress, and effect of fatigue, are available for use in clinical situations and can aid in the evaluation of intervention strategies (Piper et al., 1998).

# ■ HISTORY AND PHYSICAL EXAMINATION

It may be necessary to ask about fatigue during an initial history and follow-up visits with patients. As previously noted, fatigue may be viewed as inevitable by patients and families or may not be noticed until more distressing symptoms have been relieved (Neuenschwander & Bruera, 1998).

The clinician must look for potential causes and associations for fatigue. For example, questioning about nighttime medications may uncover the cause of morning fatigue (Portenoy & Miaskowski, 1998). A review of all medications is essential in order to ascertain which might be causing drowsiness or fatigue.

# ■ DIAGNOSTICS

The extent of laboratory or radiologic investigations must be decided on a case-by-case basis. Tests may be costly and burdensome and should only be pursued when the cause is uncertain and there is a potential to make a change in treatment (Portenoy & Miaskowski, 1998). It is necessary to have a good understanding of the patient's goals and degree of distress caused by the fatigue.

Laboratory tests for hematologic or metabolic problems may be helpful. Several diagnostic evaluations are considered in the discussion of the assessment.

# ■ INTERVENTION AND TREATMENT

Patients may not report fatigue, believing it to be inevitable and untreatable. They may not be asked about fatigue during visits with clinicians, and its effect may be underestimated or ignored completely (Cella et al., 1998). Expectations for improvement should be discussed. Fatigue may not be reversible, and this possibility should be compassionately communicated. On the other hand, knowing that chemotherapy-related fatigue is short-term can in itself be therapeutic (Portenoy & Miaskowski, 1998).

The goal of care is to "reverse the reversible." For example, treatments are available for anemia (transfusions or erythropoietin), infections (antibiotics), or hypercalcemia (bisphosphates or hydration). Reversible causes of fatigue may coexist with irreversible causes, and the goal of care may be to improve function and minimize fatigue rather than to eliminate it (Cella et al., 1998; Neuenschwander & Bruera, 1998). Determining goals should be a collaborative process for the patient and practitioner. Many possible treatments for fatigue can be tiring and a trial-and-error process can be frustrating (Portenoy & Miaskowski, 1998). The aim often is to help patients have enough energy to do the things they find to be most important (Clark & Lacasse, 1998).

The following interventions may be helpful:

- Treat underlying problems such as dehydration, hypercalcemia, and hypoxia (Cella et al., 1998)
- Suggest keeping a diary to record actions and activities that increase or decrease fatigue, as an aid in planning daily and weekly activities (Clark & Lacasse, 1998).
- Teach energy conservation techniques, such as sitting instead of standing and using assistive devices such as bath chairs, raised toilet seats, or wheelchairs. Consider consultations with physical or occupational therapists.
- Encourage a balance between rest and exercise. Further research is needed to determine the role of exercise in cases of pathologic fatigue, but it is clear that excessive rest may be as fatigue-inducing as excessive exercise (Neuenschwander & Bruera, 1998; Portenoy & Miaskowski, 1998):
  - Base exercise on the individual patient's age, gender, physical condition, previous habits, and other medical concerns.

- Suggest exercises that use the large muscle groups, such as walking, swimming, and cycling.
- Take into account contraindications to exercise, including cardiac abnormalities, recurrent unexplained pain or nausea, extreme fatigue, and cyanosis (Portenoy & Miaskowski, 1998).
- Encourage good sleep habits such as napping earlier in the day, not napping in the evening, establishing a bedtime routine, using relaxation exercises, and avoiding stimulants (Portenoy & Miaskowski, 1998).

## Pharmacology

To avoid unnecessary medications and polypharmacy Portenoy and Miaskowski (1998) offer the following suggestions:

- Reduce or discontinue medications known to cause fatigue:
  - Antiemetics
  - Hypnotics (sleeping pills may increase sleep while compounding the problem of daytime fatigue [hangover effect]; assess whether sleep is restorative or nonrestorative)
  - Anxiolytics
  - Antihistamines ($H_1$ or $H_2$ blockers)
  - Analgesics (in the presence of distressing fatigue, try reducing the daily dose by 25%)
- Use antidepressants for patients with major depression who are experiencing fatigue. Consider using one of the selective serotonin reuptake inhibitors (SSRIs) that are less sedating than other classes of antidepressants.
- Psychostimulants may be helpful in treating opioid-related fatigue and depression in elderly and medically ill patients. However, these medications may also cause insomnia, anxiety, anorexia, confusion, and tachycardia:
  - Methylphenidate (Ritalin) (Walker and colleagues [1998] suggest starting with a morning trial dose of 5 to 10 mg PO; because this medication has a short half-life, beneficial effects are apparent within 24 hours; if the patient shows improvement, suggest 10 mg with breakfast and 5 mg with lunch; avoid doses after noon to prevent sleeplessness at night)—these recommendations are for immediate-release medication; for sustained-release, 5 to 10 mg daily is recommended
  - Pemoline (Cylert) (this medication is helpful in treating fatigue related to multiple sclerosis, but is also associated with liver toxicity; consider using pemoline only if treatment with methylphenidate is unsuccessful)
  - Erythropoietin (research supports that erythropoietin increases hematocrit and improves energy and quality of life; however it is extremely expensive and further research is needed to justify its use when anemia-related fatigue is mild or when life expectancy is short)
  - Corticosteroids (the stimulant effect of corticosteroids is often helpful for persons with advanced disease and multiple symptoms; Dexamethasone, 1 to 2 mg twice daily, or prednisone, 5 to 10 mg twice daily, may be used)

## Complementary Therapies

There are several other interventions that may assist in alleviating fatigue or coping with the distress of fatigue. These include but are not limited to the following:

- Stress management
- Visual imagery
- Distraction to reduce boredom (i.e., hobbies, gardening, music)
- Hot baths

## ■ PATIENT AND FAMILY EDUCATION

Patients and families may need coaching and support to let go of certain activities in order to save energy for whatever is most important. Delegation is a difficult task for many people, especially women and mothers, to learn. There may be a need to set limits on visitors and some social activities. Fatigue is not usually influenced quickly (Clark & Lacasse, 1998). In spite of these potential losses acceptance of limitations can lead to adaptation (Walker et al., 1998).

Patients and families may associate fatigue with a worsening of the disease and may be reassured by alternative explanations for this symptom and encouraged by the possibilities for improvement. They should have an understanding of the nature of the symptom, options for therapy, and expected outcomes (Portenoy & Miaskowski, 1998).

## ■ EVALUATION AND PLAN FOR FOLLOW-UP

The effect of fatigue and goals of care change over time (Portenoy & Miaskowski, 1998). Treatment of fatigue requires persistence and close follow-up. Success in the management of fatigue is highly individualized and correlated with each person's goals (Clark & Lacasse, 1998).

✔ **CASE STUDY** Joan is a 34-year-old mother of two children, 10-year-old Ben and lively 6-year-old Jackie. Her husband, Bill, is very supportive. Joan was diagnosed with colon cancer 4 years ago and was treated with a resection, colostomy, and radiation treatments. Unfortunately an abdominal computed tomography (CT) scan 1 year ago revealed liver metastases. Chemotherapy failed to help, and Joan knows that her time is limited. She is determined to be at home for as long as possible. Problems with pain and nausea are under reasonable control. You visit Joan at home one afternoon. Bill has taken the kids out to a movie, and Joan begins by telling you that she is just feeling "exhausted." She adds that she has not been sleeping at night or, rather, has to wake up to take her pain medicines every 4 hours. The nurse identifies the following contributing factors to Joan's fatigue and initiates corrective actions:

- She is on a short-acting pain medication with a stable pain problem:
  - Switch to a long-acting preparation to facilitate sleep at night.
- She has been trying to keep the environment as "normal" as possible "for the children" by trying to do all the cooking and cleaning herself:
  - Encourage Joan to consider hiring a housekeeper or asking for more help from family and friends.
  - Review energy conservation techniques with Joan.
  - Consult an occupational therapist for additional instruction in tools and techniques for energy conservation in daily activities.
- Joan has been "too tired to eat":
  - Review nutritional intake.
  - Consider liquid supplements.
  - Consider consultation with a nutritionist.
- Joan is concerned about her fatigue and her ability to continue fulfilling her role and mother and wife.
  - Discuss Joan's goals and expectations.
  - Help Joan to adjust to her limitations.
  - Assist Joan to identify the underlying meaning of her "chores" as mother and wife and other ways to fulfill these roles.
  - Consult a counselor or social worker to provide additional counseling and support.

## References

AARONSON, L. S., Teel, C. S., Cassmeyer, V., Neuberger, G. B., Pallikkathayil, L., Pierce, J., Press, A. N., Williams, P. D., & Wingate, A. (1999). Defining and measuring fatigue. *Image: Journal of Nursing Scholarship, 31*(1), 45-50.

CELLA, D., Peterman, A., Passik, S., Jacobsen, P., & Breitbart, W. (1998). Progress toward guidelines for the management of fatigue. *Oncology, 12*(11A), NCCN Proceedings, 369-377.

CLARK, P. M., & Lacasse, C. (1998). Cancer-related fatigue: Clinical practice issues. *Clinical Journal of Oncology Nursing, 2*(2), 45-53.

ENGSTROM, C. A., Strohl, R. A., Rose, L., Lewandowski, L., & Stefanek, M. E. (1999). Sleep alterations in cancer patients. *Cancer Nursing, 22*(2), 143-148.

FERRELL, B. R., Grant, M., Dean, G. E., Funk, B., & Ly, J. (1996). "Bone tired": The experience of fatigue and its impact on quality of life. *Oncology Nursing Forum, 23*, 1539-1549.

GLAUS, A. (1998). *Fatigue in patients with cancer: Analysis and assessment.* New York: Springer.

NEUENSCHWANDER, H., & Bruera, E. (1996). Asthenia-cachexia. In E. Bruera & I. Higginson (Eds.), *Cachexia-anorexia in cancer patients* (pp. 57-75). Toronto: Oxford University Press.

NEUENSCHWANDER, H., & Bruera, E. (1998). Asthenia. In D. Doyle, G. W. C. Hanks, & N. MacDonald (Eds.), *Oxford textbook of palliative medicine* (2nd ed.) (pp. 573-581). New York: Oxford University Press.

PIPER, B. F., Dibble, S. L., Dodd, M. J., Weiss, M. C., Slaughter, R. E., & Paul, S. M. (1998). The revised Piper fatigue scale: Psychometric evaluation in women with breast cancer. *Oncology Nursing Forum, 25,* 677-684.

PORTENOY, R. K., & Miaskowski, C. (1998). Assessment and management of cancer-related fatigue. In A. M. Berger, R. K. Portenoy, & D. E. Weissman (Eds.), *Principles and practice of supportive oncology* (pp. 109-118). Philadelphia: Lippincott-Raven.

TIESINGA, L. J., Dassen, T. W. N., & Halfrens, R. J. (1996). Fatigue: A summary of definitions, dimensions, and indicators. *Nursing Diagnosis, 7*(2), 51-62.

WALKER, P., Schleinich, & Bruera, E. (1998). Asthenia. In N. MacDonald (Ed.), *Palliative medicine: A case-based manual* (pp. 29-33). Toronto: Oxford University Press.

WINNINGHAM, M. L., Nail, L. M., Burke, M. B., Brophy, L., Cimprich, B., Jones, L. S., Pickard-Holley, S., Rhodes, V., St. Pierre, B., Beck, S., Glass, E. C., Mock, V. L., Mooney, K. H., & Piper, B. F. (1994). Fatigue and the cancer patient: The state of the knowledge. *Oncology Nursing Forum, 21,* 23-36.

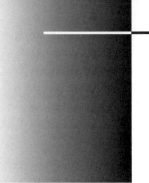

C H A P T E R **26**

# *Hiccups*

PATRICIA H. BERRY

## ■ DEFINITION AND INCIDENCE

We all experience hiccups. Short episodes are common in healthy individuals and are usually self-limited or responsive to simple measures. Hiccups can produce problems when they are prolonged or intractable. Indeed in such cases they can interrupt talking, eating, and sleeping and eventually lead to weight loss, total exhaustion, anxiety, and depression (Wilcock & Twycross, 1996). In patients at the end of life hiccups can interfere with the ability to interact with others and participate in chosen activities that all affect quality of life.

Hiccups (singultus) is an abnormal respiratory reflex characterized by a spasm of the diaphragm, combined with sudden inspiration of air and closure of the epiglottis, resulting in the characteristic sound. Less often the accessory muscles of respiration are involved, including the intercostal and abdominal muscles (Twycross & Regnard, 1998). Although hiccups are frequently observed in end-stage illness, the incidence is unknown (Rousseau, 1994).

## ■ ETIOLOGY AND PATHOPHYSIOLOGY

The more than 100 causes of hiccups are of six types:
1. Disorders affecting the peripheral branches of the phrenic and vagal nerves, such as gastric and abdominal distension (having a variety of causes, including bowel obstruction and intraabdominal hemorrhage), excessive ingestion of food, sudden changes in the gastric temperature, esophageal reflux or obstruction, pleuritis, pericarditis, pulmonary edema, pneumonia, and mediastinal or cervical tumors.
2. Central nervous system disorders, such as intracranial tumors, head injury, and stroke.
3. Metabolic and drug-induced causes, such as renal failure or insufficiency, hypocalcemia, hyponatremia, and alcohol abuse, some of which are precipitated by barbiturates, benzodiazepines, and parenteral corticosteroids.
4. Infectious disorders (infrequent), including meningitis, abscess, tuberculosis, and influenza.

5. Psychogenic disturbances, such as anxiety, emotional stress, and excitement.
6. Idiopathic causes, when a causative factor is not identified; because extensive evaluation is often unwarranted in a terminally ill patient, cause is often unknown (Rousseau, 1994; Rousseau, 1999; Twycross & Regnard, 1998).

In patients near death, however, gastric distension is most likely the underlying cause of hiccups, accounting for 95% of cases (Twycross, 1997).

As discussed, the pathophysiologic process underlying hiccups is irritation of the vagal and phrenic nerves, including their peripheral branches. For centrally mediated hiccups an interaction of the respiratory center, phrenic nerve nuclei, medullary formation, and hypothalamus is proposed as the underlying cause (Kolodzik & Eilers, 1991; Rousseau, 1994).

## ■ ASSESSMENT AND MEASUREMENT

A complete evaluation for hiccups should be based on the disease trajectory—less evaluations are required as the patient comes closer to death (Rousseau, 1994).

## ■ HISTORY AND PHYSICAL EXAMINATION

Underlying medical diagnoses often suggest the cause of hiccups. The history and physical examination should be directed to rule out the causes discussed. In addition the following aspects of the history and physical examination should be considered:

- Length of the episode and its effect on the patient's quality of life
- Review of medications
- Measures, if any, the patient has used in an attempt to relieve the hiccups

## ■ DIAGNOSTICS

Diagnostic tests often do not yield a cause for hiccups. However, an x-ray study may be beneficial if the patient's functional status is adequate.

## ■ INTERVENTION AND TREATMENT

As discussed, treatment for hiccups in end-stage illness is often questionable. However, if an underlying cause is identified and the treatment is consistent with the goals of care and desires of the patient and family, treatment is appropriate. For example if the underlying cause is related to pneumonia, treating the pneumonia with the intent of providing comfort—in this case, relief of distressing hiccups—is entirely appropriate. In addition, if medications are identified as a possible cause, discontinuing the offending medication and/or substituting another may also be appropriate.

## Pharmacologic

The pharmacologic approaches to hiccups can be organized into several categories: phrenic and/or vagal stimulation, reduction of gastric distension, muscle relaxation, and central suppression of the hiccup reflex. If the underlying cause is identified, these categories, summarized in Table 26-1, may guide intervention.

## Complementary

Nonpharmacologic interventions for hiccups are numerous. Although it may be appropriate to try these approaches, most patients and families request help with troubling hiccups after trying such attempts. These are summarized in Table 26-2.

## ■ PATIENT AND FAMILY EDUCATION

Hiccups can be a distressing symptom for both patient and family. As with all symptoms patients and families should be taught about the probable underlying cause and proposed treatment plan(s) and urged to contact their health care provider if the planned interventions are not effective. They also

### TABLE 26-1

#### Pharmacologic Treatment of Hiccups

| Suspected Underlying Cause | Recommended Treatment |
|---|---|
| Phrenic or vagal stimulation | Nebulized normal saline solution (0.9%), 2 ml over 5 minutes<br>Cisapride, 10-20 mg PO qid* |
| Gastric distension | Antiflatulent, such as simethicone, 10 ml PO qid<br>Metoclopramide, 10 mg PO qid* |
| Need for muscle relaxation | Cisapride, 10-20 mg PO qid*<br>Baclofen, 5-20 mg PO bid or tid<br>Nifedipine, 10-20 mg PO q8h |
| Central causes (may also be tried when preceding measures are not effective or inappropriate) | Chlorpromazine, 10-50 mg IV, IM, PR, or PO tid-qid[†]<br>Haloperidol, 1-4 mg SC or PO tid<br>Carbamazepine, 200 mg PO tid<br>Valproic acid, 15 mg/kg/day in divided doses<br>Amitriptyline, 10 mg tid[†]<br>Midazolam, 10-60 mg/day by SC infusion *if all else fails* (Wilcock & Twycross, 1996) |

From Loft, L. M., & Ward, R. F. (1992). Hiccups: A case presentation and etiologic review. *Archives of Otolaryngology and Head and Neck Surgery, 118,* 1115-1119; Rousseau, P. (1994). Hiccups in terminal disease. *American Journal of Hospice and Palliative Medicine, 11*(6), 7-10; Twycross R. (1997). *Symptom management in advanced cancer* (2nd ed.). Oxon, UK: Radcliffe Medical Press.
*Contraindicated in bowel obstruction.
† Caution advised for elderly or debilitated patients.

| TABLE 26-2 | |
| --- | --- |

### Nonpharmacologic Interventions for Hiccup

| Mode of Action | Treatment Options |
| --- | --- |
| Stimulating the phrenic and/or vagal nerve | Rapidly ingesting two heaping teaspoons of sugar |
| | Gargling or sipping ice water |
| | Swallowing dry bread |
| | Drinking from the wrong side of a cup |
| | Biting on a lemon |
| | Rubbing the back of the neck |
| Increasing $P_{CO_2}$ affects the central inhibition of hiccups | Rebreathing from a paper bag |
| | Holding the breath |
| Reducing gastric distension | Drinking peppermint water (causes relaxation of the cardiac sphincter and thus allows belching)* |

From Rousseau, P. (1994). Hiccups in terminal disease. *American Journal of Hospice and Palliative Medicine, 11*(6), 7-10; Twycross R. (1997). *Symptom management in advanced cancer* (2nd ed.). Oxon, UK: Radcliffe Medical Press.
*Peppermint water and metoclopramide should not be used concurrently.

need to be reassured that control of distressing symptoms is the highest priority in their plan of care, in keeping of course with the wishes and goals of the patient and family. The consequences of no treatment should be part of the overall goal-setting discussion.

## ■ EVALUATION AND PLAN FOR FOLLOW-UP

Treatment is judged successful when the hiccups are resolved (in terms of patient-determined goals) or do not recur. In some cases several trials and combinations of different interventions may occur before the symptom is resolved to the patient's and family's satisfaction. Although there is little in the literature regarding hiccups in end-of-life care, it is reasonable to expect them to occur as the patient status changes. Therefore continual patient evaluation and inquiries about new or recurrent symptoms and their management are important factors.

### ✔ CASE STUDY

Mrs. B. is a 61-year-old woman with a history of metastatic breast cancer to the lung, the liver, and possibly the brain. She reports a 3-week history of hiccups unresponsive to nonpharmacologic treatments. Her hiccups interfere with her ability to visit with others or go out to enjoy an occasional movie or play. She also reports a lack of appetite, nausea, and a feeling of dread that she will not be able to manage hiccups. Her other medications include sustained-release morphine for pain and breathlessness, metoclopramide for abdominal distension and nausea, and stool softeners and laxatives. Her last bowel movement occurred 9 days ago.

The advanced practice nurse (APN) suspects that her hiccups are partly due to obstipation; however, after that is corrected and additional stool softener and laxative medications are added to her regimen, hiccups persist. Chlorpromazine, 25 mg PO tid, is initiated, but it makes Mrs. B. too drowsy to interact with her husband, children, and grandchildren—something she really values. Baclofen, 5 mg PO bid, is initiated but is not effective. When the dose is increased to 10 mg tid, it produces complete relief.

Mrs. B. remains free of her distressing hiccups until her death 2 months later.

## References

KOLODZIK, P. W., & Eilers, M. A. (1991). Hiccups (singultus): Review and approach to management. *Annals of Emergency Medicine, 20,* 565-573.

LOFT, L. M., & Ward, R. F. (1992). Hiccups: A case presentation and etiologic review. *Archives of Otolaryngology and Head and Neck Surgery, 118,* 1115-1119.

ROUSSEAU, P. (1994). Hiccups in terminal disease. *American Journal of Hospice and Palliative Medicine, 11*(6), 7-10.

ROUSSEAU, P. (1999). Evaluation and management of gastrointestinal symptoms. In R. S. Schonwetter, W. Hawke, & C. F. Knight (Eds.), *Hospice and palliative medicine: Core curriculum and review syllabus* (pp. 85-92). Dubuque, IA: Kendall/Hunt.

TWYCROSS R. (1997). *Symptom management in advanced cancer* (2nd ed.). Oxon, UK: Radcliffe Medical Press.

TWYCROSS R., & Regnard, C. (1998). Dysphagia, dyspepsia, and hiccup. In D. Doyle, G. W. C. Hanks, & N. MacDonald (Eds.), *Oxford textbook of palliative medicine* (2nd ed.) (pp. 499-512). New York: Oxford University Press.

WILCOCK, A., & Twycross, R. (1996). Midazolam for intractable hiccup. *Journal of Pain and Symptom Management, 12,* 59-61.

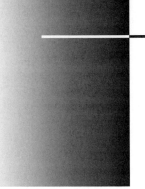

CHAPTER 27

# Nausea and Vomiting

JULIE GRIFFIE, SANDY MCKINNON

## ■ DEFINITION AND INCIDENCE

*Nausea* is defined as an unpleasant feeling of needing to vomit. Autonomic symptoms such as pallor, cold sweat, salivation, tachycardia, and diarrhea often accompany this symptom, as well as possibly far-reaching effects ranging from mild discomfort to malnutrition (Jablonski, 1993). Additional distressing gastrointestinal sensations include the following:

- Retching—spasmodic movements of the diaphragm and abdominal muscles that may lead to vomiting
- Vomiting—a complex process of the involuntary reflux expulsion of gastric contents through the mouth

Nausea and vomiting affect 40% to 70% of patients with advanced cancer and can seriously diminish quality of life for people who have acquired immunodeficiency syndrome (AIDS) and liver or renal failure (Fallon, 1998). Symptoms are more common in women, patients less than 65 years of age, and patients who have cancer of the breast or stomach (Baines, 1999).

## ■ ETIOLOGY AND PATHOPHYSIOLOGY

Successful treatment of nausea or vomiting requires that we understand the underlying processes involved. However, unlike in the treatment of pain, there are no generally accepted management guidelines available (Mannix, 1998). There may be multiple causes for nausea and vomiting, so initial identification and treatment of the major triggering factors are recommended (Twycross & Back, 1998).

The vomiting center (VC) coordinates the emetic reflex. It is located in the brain stem and is within the blood-brain barrier. The VC is a diffuse, interconnected neural network that produces the vomiting reflex (Mannix, 1998; Twycross & Back, 1998). Afferent nerves from at least five areas arrive at the VC and can stimulate nausea and vomiting (Figure 27-1):

- The chemoreceptor trigger zone (CTZ) is located in the area postrema of the fourth ventricle in the brain stem. The CTZ is in close proximity to

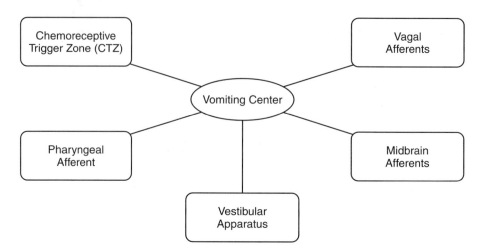

**FIG. 27-1** Physiologic Mechanisms of Nausea and Vomiting

the VC but is outside the blood-brain barrier. Thus, it is exposed to emetogenic substances in the systemic circulation such as calcium ions, urea, morphine, and digoxin. These substances probably stimulate dopamine-type 2 (D2) receptors in this area, leading to nausea and vomiting (Twycross & Back, 1998).

- The vagus nerve is the major afferent neural pathway from the body to the VC. The vagal afferents are stimulated by chemoreceptors and mechanoreceptors in the gastrointestinal (GI) tract, serosa, and viscera (Twycross & Back, 1998). Cell destruction by chemotherapy and radiation therapy, gastric lining irritation by other medications, compression or obstruction by tumors, and slowed activity of the GI tract may all stimulate the vagus nerve and cause nausea and vomiting.
- In a similar way pharyngeal afferents can stimulate the VC. Pharyngeal irritation from *Candida* sp., tenacious sputum, and coughing can lead to vomiting when the VC is activated by the glossopharyngeal nerves (Mannix, 1998).
- The vestibular apparatus is the motion sensor of the body and also sends messages to the VC. It is the primary mechanism involved in motion sickness. Persons with a history of motion sickness may be more prone to nausea and vomiting that result from chemotherapy treatments (Fallon, 1998). Persons who have brain tumors or metastasis may also experience nausea and vomiting associated with a dizzy feeling that may involve the vestibular apparatus.
- Midbrain afferents may also stimulate the VC. This is the mechanism underlying the nausea and vomiting associated with anxiety and

| BOX 27-1 | *Common Causes of Nausea and Vomiting in Palliative Care* |
|---|---|

**GASTROINTESTINAL**
*GI obstruction
*Constipation
*Gastritis
*Gastric stasis
Squashed stomach syndrome
GI infection
Carcinomatosis
Extensive liver metastasis

**PHARYNGEAL IRRITATION**
*Candida* spp. infection
Thick sputum
Cough

**CENTRAL NERVOUS SYSTEM**
*Increased intracranial pressure
Posterior fossa tumors or bleeding
Meningitis, infectious or neoplastic

**MEDICATIONS**
*Opioids
Antibiotics

Chemotherapy
Corticosteroids
Digoxin
Nonsteroidal antiinflammatory
    drugs (NSAIDs)
Iron

**METABOLIC**
Hypercalcemia
Liver failure
Renal failure

**PSYCHOLOGIC/EMOTIONAL**
Anxiety
Pain
Conditioned response (anticipatory
    nausea)

**SITUATIONAL**
Odors
Inadequate mouth care

stress (e.g., anticipatory nausea with chemotherapy). Brain tumors and increased intracranial pressure also cause stimulation of midbrain afferents, leading to nausea and vomiting.

Box 27-1 lists common causes of nausea and vomiting in the palliative care setting. The causes most frequently identified in persons with end-stage diseases are identified by an asterisk.

# ■ ASSESSMENT AND MEASUREMENT

The causes of vomiting can usually be found through a detailed history and physical examination. Nausea should be evaluated separately from vomiting. The following are appropriate assessment questions:

## Temporal Characteristics

- When did it start?
- Is there a pattern (specific times of the day)?
- Is it continuous or intermittent?
- If it is intermittent, what is the frequency and length of episodes?
- Does nausea precede vomiting, or does vomiting occur without warning?

- What makes it better/worse?
  - Is it affected by movement?
  - Is it better or worse with eating?
- What have you tried to treat the nausea?
  - Pharmacologic interventions, including prescription, over-the-counter, and herbal or natural remedies
  - Nonpharmacologic interventions
- Have the bowels moved in the last 24 hours? When was the last bowel movement?
- What medications have been used in the last 24 hours?
- What other medications have been tried for this episode of nausea?
- What does the patient feel the cause is?
- What is the content of vomitus: food, bile, or feces?
- What is the volume of emesis (large volume suggests gastric stasis)?
- How distressing is the nausea to the patient on a visual analogue scale of 0 to 10?
- How distressing is the vomiting to the patient on a visual analogue scale of 0 to 10?
- What is the patient's goal for comfort?
- Are there any associated symptoms such as anxiety, pain, or cough that may require simultaneous intervention?

## ■ HISTORY AND PHYSICAL EXAMINATION

The history and physical examination include reviewing patients' medical and nursing diagnoses and making a targeted systems assessment:
- Consider medical diagnoses, especially disease processes with a potential to cause nausea and vomiting, such as GI or genitourinary (GU) malignancies, primary or metastatic brain tumors, liver failure, and renal failure.
- Determine the treatment history:
  - Identify past or recent treatment with chemotherapy or radiation therapy.
  - Identify any surgical procedures affecting the GI system.
  - Evaluate the patient's past experiences with nausea and vomiting and effectiveness of interventions for that nausea and vomiting.
  - Review current medications that may contribute to nausea.
- Conduct a general physical examination:
  - Note any recent weight change.
  - Check for fever to rule out infection.
  - Check for signs of dehydration.
  - Ask about intake versus output.
  - Check for orthostatic hypotension.
  - Assess hydration status by examining mucous membranes and skin turgor.
  - Note signs of oral or pharyngeal infection or irritation.

- Perform an abdominal examination:
  - Auscultate bowel sounds and identify whether they are present or absent, hyperactive or hypoactive.
  - Palpate, noting hepatomegaly, ascites, tumor masses, gastric or bowel distension.
  - Perform a digital rectal examination, as appropriate, to check for constipation or impaction.
  - Assess for any abdominal pain or discomfort.
- Perform a neurologic examination:
  - Check fundi for papilledema.
  - Identify any changes in orientation or level of consciousness.

## ■ DIAGNOSTICS

On the basis of the findings of the physical examination the following tests may be appropriate for identifying the cause of nausea and vomiting and for guiding treatment planning.

### Laboratory Studies

- Serum sodium to identify dehydration
- Blood urea nitrogen (BUN) and creatinine to identify renal dysfunction
- Calcium (corrected for albumin) to identify hypercalcemia

### Radiographic Studies

- Brain scanning, computed tomography (CT), or magnetic resonance imaging (MRI) to identify brain tumors and/or abdominal abnormalities
- Abdominal radiography to rule out obstruction by tumor or stool

## ■ INTERVENTION AND TREATMENT

Whenever possible the goals of palliative care are to identify and treat the underlying cause of the symptom. Thus the treatment of nausea and vomiting is dependent upon selection of appropriate medications/interventions according to the suspected cause of nausea and vomiting in the individual patient (World Health Organization, 1998). Table 27-1 identifies some potential causes of nausea and vomiting and provides suggested interventions for each. Specific medications and doses are identified in Table 27-2. It is important to consider that individuals may have more than one cause of nausea and vomiting.

Antiemetics are considered the drug of choice yet often prove ineffective, most likely due to an inadequate dose, incomplete diagnosis, or incorrect diagnosis (Lichter, 1993). If the cause of nausea and vomiting is multifactorial, select the most potent antiemetic against each of the recognized or probable causes rather than one multipurpose agent. Compounding pharmacists may

## TABLE 27-1

### Interventions for Nausea and Vomiting

| Causes | Intervention |
|---|---|
| Motion/dizziness | Antihistamines |
|  | Anticholinergics |
| Anxiety | Benzodiazepines |
|  | Relaxation techniques |
| Increased intracranial pressure (ICP) | Corticosteroids |
| Gastric status | Cholinergic/prokinetic |
| Stimulation of CTZ (medications, uremia) | Dopamine antagonists |
|  | Serotonin antagonists |
| Constipation | Laxatives/stool softeners |
|  | Enemas |
| Bowel obstruction | Corticosteroids |
|  | Surgery (if appropriate) |
|  | Gastric decompression (nasogastric or gastric tube) |
|  | Antisecretive agents (e.g., octreotide) |
| Hypercalcemia | Hydration |
|  | Bisphosphonates |

From Baines, M. J. (1998). The pathophysiology and management of malignant intestinal obstruction. In D. Doyle, G. Hanks, & N. MacDonald (Eds.), *Oxford textbook of palliative medicine* (2nd ed.) (pp. 526-534). London: Oxford University Press; Ferris, R., Kerr, I., Sone, M., & Marcuzzi, M. (1991). Transdermal scopolamine use in the control of narcotic induced nausea. *Journal of Pain and Symptom Management, 6,* 389-393; Lichter, I. (1993). Which antiemetic? Journal of Palliative Care, 9, 42-50; Weissman, D. E., & Ambuel, B. (1999). *Improving end of life symptom care: A resource manual for physician education* (2nd ed.). Milwaukee: Medical College of Wisconsin.

prepare combination antiemetics in suppository, oral suspension, or transdermal form. Common combinations include the following:

- Diphenhydramine, dexamethasone, and metoclopramide
- Diphenhydramine, lorazepam, and haloperidol

## Nonpharmacologic Interventions

- Complementary therapies:
  - Acupuncture (when a trained therapist is available and the patient/family is interested; may be helpful)
  - Acupressure (application of pressure to the anterior surface of the wrist, three finger-breadths proximal to the distal skin crease, between the tendons of palmaris longus and flexor carpi radialis may be effective; this can be done manually or with a commercial wrist band sold in pharmacies for motion sickness)
  - Relaxation therapy
  - Distraction
- Food and eating pattern interventions:
  - Recommendation of six to eight small meals a day, instead of three large meals

## TABLE 27-2

### Medications for the Treatment of Nausea and Vomiting

| Specific Medications | Recommended Dosing Schedule |
|---|---|
| **DOPAMINE ANTAGONISTS** | |
| Prochlorperazine (Compazine) | PO, IV, IM 10 mg q6h; PR 25 mg supp q12h |
| Chlorpromazine (Thorazine) | PO, IV, IM 25-50 mg q6h; PR 25 mg supp PR q6h; or continuous infusion |
| Haloperidol (Haldol) | PO, IV, SC, IM 0.5-2 mg q6h |
| Droperidol (Inapsine) | IV, IM 0.5-2.5 mg q6h |
| Thiethylperazine (Torecan) | IV, PO 10 mg q8h |
| Promethazine (Phenergan) | IV, PO 25 mg q6h; PR 12.5-50 mg supp q6h |
| Metoclopramide HCl (Reglan) | PO 10 mg $\frac{1}{2}$ hr ac, hs |
| **SEROTONIN ANTAGONISTS*** | |
| Ondansetron (Zofran) | IV 10 mg q8h; PO 4-8 mg q8h |
| Granisetron (Kytril) | IV 10 $\mu$g/kg qd; PO 1 mg qd or bid |
| Dolasetron mesylate (Anzemet) | IV or PO 100 mg qd |
| **PROKINETIC DRUGS†** | |
| Metoclopramide HCl (Reglan) | PO 10 mg $\frac{1}{2}$ hr ac, hs |
| **CORTICOSTEROIDS** | |
| Dexamethasone | Dose and schedule are empiric; PO or IV 4-10 mg q6h |
| **BENZODIAZEPINES** | |
| Lorazepam (Ativan) | PO or IV 0.5-2.0 mg q6h |
| **CANNABINOIDS** | |
| Dronabinol (Marinol) | PO 2.5-10 mg q6h |
| **ANTIHISTAMINES** | |
| Diphenhydramine (Benadryl) | PO or IV 25-50 mg q6h |
| Hydroxyzine (Vistaril) | PO or IM 25-50 mg q6h |
| **ANTISECRETORY AGENTS** | |
| Octreotide acetate (Sandostatin) | 300-600 $\mu$g/24 hr; used in intestinal obstruction to reduce gastrointestinal secretions and motility (Baines, 1998) |

*Because of the significantly higher cost of these medications, they are used when other antiemetic regimens are ineffective.
†Caution: Prokinetic medications (drugs that accelerate gastrointestinal transit with a meurohumoral mechanism [Twycross, Wilcock, & Thorp, 1998]) should not be used in complete bowel obstruction.

*Continued*

| TABLE 27-2 | |
|---|---|
| *Medications for the Treatment of Nausea and Vomiting—cont'd* | |
| **Specific Medications** | **Recommended Dosing Schedule** |
| **DRUGS THAT CAN BE ADMINISTERED AS CONTINUOUS INFUSIONS** | |
| Haloperidol (Haldol) (dopamine antagonist) | SC or IV |
| Metoclopramide HCl (Reglan) (prokinetic) | SC or IV |
| | Can be run simultaneously with morphine or hydromorphone in the same pump (haloperidol in D5W only) (Storey, Hill, St. Louis, & Tarver, 1990) |
| Chlorpromazine (Thorazine) | IV (Weissman, 1999) |
| **DRUGS AVAILABLE IN INTENSOL CONCENTRATIONS FOR SUBLINGUAL ADMINISTRATION** | |
| Haloperidol (Haldol) | 2mg/ml |
| Lorazepam (Ativan) | 2mg/ml |

- Selection of foods that do not have strong odors
- Eating of foods at cool temperatures instead of hot
- Encouragement of patient to sit up or recline with head raised for a least 1 hour after eating.
- Encouragement to eat slowly.

## Special Consideration for Bowel Obstruction

Persons with tumors in or around the bowel are at risk for bowel obstruction. Malignant obstructions may present acute symptoms but more often have a slow, insidious onset (Baines, 1998). Symptoms include vomiting, colicky abdominal pain, and constipation or diarrhea.

- Review with the physician the appropriateness of surgical consultation:
  - Factors associated with poor surgical or postoperative outcomes include advanced age, poor nutritional status, poor functional status, presence of ascites, previous radiation therapy to the abdomen/pelvis, presence of multiple bowel obstructions, obstruction of the small bowel, and the presence of diffuse peritoneal carcinomatosis (Baines, 1998).
- Nasogastric drainage or percutaneous gastrostomy is indicated only for vomiting or abdominal distension caused by gastric stasis/obstruction or bowel obstruction that is refractory to more conservative management of these symptoms. Remember that the goal is comfort. If the nasogastric (NG) tube causes more discomfort than the nausea or distension, it is not a good palliative intervention. When a nasal gastric (NG) or percuta-

neous endoscopic gastrostomy (PEG) tube is indicated, it should be used only until the distension is resolved.
- Symptomatic interventions are aimed at managing the discomforts associated with obstruction:
  - Treat visceral pain aggressively with opioids.
  - Treat colicky spasm pain with anticholinergics.
  - Treat nausea with antiemetics. There are no well-controlled studies that identify the best antiemetics. Haloperidol is often used as first-line treatment (Baines, 1998). Metoclopramide is often avoided in complete bowel obstruction because of potential for increased colicky pain, fistula formation, or bowel perforation (Baines, 1998). However if the patient is passing flatus, metoclopramide is safe and effective (Twycross, 1997).
  - Consider corticosteroids to decrease inflammation in the bowel and to produce an antiemetic effect.
  - Administer antisecretory agents, such as octreotide. A prospective study demonstrated that persons with bowel obstruction who received octreotide had fewer episodes of vomiting, less intense nausea, and less pain (Mercadante, Ripamonti, Casuccio, Zecca, & Groff, 2000). Although it is expensive, if this intervention decreases the need for antiemetics, analgesics, and hospitalization, it may be cost-effective.
  - Restrict oral fluids and/or discontinue intravenous (IV) fluids to decrease GI fluid output and vagal stimulation, with regard to the patient's wishes.
  - Discontinue laxatives.

## ■ PATIENT AND FAMILY EDUCATION

To decrease the incidence of nausea and vomiting and treat it effectively, the following information is taught to patients and their family caregivers:
- Encourage monitoring for patterns and frequency of nausea and vomiting episodes.
- Inform them to notify their health care provider when:
  - More than three episodes of vomiting occur in a day.
  - Vomiting occurs soon after oral administration of medication.
- Instruct them on the proper dose and administration of antiemetics.
- Teach them to avoid eating or drinking for 1 to 2 hours after vomiting and to encourage fluid intake. A liquid diet for 24 hours may allow the GI tract to rest and allow the antiemetics a chance to work.
- Tell patients and caregivers that the patient should choose when and what to eat.
- Oral medication and oral hygiene measures may contribute to nausea.
- Teach good treatment of pain, anxiety, and cough as these symptoms can contribute to nausea and vomiting.

- As with all treatments at the end of life, emphasize that the treatment of nausea and vomiting is a patient choice. The consequences of no treatment should be part of the overall goal-setting discussion with the patient.

## ■ EVALUATION AND PLAN FOR FOLLOW-UP

Success of the therapy regimen should be determined by evaluating mutually established goals with the patient, such as "one episode of nausea and emesis per day." In general patients are usually satisfied if nausea is controlled and vomiting is limited to once a day.

---

✔ **CASE STUDY**

Mr. B. is a 78-year-old gentleman who has advanced prostate cancer. He enters the clinic for control of nausea. He has been under treatment for the past 7 years and now has uncontrolled disease with widespread metastatic sites of cancer, including the bladder. He has nephrectomy tubes in place. Three months ago he underwent a colostomy for blockage of his lower bowel. Mr. B. is receiving leuprolide acetate injections every 3 months. He has not had radiation therapy in the past year. He reports a weight loss of 30 pounds over the last 4 months. When asked what the physicians told him about his disease status, he states, "They told me 6 to 9 months, 6 months ago."

You obtain the following assessment data regarding Mr. B.'s nausea: The nausea is constant and began after the colostomy was placed. It has gradually increased in intensity and now has accompanying episodes of emesis, about every third day. His emesis consists of small amounts of digested food. He reports that eating large amounts of food makes it worse. He cannot name anything that makes it worse or makes it better! The colostomy is functioning. Bowel sounds are normal and laboratory values are normal.

Mr. B. has not taken anything for the nausea. He reports trying to avoid any extra pills but now feels he no longer can avoid medications. His only medication, besides the every-3-month leuprolide acetate injection, is clonidine (Catapres) daily. He does not take any over-the-counter medications. Mr. B. states that he does not want to undergo any further evaluation tests if they can be avoided.

In determining the best pharmacologic choices, you consider that the nausea is constant, the cause is not known, and there are no signs or symptoms of intestinal obstruction. A dopamine antagonist is perhaps the best beginning point to provide broadest coverage of causes. Prochlorperazine, 10 mg PO q6h around the clock, is an appropriate starting regimen.

This patient will likely benefit from nonpharmacologic interventions as well. Suggest small meals. Assure Mr. B. that there are a number of approaches to therapy and that any medications are easily adjusted to find the best medication and dose for him. Allow time for Mr. B. to talk about his statement "They told me 6 to 9 months, 6 months ago," as this may open a wide variety of emotional concerns that need to be addressed.

Mr. B. and his family are given the following instructions:

- Start the prochlorperazine, 10 mg PO q6h around the clock
- Keep a record of episodes of nausea and emesis and note any relationship to time of last meal.
- Contact health care provider if no relief in intensity of nausea occurs in 3 days (mutually agreed upon goal).

## References

BAINES, M. J. (1998). The pathophysiology and management of malignant intestinal obstruction. In D. Doyle, G. Hanks, & N. MacDonald (Eds.), *Oxford textbook of palliative medicine* (2nd ed.) (pp. 526-534). London: Oxford University Press.

BAINES, M. J. (1999). Nausea, vomiting, and intestinal obstruction. In M. Fallon & B. O'Neill (Eds.), *ABC of palliative care* (pp. 16-18). London: BMJ Books.

FALLON, B. G. (1998). Nausea and vomiting unrelated to cancer treatment. In A. Berger, R. Portenoy, & D. E. Weissman (Eds.), *Principles and practice of supportive oncology* (pp. 179-189). Philadelphia: Lippincott-Raven.

FERRIS, R., Kerr, I., Sone, M., & Marcuzzi, M. (1991). Transdermal scopolamine use in the control of narcotic induced nausea. *Journal of Pain and Symptom Management, 6,* 389-393.

JABLONSKI, R. (1993). Nausea: The forgotten symptom. *Holistic Nursing Practice, 7,* 64-72.

LICHTER, I. (1993). Which antiemetic? *Journal of Palliative Care, 9,* 42-50.

MANNIX, K. F. (1998). Palliation of nausea and vomiting. In D. Doyle, G. Hanks, N. MacDonald (Eds.), *Oxford textbook of palliative medicine* (2nd ed.) (pp. 489-499). London: Oxford University Press.

MERCADANTE, S., Ripamonti, C., Casuccio, A., Zecca, E., & Groff, L. (2000). Comparison of octreotide and hyoscine butylbromide in controlling gastrointestinal symptoms due to malignant inoperable bowel obstruction. *Supportive Care in Cancer, 8,* 188-192.

STOREY, P., Hill, H., St. Louis, R., & Tarver, E. (1990). Subcutaneous infusions for control of cancer symptoms. *Journal of Pain and Symptom Management, 5,* 33-41.

TWYCROSS, R. (1997). *Symptom management in advanced cancer* (2nd ed.). Oxon, UK: Radcliffe Medical Press.

TWYCROSS, R., & Back, O. (1998). Nausea and vomiting in advanced cancer. *European Journal of Palliative Care, 5,* 39-45.

TWYCROSS, R., Wilcock, A., & Thorp, S. (1998). *Palliative care formulary.* Oxon, UK: Radcliffe Medical Press.

WEISSMAN, D. E., & Ambuel, B. (1999). *Improving end of life symptom care: A resource manual for physician education* (2nd ed.). Milwaukee: Medical College of Wisconsin.

WORLD Health Organization (1998). *Symptom relief in terminal illness.* Geneva, Switzerland: Author.

C H A P T E R **28**

# *Pain*

JULIE GRIFFIE, SANDY MCKINNON, PATRICIA
H. BERRY, DEBRA E. HEIDRICH

**T**he assessment and management of pain are central to high-quality end-of-life care. This overview of pain includes its definition, incidence, cause, assessment, and management, as well as the special issues associated with managing pain in a person with a current or past history of substance abuse. We strongly encourage the reader to invest in another reference that is devoted entirely to pain. Margo McCaffery and Chris Pasero's 1999 book, *Pain: Clinical Manual* (2nd ed.), published by Mosby, is an excellent reference. There are also several resources for pain management on the internet, including the American Pain Society (http://www.ampainsoc. org), City of Hope Pain/Palliative Care Resource Center Website (http:// mayday.coh.org), and The Resource Center for Pain Medicine and Palliative Care at Beth Israel Medical Center (http://www.stoppain.org). Likewise, we urge the reader to identify resources regarding pain and its management available in your community. For example, is there access to persons experienced in treating pain patients with chemical dependency or a history of addiction? Is there a pain specialist available for consultation about the treatment of difficult pain syndromes or refractory pain? Does the local pharmacy stock commonly used pain medications? Is there a drug information center or a specialist in drug interactions available?

## ■ DEFINITION AND INCIDENCE

The International Association for the Study of Pain (IASP) defines *pain* as an unpleasant sensory and emotional experience associated with actual or potential tissue damage or described in terms of such damage (IASP, 1979). Pain, however, is a highly personal and subjective experience. McCaffery (1968) proposed the definition most applicable to clinical practice: "Pain is whatever the experiencing person says it is, existing whenever he/she says it does." The patient's self-report of pain is its single most reliable indicator. In other words, the patient's report must be accepted at face value (American Pain Society, 1999; Jacox et al., 1994).

The deleterious physical, psychosocial, emotional, spiritual, and financial effects of uncontrolled pain contribute markedly to suffering and decreased quality of life. Physical effects include reduced functional ability, including walking and other basic activities of daily living (ADLs); decreased strength and endurance; nausea; anorexia; insomnia; and impaired immune response (Cousins, 1994; Desbiens, Mueller-Rizner, Connors, & Wenger, 1997; Keller, Weiss, Schliefer, Miller, & Stein, 1981; Liebeskind, 1991; Serlin, Mendoza, Nakamura, Edwards, & Cleeland, 1995; Sklar & Anisman, 1979; Sydow, 1988; Visintainer, Volpocelli, & Seligman, 1982; Wattine, 1988). Pain also interferes with social and intimate relations, causing isolation and inability to work or attend to important issues. It increases caregiver burden and diminishes important social supports for both the patient and the family. Uncontrolled pain increases fear and anxiety and fosters depression, feelings of despair, and even consideration of suicide or physician-assisted suicide (BenDebba, Torgerson, & Long, 1997; Casten, Parmalee, Kleban, Lawton, & Katz, 1995; Foley, 1991; McCaffery & Pasero, 1999; Snelling, 1994; Taylor, Ferrell, Grant, & Cheyney, 1993). Finally some pain medications and other treatment regimens are expensive, causing economic stress at a particularly vulnerable time.

Pain may be classified based on duration or by inferred pathophysiology. The interventions selected to treat pain will be influenced by both of these types of classification (McCaffery & Pasero, 1999). These classifications are as follows:

- Types of pain based on duration:
  - Acute pain is relatively brief in duration. There is a recognized cause of the pain and the pain diminishes as healing takes place. With acute pain, there are often observable autonomic signs of discomfort (e.g., increased pulse rate and blood pressure) and nonverbal signs (e.g., tense muscles, facial grimace).
  - Chronic pain is described as pain that persists after the initial injury. It is perceived as irreversible and meaningless. Due to physiologic and behavioral adaptation, there are few or no autonomic or nonverbal signs of discomfort.
- Types of pain based on inferred pathophysiology:
  - Nociceptive pain arises from direct stimulation of the afferent nerves in the skin, soft tissue, or viscera. This type of pain may be further classified as somatic pain, caused by stimulation of nociceptors in the skin, joints, muscle, bone, or connective tissue; or visceral pain, caused by stimulation of nociceptors in the visceral organs.
  - Neuropathic pain results from abnormal processing of sensory input due to nerve damage. This type of pain may be further classified as centrally generated pain or peripherally generated pain.

The sensations the patient experiences may be different with each type of pain. Table 28-1 identifies common descriptors for each type of pain and gives examples of each. Patients may experience several different types of pain at the same time; some of these pains may be somatic, some visceral, some neuropathic, and some mixed. Because interventions are based on the type and severity of pain, thorough assessment of each site of pain is critical to appropriate pain management.

The term *breakthrough pain* refers to yet another pain experience. Portenoy & Hagen (1990) define breakthrough pain as a "transitory exacerbation of

## TABLE 28-1

### Classifications and Examples of Pain

| Pain Type | Subtype | Descriptors | Examples |
|---|---|---|---|
| Nociceptive | Somatic | ■ Aching<br>■ Throbbing<br>■ Well-localized | Acute somatic pain:<br>■ Surgical incisions<br>■ Muscle or joint sprain<br>Chronic somatic pain:<br>■ Arthritis<br>■ Metastatic cancer to the bone |
| Nociceptive | Visceral | ■ Aching<br>■ Gnawing<br>■ Deep and squeezing<br>■ Intermittent cramping<br>■ Poorly localized; referred | Acute visceral pain:<br>■ Angina<br>■ Bladder irritation (e.g., infection)<br>■ Acute bowel obstruction<br>Chronic visceral pain:<br>■ Pancreatic cancer<br>■ Metastatic cancer to the liver |
| Neuropathic: Centrally generated | Deafferentation | ■ Burning<br>■ Aching<br>■ Lancinating<br>■ Pricking<br>■ Lacerating<br>■ Pressing | ■ Phantom limb pain (may have both central and peripheral mechanisms)<br>■ Spinal cord injury |

Adapted from Boivie, J. (1999). Central pain. In P. D. Wall & R. Melzack (Eds.), *Textbook of pain* (4th ed.) (pp. 879-941). New York: Churchill Livingstone; Cousins, M., & Powers, I. (1999). Acute and postoperative pain. In P. D. Wall & R. Melzack (Eds.), *Textbook of pain* (4th ed.) (pp. 474-491). New York: Churchill Livingstone; Jensen, T. S., & Nikolajsen, L. (1999). Phantom pain and other phenomena after amputation. In P. D. Wall & R. Melzack (Eds.), *Textbook of pain* (4th ed.) (pp. 799-814). New York: Churchill Livingstone; McCaffery, M., & Pasero, C. (1999). *Pain: Clinical manual* (2nd ed.). St. Louis: Mosby; Scadding, J. W. (1999a). Complex regional pain syndrome. In P. D. Wall & R. Melzack (Eds.), *Textbook of pain* (4th ed.) (pp. 835-849). New York: Churchill Livingstone; Scadding, J. W. (1999b). Peripheral neuropathies. In P. D. Wall & R. Melzack (Eds.), *Textbook of pain* (4th ed.) (pp. 815-834). New York: Churchill Livingstone.

*Continued*

## TABLE 28-1

### Classifications and Examples of Pain—cont'd

| Pain Type | Subtype | Descriptors | Examples |
|-----------|---------|-------------|----------|
| Neuropathic: Centrally generated | Sympathetically maintained | ▪ Burning<br>▪ Hyperalgesia<br>▪ Allodynia<br>▪ Accompanied by excessive sweating and vasomotor changes | ▪ Complex regional pain syndromes |
| Neuropathic: Peripherally generated | Polyneuropathies | ▪ Deep aching<br>▪ Superficial burning, stinging, or prickling<br>▪ Shocklike; lancinating<br>▪ Pain felt along distribution of many peripheral nerves | ▪ Diabetic neuropathy<br>▪ Drug-induced neuropathy (e.g., due to vinca alkaloid chemotherapy) |
| Neuropathic: Peripherally generated | Mononeuropathies | ▪ Burning<br>▪ Severe aching<br>▪ Intermittent staging or electric shock–like<br>▪ Pain along distribution of single nerve or dermatome | Mononeuropathies:<br>▪ Nerve root compression<br>▪ Trigeminal neuralgia<br>Multiple mononeuropathies:<br>▪ Postherpetic neuralgia |

pain that occurs on a background of otherwise stable pain in a patient receiving chronic opioid therapy (p. 273)." Breakthrough pain varies widely according to the following features and must be assessed thoroughly:

- Temporal characteristics:
  - Time from first perception to maximum intensity—Paroxysmal breakthrough pain reaches maximal intensity within 3 minutes; gradual breakthrough pain reaches maximal intensity in greater than 3 minutes.
  - Frequency of occurrence—The number of episodes in a 24-hour period can vary widely. Portenoy & Hagen (1990) reported that, in a group of 41 participants with breakthrough pain, the median number of episodes in this time period was 4; the range, however, was 1 to 3600 episodes per day.
  - Duration—Breakthrough pain can last anywhere from minutes to hours.
- Severity: Most breakthrough pain is severe to excruciating in intensity.

- Location: The location of pain may be the same as the underlying pain syndrome that is being treated or may involve an entirely different site.
- Precipitating event: Some breakthrough pain is associated with end-of-dose failure of routine analgesic, some pains are associated with precipitating events, and some are idiopathic.
- Pathophysiology: Breakthrough pain may be somatic, visceral, neuropathic, or mixed.

The experience of pain is the product of complex physical, cognitive, emotional, and social processes. Although pain is usually associated with tissue damage, its intensity is not always proportional to the extent of the damage (Jacox et al., 1994). Many factors mediate the subjective experience of pain, such as type and stage of disease, personal history, and personality characteristics (Foley, 1998).

Many illnesses in the terminal phase can produce severe pain, including cancer, acquired immunodeficiency syndrome (AIDS), multiple sclerosis, and sickle-cell disease (Payne & Gonzales, 1998). Pain control at the end of life remains an important, yet often neglected issue. Data from the SUPPORT study showed a high incidence of uncontrolled pain (from 74% to 95%) in very ill and dying hospitalized adults in spite of planned interventions from nurses encouraging physicians to attend to pain control (SUPPORT Study Principal Investigators, 1995). Table 28-2 summarizes the incidence of pain in the most common end-stage illnesses.

## ■ ETIOLOGY AND PATHOPHYSIOLOGY
### Etiology

The "unpleasant sensory experience" in the definition of pain arises from the transmission of pain stimuli through the peripheral and central nervous systems. Pain may be caused by direct effects of the disease process or by treatments aimed at mediating the disease such as surgery, chemotherapy, or radiation therapy. Refer to Table 28-1 for a brief discussion of the cause of each pain type.

### Pathophysiology

There are two major classifications of pain, based on physiologic characteristics: nociceptive pain and neuropathic pain. Each of these has two subtypes, as identified in Figure 28-1.

Nociceptive pain occurs when a pain stimulus is generated from either somatic or visceral structures. Pain from somatic structures, including bone, joints, muscle, skin, and connective tissue, is usually described as "aching" or "throbbing," and the patient can often point to the exact area where the painful stimulus is occurring (i.e., it is well localized). Stimuli from visceral tissues—mainly thoracic, abdominal, and pelvic organs—cause pain that is described as gnawing and aching. This pain may or may not be well localized; in fact, visceral pain may be felt in areas other than the original site, a phenomenon

## TABLE 28-2

### The Incidence of Pain in Common Advanced Illnesses

| Disease Process | Incidence | Examples |
|---|---|---|
| Advanced cancer | 64%-80% | Acute:<br>■ Tests and procedures<br>■ Acute infections<br>■ Flare response to medications<br>■ Spinal cord compression<br>Chronic:<br>■ Primary malignancy or metastasis to bone, liver, pancreas, brain, spinal cord<br>■ Chemotherapy-related neuropathies<br>■ Postherpetic neuropathy<br>■ Postsurgical pain syndromes<br>■ Postradiation plexopathies |
| AIDS | 30%-97% with 25% neuropathic, 44% somatic, 14% visceral, 17% idiopathic | ■ Headache due to meningitis<br>■ Neuropathies: HIV-related, medication-related, postherpetic<br>■ Abdominal pain due to infection and diarrhea<br>■ Arthralgia and myalgia<br>■ Esophagitis due to infections |
| Multiple sclerosis | 42%-65% | ■ Trigeminal neuralgia<br>■ Musculoskeletal pain<br>■ Dysesthetic pain (likely centrally-generated) |
| Cerebrovascular disease | 8% | ■ Central poststroke pain syndrome |
| Diabetes | 10%-32% | ■ Diabetic neuropathy (centrally generated)<br>■ Cranial nerve palsies (mononeuropathy) |

Adapted from Boivie, J. (1999). Central pain. In P. D. Wall & R. Melzack (Eds.), *Textbook of pain* (4th ed.) (pp. 879-941). New York: Churchill Livingstone; Cousins, M., & Powers, I. (1999). Acute and postoperative pain. In P. D. Wall & R. Melzack (Eds.), *Textbook of pain* (4th ed.) (pp. 474-491). New York: Churchill Livingstone; Jensen, T. S., & Nikolajsen, L. (1999). Phantom pain and other phenomena after amputation. In P. D. Wall & R. Melzack (Eds.), *Textbook of pain* (4th ed.) (pp. 799-814). New York: Churchill Livingstone; McCaffery, M., & Pasero, C. (1999). *Pain: Clinical manual* (2nd ed.). St. Louis: Mosby; Scadding, J. W. (1999a). Complex regional pain syndrome. In P. D. Wall & R. Melzack (Eds.), *Textbook of pain* (4th ed.) (pp. 835-849). New York: Churchill Livingstone; Scadding, J. W. (1999b). Peripheral neuropathies. In P. D. Wall & R. Melzack (Eds.), *Textbook of pain* (4th ed.) (pp. 815-834). New York: Churchill Livingstone.

known as *referred pain*. Figure 28-2 illustrates some commonly reported sites where pain may be referred from visceral organs.

Neuropathic pain is not as clearly understood as nociceptive pain. Peripherally generated neuropathic pains involve abnormal processing of sensory input from the peripheral nerves and may be described as

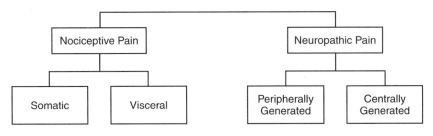

**FIG. 28-1** Types of pain.

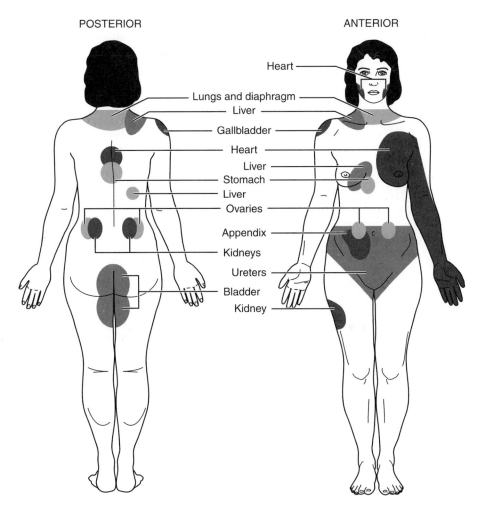

**FIG. 28-2** Commonly reported sites where pain may be referred from visceral organs. From Brockrath, M. (1985). *Fundamentals. Nursing Now* (p. 18). Springhouse, PA). Springhouse Corporation.

"aching," "burning," "tingling," or "shocklike." Centrally generated neuropathic pains involve abnormal processing of sensory input at the spinal cord level, leading to hyperexcitability. This causes an abnormal continuation of pain impulses, even in the absence of further pain stimuli or an abnormal processing of stimuli such that normally nonpainful stimuli are perceived as painful (allodynia). Neuropathic pain syndromes can be difficult to treat.

**Nociceptive pain processes.** There are four processes involved in nociceptive pain: transduction, transmission, perception, and modulation. Transduction occurs when the pain fibers of the tissues are exposed to mechanical, thermal, or chemical stimuli, causing actual tissue damage. The damaged tissue releases substances that stimulate or sensitize the pain fibers (see Table 28-3). In the presence of sufficient stimulation the nerve membrane becomes permeable to sodium, leading to depolarization. An efflux of potassium causes repolarization. Repeated depolarization and repolarization generate an impulse and transduction is complete (Fields, 1987; McCaffery & Pasero, 1999; Wilke, 1995).

The second phase of nociception is transmission of the impulse from the site of injury to the spinal cord, up to the brain stem, and out to the thalamus and cortex. Nociceptive fibers carry the impulse to the dorsal horn of the spinal cord, where these fibers end. In order to transmit the impulse to dorsal horn neurons, neurotransmitters are required. These neurotransmitters include adenosine triphosphate, glutamate, and substance P (Fields, 1987; McCaffery & Pasero, 1999).

One of several receptors involved in this process is the N-methyl-D-aspartate (NMDA) receptor. Glutamate, an excitatory neurotransmitter, normally binds to the NMDA receptor, facilitating the transmission of the pain impulse (Fields, 1987). Interference with this process can inhibit the transmission of pain.

---

**TABLE 28-3**

*Substances Released in Response to Tissue Injury*

| Stimulate Pain Fiber | Sensitize Pain Fiber |
| --- | --- |
| Bradykinin | Leukotrienes |
| Serotonin | Prostaglandins |
| Histamine | Substance P |
| Potassium | |
| Norepinephrine | |

From Fields, H. L. (1987). *Pain.* New York: McGraw-Hill; Aimone, L. D. (1992). Neurochemistry and modulation of pain. In R. S. Sinatra, A. H. Hord, B. Ginsberg, & L. M. Preble (Eds.), *Acute pain: Mechanisms and management* (pp. 29-43). St. Louis: Mosby Year Book; Wilke, D. J. (1995). Neural mechanisms of pain: A foundation for cancer pain assessment and management. In D. B. McGuire, C. H. Yarbro, & B. R. Ferrell (Eds.), *Cancer pain management* (2nd ed.) (pp. 61-87). Boston: Jones & Bartlett.

Once transmitted across the synaptic space in the dorsal horn, the impulse is transmitted through several different ascending pathways to the brain stem, thalamus, and higher brain centers. This ends the transmission phase of nociception and begins the phase of perception. Precisely where pain is perceived in the brain is not clear, but this is thought to occur at several cerebral levels. Processing by the somatosensory cortex allows an individual to localize and characterize the pain. The emotional and behavioral responses to pain occur when the pain stimulus is processed in the limbic system. The reticular activating system is responsible for the autonomic responses to pain (Fields, 1987; McCaffery & Pasero, 1999; Wilke, 1995).

The fourth process in nociception is modulation. This involves the descending pathways from the brain to the dorsal horn of the spinal cord. Substances that inhibit the transmission of pain may be released by these descending fibers. Among these substances are endogenous opioids (enkephalin), serotonin, norepinephrine, gamma-aminobutyric acid (GABA), alpha$_2$-adrenergic substances, and neurotensin (Fields, 1987).

**Neuropathic pain processes.**   As mentioned, neuropathic pain processes are not as clearly understood but involve abnormal processing of sensory input. The peripheral neuropathic pains may be caused by injury to the nerve that causes a spontaneous generation of an action potential (Coderre & Melzack, 1992). An example of a peripheral neuropathic pain is that caused by neurotoxic chemotherapy agents. The resulting nerve damage may cause this spontaneous generation of the painful stimulus even after the discontinuation of the offending medication.

Centrally generated neuropathic pain may occur as a result of repetitive transmission of nociceptive signals to the dorsal horn, causing changes in the processing of these impulses. Hypersensitivity and hyperexcitability result. The NMDA receptors are proposed to be involved in this process (Coderre & Melzack, 1992; Wilke, 1995). Prevention and prompt treatment of pain may prevent these dorsal horn changes.

**Physiologic rationale for pain medications.**   Medications used to treat pain are discussed in detail in the "Intervention and Treatment" section of this chapter. It is important to understand the rationale for the use of these medications, which is based on the physiologic characteristics of pain. Most medications used to manage pain function by interrupting transduction or transmission or by enhancing modulation, as summarized in Table 28-4.

## Myths and Misconceptions about Pain

The treatment of pain is wrought with myths, misconceptions, and erroneous beliefs. Understanding these myths and correcting them are essential to the assessment and treatment of pain. Unfortunately these issues are quite common among patients, families, health care professionals, and the general public.

## TABLE 28-4

### The Physiologic Rationale for Pain Medications

| Medication Class | Mechanism of Action |
| --- | --- |
| NSAIDs | Block production of prostaglandins |
| Anticonvulsants | Block influx of sodium ions, preventing depolarization and generation of an action potential |
| Local anesthetics | Block influx of sodium ions, preventing depolarization and generation of an action potential |
| Corticosteroids | Block production of prostaglandins |
| Opioids | Bind with opioid receptors and block release of substance P |
| NMDA receptor antagonists | Inhibit binding of excitatory amino acids, such as glutamate, preventing transmission |
| Tricyclic antidepressants | Prevent reuptake of serotonin and norepinephrine |
| GABA agonists | Enhance release of GABA |
| Alpha-adrenergic agonists | Inhibit release of substance P |

From McCaffery, M., & Pasero, C. (1999). *Pain: Clinical manual* (2nd ed.). St. Louis: Mosby.

Recall the pain content in your undergraduate and graduate programs. Likely you did not receive education about pain assessment or management; consequently we find this to be an area in which clinicians need substantial self-education. So we return to the basics here, including a review of the erroneous beliefs and attitudes that prevent patients and families from reporting pain and using analgesics and the erroneous beliefs and attitudes held by health care professionals. We also define addiction, tolerance, and physical dependence, and iatrogenic opioid pseudoaddiction.

Understanding why patients and families may hesitate to report pain and use analgesics is essential to the successful treatment of pain and an improved quality of life. Ward and colleagues (Ward et al., 1993) have identified eight barriers; lack of adequate pain control in cancer patients at all stages of illness is related to their concerns about reporting pain and using analgesics (Ward et al., 1993; Ward & Hernandez, 1994). These barriers can serve as a departure point for discussing effective pain management with patients and families:

1. Fear of opioid side effects
2. Fear of addiction
3. Belief that increasing pain signifies disease progression
4. Fear of injections
5. Concern about drug tolerance
6. Belief that "good" patients do not complain about pain
7. Belief that reporting pain may distract the physician from treating or curing the cancer
8. Fatalism, the belief that pain is inevitable with cancer and that it cannot be relieved

Likewise, health care professionals retain erroneous attitudes and beliefs about pain and the use of medications that negatively affect pain assessment and management:

1. *The patient's self report of pain is not to be believed; health care professionals are the best judge of pain.* The patient's report of pain must be accepted; there are no diagnostic or "objective" tests for pain. Pain is whatever the experiencing person says it is, existing whenever he or she says it does (McCaffrey, 1968). History is 80% of the diagnosis: the patient's subjective report of pain is more important to an accurate diagnosis, since there are no physical examination techniques or diagnostic tests to confirm pain history. The patient's report must be accepted.

2. *Addiction to pain medication is common.* Addiction, when pain medications are used for the treatment of pain, is extremely rare (Weissman, Burchman, Dahl, & Dinndorf, 1994). There is much confusion over the meanings and application of addiction, tolerance, and physical dependence. They are defined as follows:

   ▪ *Addiction* is overwhelming involvement with obtaining and using a drug for its psychic benefits, not for medical reasons; behavior is compulsive and subject to relapse. Quality of life is not improved; however, use continues despite harm and is out of control.

   ▪ *Tolerance* occurs after repeated administration of an opioid when a given dosage begins to lose its effectiveness—first in duration of action, second in overall effectiveness.

   ▪ *Physical dependence* is the condition in which, after repeated administration of an opioid, withdrawal symptoms occur when it is not taken. Signs and symptoms of abstinence syndrome (withdrawal) include anxiety, irritability, lacrimation, rhinorrhea, sweating, nausea, vomiting, cramps, insomnia, and, rarely, multifocal myoclonus.

   Requests for pain medication because pain is uncontrolled are often mistaken for addiction. This is referred to as opioid pseudoaddiction.

   ▪ *Opioid pseudoaddiction* is an iatrogenic (meaning "health care system–acquired") syndrome in which certain behavioral characteristics of psychologic dependence develop as a consequence of inadequate pain treatment (Weissman & Haddox, 1989).

3. *Respiratory depression is a frequent, serious complication with opioid use.* Respiratory depression is feared and misunderstood by patients, families, and health care professionals. Tolerance develops rapidly to respiratory depression; thus it is rarely a problem except in the opioid naïve patient. Keep in mind that respiratory rate alone is not an indicator of respiratory depression; careful assessment of the whole patient, not just respiratory rate, is required. Most importantly, adequate pain management does not shorten life or hasten death.

There are other barriers to adequate pain management including our "antidrug" culture and perceived regulatory barriers that vary state to state.

Such restrictions include triplicate prescription programs or other systems that monitor prescribing patterns or a lack of laws facilitating pain management in end-stage illness, including partial filling of scheduled medications. Familiarize yourself with your own state's nurse practice act, regulations, and controlled substances laws.

## ■ ASSESSMENT AND MEASUREMENT

If pain is not assessed, appropriate management is impossible. Pain is a multidimensional human experience and thus requires a comprehensive, holistic evaluation. Each new pain report requires a systematic assessment, appropriate treatment, and follow-up. A complete pain assessment includes the following:

- Site: The patient identifies primary sites as well as sites of radiation on his or her body or a diagram. Remember also that the patient may have more than one site of pain, and it may be helpful to number pains to organize assessment, interventions, and evaluations.
- Character: Use the patient's own words; a careful description will lead to the diagnosis of pain type, and therefore use of appropriate analgesics (i.e., *sharp, shooting* describes neuropathic pain syndromes).
- Onset: When did it start? Did (or does) a specific event trigger the pain? Carefully distinguish between new and preexisting pain (i.e., arthritis, chronic low back pain syndromes).
- Duration and frequency: How long has the pain persisted? Is it constant or intermittent?
- Intensity: Intensity is commonly defined on a scale, most frequently of 0 to 10, as this intensity scale has been validated in international populations and based on function, defining pain that is mild, moderate, and severe (Serlin et al., 1995). However, the pain intensity measure must be adapted to the patient and you should have an alternate scale available for patients unable or unwilling to use the 0 to 10 scale. For example, some patients prefer a verbal descriptor scale or a modification of a smile/sad scale. Regardless you must adapt the intensity rating method to the patient. Record pain intensity "now," at its "worst," and at its "least." Other intensity scales are available as well. Note that ratings of pain intensity are the most important pain assessment data to collect if time is short; pain intensity directly correlates with interference with the patient's quality of life.
- Exacerbating factors: What times, activities, or other circumstances make the pain worse?
- Associated symptoms: What other symptoms occur before, with, or after the pain?
- Alleviating factors: What makes the pain better? Which treatments have been successful in the past and which unsuccessful? Include a thorough medication history, especially for the past 24 hours.

- Effect on quality of life: How does the pain affect the patient's ability to perform the activities of daily living? How does the pain affect relationships with close others? What does the pain mean to the patient and family? How has this pain affected them? How much do the patient and family know about pain? Do they have the expectation that it can be relieved? Are there emotional or spiritual components to the pain? Does unrelieved pain lead to increased fear or anxiety, or to fears that death is imminent?
- The patient's goal for relief: Consider using either a pain intensity score or a functional goal, for example, the ability to walk without pain.
- Physical examination: Observe the site of the pain, and validate with the patient the pain's location. Note skin color, warmth, irritation, integrity, and any other unusual findings (Berry et al., 1999).
- Other effects of pain: Assess for the presence of depression, anxiety, and other emotional aspects of the pain or the experience or perception of the pain.

There are multiple pain assessment forms and scales available. Figure 28-3, one example, presents a 0 to 10 scale and other alternate scales.

## Assessment of the Cognitively Impaired

Assessment of patients who lack verbal skills because of cognitive impairment requires astute observation of behavior. Nonverbal behavior, vocalizations, changes in functional level or activities of daily living, and caregiver reports should be used as aspects of pain assessment in the older person (American Geriatrics Society Panel on Chronic Pain in Older Persons, 1998). A change in behavior is the gold standard for suspecting pain or discomfort in a cognitively impaired person. Kovach et al. (1999) suggests the following protocol for assessing discomfort in patients with dementia who exhibit a change in behavior:

- Physical assessment for a cause of discomfort/pain. If a cause is found, treatment is initiated.
- Review of the patient's history for possible causes of pain through medical records and family members.
- Trial of nonpharmacologic interventions appropriate to the circumstances; levels of environmental stimuli should also be evaluated and adjusted for the patient's comfort.
- If the preceding steps are unsuccessful, a trial of a nonopioid analgesic is indicated.
- If the nonopioid is unsuccessful, choose a stronger medication, using the WHO analgesic ladder as a guide (Figure 28-4); for example, a smaller dose of an opioid in combination with acetaminophen such as hydrocodone (World Health Organization, 1990).

The importance of including a caring approach and the use of nonpharmacologic interventions that enhance the dignity and self-esteem of the individual cannot be stressed enough in the care of persons with cognitive impairment.

## INITIAL PAIN ASSESSMENT

**A**

**LOCATION**
*Mark site A, B, or C*

| PATIENT NAME | MEDICAL RECORD NUMBER |
|---|---|
| DATE | RN SIGNATURE |

Pain Intensity Rating Scale:

```
     0  1  2  3  4  5  6  7  8  9  10
No  |__|__|__|__|__|__|__|__|__|__|     Worst
Pain                                     Possible
                                         Pain
```

| Patient's Rating of Pain Intensity: | Site A | Site B | Site C |
|---|---|---|---|
| Scale used:    Present: | | | |
| ☐ 0-10 (preferred) | | | |
| ☐ Smile-Sad    At Worst: | | | |
| ☐ Verbal    At Best: | | | |
| Pain Characteristics  Describe: | Describe: | Describe: | Describe: |

Cues:
Aching, deep, dull, gnawing, sharp, stabbing
Crampy, pressure, squeezing
Burning, numb, radiating, shooting, stabbing, tingling, touch sensitive

History of pain management:

What relieves pain?

What have you done in the past when you've had pain?

How does the pain affect your day-to-day life and activities?

How do you feel about taking pain medications?

Physical findings at the site of pain:

Present pain medication and effectiveness:

**PATIENT'S PAIN CONTROL GOAL**
☐ Sleep comfortably
☐ Comfort at rest
☐ Comfort with movement
☐ Total pain control
☐ Stay alert
☐ Perform activity:
☐ Other:

**PATIENT'S PAIN INTENSITY GOAL**
0  1  2  3  4  5  6  7  8  9  10

Start Pain Management Flowsheet if:
• Pain score is 5 or greater *or*
• Patient is taking analgesics *or*
• Pain score is greater than patient's goal

**FIG. 28-3** **A,** Initial Pain Assessment. **B,** FACES pain rating scale. *A* is adapted from an assessment form developed by the University of Wisconsin Hospital and Clinics Home Health Agency, Madison, WI. *B* is modified from Wong DL, Hockenberry-Eaton M, Wilson D et al (Eds.) (2001). *Wong's Essentials of Nursing,* ed. 6, St. Louis, Mosby.

Pain Rating Scales

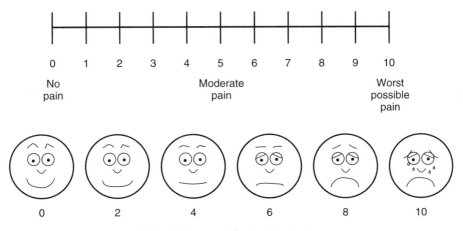

B

FIG. 28-3, cont'd   B, Pain Scales.

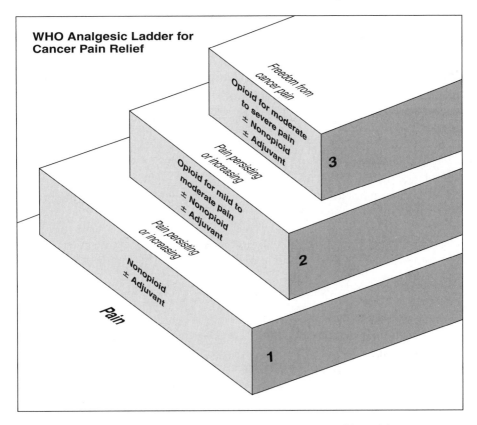

FIG. 28-4   The WHO three-step analgesic ladder. From World Health Organization (1996). *Cancer pain relief*, ed. 2, Geneva, Author.

# ■ HISTORY AND PHYSICAL EXAMINATION

Physical examination, appropriate to each location of the pain determined in the assessment, should be performed. Additional history may be suggested by physical findings.

# ■ DIAGNOSTICS

Radiologic examinations may be appropriate to direct treatment of the underlying cause of pain within the patient's goals of care. As discussed in the previous chapters, decisions to pursue further diagnostics are based upon the patient's place on the disease trajectory and the goals of care.

Laboratory evaluation may or may not be appropriate. In any case, the most recent laboratory values should be reviewed. Blood urea nitrogen (BUN) and creatinine levels may be indicated to ascertain renal function prior to initiation of opioid therapy if renal insufficiency is suspected. Likewise, liver functions may also be indicated if hepatic insufficiency is suspected. A vitamin $B_{12}$ level may be determined to rule out a $B_{12}$ deficiency in the patient who has neuropathic pain.

# ■ INTERVENTION AND TREATMENT
## Basic Principles of Pain Management

The following principles serve as a guide to the basics of pain management (Berry et al., 1999; Dahl, 2000):

1. Document the pain assessment data so the pain syndrome can be identified and appropriately treated.
2. Match the choice of drug with the intensity and type of pain.
3. Give adequate doses. Titrate to the dose that relieves pain without incurring intolerable side effects
4. Use the oral route whenever possible. If the patient is unable to take oral (PO) medications, buccal, sublingual, rectal, and transdermal routes are considered before parenteral routes. The intramuscular (IM) route is avoided.
5. Continuous pain calls for treatment with a scheduled sustained-release or long-acting opioid and a short-acting medication for breakthrough pain.
6. Use an adequate rescue dose for breakthrough pain: 10% to 20% of the 24-hour dose every 1 to 2 hours is the customary rescue dose.
7. To calculate the rescue dose when fentanyl (Duragesic-25, -50, -75, or -100) is used, divide the total patch dose by three; this is the appropriate dose of morphine sulfate immediate release (MSIR). The dosage of other breakthrough medications can be determined from that point.
8. Increase the baseline dose if the patient needs more than three rescue doses in 24 hours.

9. If an increase in the baseline dose is required, it can be done safely every 2 hours with immediate-release preparations, every 12 hours with long acting preparations, and every 72 hours (3 days) with a fentanyl transdermal patch.

10. Intermittent pain calls for treatment with an as needed (prn) medication. Patients and families, however, need to be educated about taking the medication when the pain is first perceived—not when it has become severe or unbearable.

11. Order only one analgesic for breakthrough pain.

12. Order only one long-acting opioid for constant pain.

13. Increase doses of opioids commensurately with the patient's report of pain:
   - For mild to moderate pain, increase by 25% to 50%.
   - For moderate to severe pain, increase by 50% to 100%.
   - Increases less than 25% are meaningless.

14. Use equianalgesic conversions when changing medications or routes.

15. Use adjuvant medications for opioid-unresponsive neuropathic pain.

16. Nonpharmacologic approaches are always a part of any pain management plan.

17. Order an appropriate preventative bowel regimen if the patient is on opioids.

Commonly used analgesics and their formulations can be found in Tables 28-5, 28-6, and 28-7. The following medications should be avoided:

- Meperidine is short acting with a duration of 2 to 3 hours; active excitatory metabolites accumulate with chronic use.
- Propoxyphene has modest analgesic efficacy and is biotransformed to potentially toxic central nervous system and cardiac metabolites.
- Agonist-antagonists (e.g., buprenorphine, butorphanol, nalbuphine, pentazocine) have a ceiling effect (i.e., above a certain dose there is no more gain in analgesia) and can generate an acute withdrawal syndrome if used with opioids.

## Selection of an Opioid Starting Dose

The starting dose of an opioid is determined by the patient's pain intensity and the results of the history and physical examination, including the patient's age, circulatory status, and hepatic and renal function. The WHO analgesic ladder (Figure 28-4) may also be used as a guide. Be aware, however, that successful pain management requires an individualized approach, frequent monitoring, and appropriate dosage escalation (as outlined in "Basic Principles of Pain Management") until the patient is comfortable.

## Equianalgesic Conversions

Understanding opioid pharmacodynamics requires an understanding of the concepts of potency and equianalgesia. Equianalgesic conversion tables must be made available. Refer to Table 28-8. Note that 10 mg of parenteral

## TABLE 28-5

### Commonly Used Nonopioid Analgesics

| Chemical Class | Generic Name | Available Forms | Starting Dose | Dosing Schedule | Maximal Daily Dose |
|---|---|---|---|---|---|
| P-Aminophenol derivatives | Acetaminophen | Tablets: 160, 325, 500, 650 mg<br>Suppository: 120, 125, 325, 600, 650 mg<br>Liquid: 160mg/5 ml, 500 mg/15 ml<br>Elixir: 120, 160, 325mg/5 ml | 2600 mg/day | q4-6h | 6000 mg |
| Salicylates | Aspirin | Tablets: 325, 500, 650, 975 mg<br>Suppository: 120, 200, 300, 600 mg | 2600 mg/day | q4-6h | 6000 mg |
| | Choline magnesium trisalicylate* | Tablets: 500, 750, 1000 mg<br>Liquid: 500 mg/5 ml | 1500 mg × 1 dose, then 1000 mg q12h | q12h | 4000 mg |
| Proprionic acids | Ibuprofen | Tablets: 100, 200, 300, 400, 600, 800 mg<br>Suspension: 40 mg/ml, 100 mg/5 ml | 1600 mg/day | q4-6h | 3200 mg |
| | Naproxen | Tablets: 250, 375, 500 mg<br>Suspension: 125 mg/ml | 500 mg/day | q8-12h | 1025-1375 mg |
| Acetic acids | Indomethacin | Capsules: 25, 50 mg<br>Extended release: 75 mg<br>Suspension: 25 mg/5 ml<br>Suppository: 50 mg | 75 mg/day | q8-12h | 150 mg |
| | Diclofenac | Tablets: 25, 50, 75, 100 mg<br>Extended release: 100 mg | 75 mg/day | q8-12h | 150 mg |
| Pyranocarboxylic acids | Nabumetone | Tablets: 500, 750 mg | 1000 mg/day | q24h | 2000 mg |
| | Etodolac | Capsules: 200, 300 mg<br>Tablets: 400, 500 mg<br>Extended release: 400, 600 mg | 600 mg/day | q6-8h | 1200 mg |
| Cyclooxygenase-2+ inhibitors | Celecoxib | Capsules: 100, 200 mg | 200 mg/day | q12-24h | 400 mg |
| | Relecoxib | Tablets: 12.5, 25 mg<br>Suspension: 12.5, 25 mg/5 ml | 12.5 mg/day | q24h | 50 mg |

Adapted from McCaffery, M., & Pasero, C. (1999). Pain: Clinical manual (2nd ed.). St. Louis: Mosby; Portenoy, R. K. (1997). Contemporary diagnosis and management of pain in oncologic and AIDS patients. Newton, PA: Handbooks in Health Care; Skidmore-Roth, L. (2001). Mosby's 2001 nursing drug reference. St. Louis: Mosby.

*Choline magnesium trisalicylate is the only NSAID that does not interfere with platelet aggregation.
+COX-2 inhibitors should be used with caution in persons with impaired renal or hepatic functioning.

| TABLE 28-6 | |
|---|---|

### Formulations of Commonly Used Combination Analgesics

| Opioid | Proprietary Name and Combination Agent |
|---|---|
| Codeine | Tylenol #2 15/300* APAP† |
| | Tylenol #3 30/300 APAP |
| | Tylenol #4 60/300 APAP |
| Hydrocodone | Lorcet HD 5/500 APAP |
| | Lorcet Plus 7.5/650 APAP |
| | Lorcet 10/650 APAP |
| | Vicodin 5/500 APAP |
| | Vicodin HP 10/650 APAP |
| | Vicodin ES 7.5/750 APAP |
| | Vicoprofen 7.5/200 ibuprofen |
| | Zydone 5/500 APAP |
| | Co-Gesic 5/500 APAP |
| | Norco 10/325 APAP |
| | Lortab 2.5/500, 5/500, 7.5/500, 10/500 APAP |
| | Lortab ASA 5/500 ASA |
| Oxycodone | Percocet 2.5/325, 5/325, 7.5/500, 10/650 APAP |
| | Percodan 4.5/325 ASA |
| | Percodan-Demi 2.25/325 ASA |
| | Roxicet 5/325, 5/500 APAP |
| | Roxilox 5/500 APAP |
| | Roxiprin 4.5/325 ASA |
| | Tylox 5/500 APAP |
| | Generic 5/325 APAP |

*Caution: The first number of the dosage listed is the milligram dosage of the opioid; the second is the milligram dosage of the nonopioid analgesic that is used in combination. Example: Percocet 2.5/325 contains 2.5 mg oxycodone, 325 mg acetaminophen.
†APAP is the pharmacologic designation for acetaminophen. The acetaminophen dosage should not exceed 4 g/24 hr. ASA is the pharmacologic designation for aspirin.

morphine sulfate has the same analgesic effect as 30 mg oral morphine sulfate. Providers should use such tables with caution, in that the dosages stated are not standard starting doses. Rather the doses on the table represent ratios of one drug to another, and one route to another. Starting doses should be based upon pain intensity combined with other information from the patient assessment. One dose can be converted to another by following a four-step procedure. Table 28-9 works through four basic steps for calculating an equianalgesic conversion.

## Common Side Effects of Opioids and Their Management

- *Sedation:* Usually clears in 1 to 3 days. If sedation persists, patients may benefit from a slight reduction in the opioid dose and an evaluation for the need to add an adjuvant medication or a stimulant such as methylphenidate. Excessive sedation is often a sign that the pain syndrome is opioid-resistant.

| TABLE 28-7 | | |
|---|---|---|

### Formulations of Commonly Used Opioid Analgesics

| Short-Acting Opioids | | |
|---|---|---|
| **Opioid** | **Formulations** | **Available Dosages** |
| Morphine | Tablet | 15, 30 mg |
| | Solutab | 10, 15, 30 mg |
| | Liquid | 10 mg/5ml, 20 mg/5 ml, 20 mg/ml |
| | Suppository | 5, 10, 20, 30 mg |
| Oxycodone | Tablet | 5, 10 mg |
| | Liquid | 5 mg/5 ml, 20 mg/ml |
| Hydromorphone | Tablet | 2, 4, 8 mg |
| (Dilaudid) | Suppository | 3 mg |

| Long-Acting Opioids | | |
|---|---|---|
| **Opioid** | **Formulations** | **Available Dosages/Intervals** |
| **MORPHINE** | | |
| Oramorph SR | Tablet | 15, 30, 60, 100 mg q8-12h (initial starting interval: 12 hr) |
| MS Contin | Tablet | 15, 30, 60, 100, 200 mg q8-12h (initial starting interval: 12 hr) |
| Kadian | Capsule | 20, 50, 100 mg q12-24h (starting interval: 24 hr) |
| **FENTANYL** | | |
| Duragesic-25, -50, -75, -100 patch | Transdermal | 25, 50, 75, 100 $\mu$g/hr q72h |
| **OXYCODONE** | | |
| OxyContin | Tablet | 10, 20, 40, 80 mg q12h |
| Hydromorphone | Tablet | Pending FDA approval |

- *Constipation:* A common but preventable side effect; regularly scheduled laxatives are almost always required; surface wetting agents in addition to a gentle laxative such as senna should be considered as a starting regimen.
- *Nausea:* Persons usually become tolerant to the emetic effect after 3 to 5 days. In the interim, use of an antiemetic is appropriate.
- *Confusion:* Evaluate for the underlying cause; eliminate nonessential central nervous system (CNS)–acting medications, if analgesia is satisfactory; and reduce the dosage of the opioid by 25%. If confusion persists, try a neuroleptic (for example, haloperidol, 0.5 to 1 mg PO bid or tid, or 0.25 to 0.5 mg SC or IV (Pasero et al., 1999).
- *Less common side effects:* Sweating, pruritus, and urinary retention.

## TABLE 28-8

### Equianalgesic Dosages of Opioids

| Drug | Parenteral | PO | Parenteral/ Oral Ratio | Duration of Action (hr)[*] |
|---|---|---|---|---|
| Morphine[+] | 10 | 30 | 1:3 | 3-4 |
| Hydromorphone (Dilaudid) | 1.5 | 7.5 | 1:5 | 3-4 |
| Oxymorphone (Numorphone) | 1 | 10 | 1:10 | 3-4 |
| Oxycodone[‡] (Roxicodone, Roxicet, Percocet) | Not available in U.S. | 20-30 | — | 3-4 |
| Codeine | 130 | 200 N/A[§] | 1:1.5 | 3-4 |
| Hydrocodone[||] (Vicodin, Vicoprofen, Lortab, Lorcet) | — | 30 | — | 3-4 |
| Propoxyphene-N 50, (Wygesic, Darvocet-N 50, -N 100) | — | N/A[¶] | — | 4-6 |
| Meperidine (Demerol HCl) | 75 | 300[#] | 1:4 | 2-3 |
| Levorphanol (Levo-Dromoran) | 2 | 4 | 1:2 | 4-8 |
| Methadone (Dolophine HCl) | 10 | 3-5[**] | — | 4-12 |
| Fentanyl (Sublimaze, Duragesic -25, -50, -75, -100h) | 0.1[††] | — | — | 1-3[††] |

[*] Duration of action is based on use of short-acting formulations.

[+] Morphine produces active metabolites (morphine 6-gluceronide [M6G] and morphine 3-gluceronide [M3G]), which accumulate more rapidly with intravenous infusions of morphine and are more likely retained and thus problematic for elderly persons and those with impaired renal function. M6G has strong analgesic, sedative, and respiratory depressant properties. M3G produces central nervous system hyperexcitability and possibly myoclonus. If you suspect this is a problem, small amounts of hydration (IV or hypodermoclysis fluids at 30-50 cc/hr) facilitates renal clearance. Hydromorphone may be a safer choice for the elderly or those with diminished renal function.

[‡] These products contain 2.25-10 mg oxycodone with some combination of aspirin or acetaminophen.

[§] NA, equianalgesic data are unavailable. Codeine doses should not exceed 1.5 mg/kg because higher doses cause increased side effects.

[||] These products contain 5, 7.5, or 10 mg hydrocodone with some combination of aspirin, acetaminophen, or ibuprofen.

[¶] Long half-life; accumulation of toxic cardiac and central nervous system metabolite (norpropoxyphene) with repetitive dosing; inappropriate for use in the elderly.

[#] Avoid multiple dosing with meperidine (no longer than 48 hrs). Accumulation of toxic metabolite normeperidine (half-life 12-16 hr) can lead to central nervous system (CNS) excitability and convulsions. Contraindicated in patients prescribed monoamine oxidase inhibitor (MAO) and in the elderly.

[**] Although many equianalgesic tables list 20 mg as the PO oral methadone equianalgesic dose, recent data suggest methadone is much more potent with repetitive dosing. Ratios of PO morphine to PO methadone may range from 4:1 to 14:1. Caution is advised.

[††] Transdermal fentanyl 100 $\mu$g/hr is approximately equivalent to 2-4 mg/hr IV morphine. A conversion factor for transdermal fentanyl that can be used for equianalgesic calculation is 17 $\mu$g/hr. The microgram/hour dose of transdermal fentanyl is approximately half of the 24-hr dose of oral morphine.

[††] Single-dose data; continual intravenous infusion causes lipid accumulation and prolonged excretion.

## TABLE 28-9

### Equianalgesic Calculation Guide

This guide illustrates one method of changing from one opioid or route of administration to another. Clinicians must be able to identify appropriate opioid doses when a patient requires a change of opioid or route of administration. Mastering this skill enables you to determine a dose of a new opioid that is approximately equal in analgesic effect to the dose of a former opioid to ensure continued pain relief.

1. Add up the total amount of current drug given in 24 hours. Remember to add in both scheduled and rescue doses. (If two or more different opioids have been taken, they must each be converted to the same drug and route.)

2. Plug numbers into the following proportion:

$$\frac{\text{Go to equianalgesic table—find dose for current drug}}{\text{Go to equianalgesic table—find dose for new drug}} = \frac{\text{Put in 24-hr dose of current drug (from step 1)}}{N \text{ (24-hr dose of the new drug)}}$$

*Shortcut tip:* Look at the left side of the proportion as a fraction. If possible reduce the fraction. This new fraction provides the ratio and applies to the relationship between the 24-hr doses and may immediately show you the value of N. If can see this, skip to step 4.

3.

$$\frac{\text{Equianalgesic table dose of current drug}}{\text{Equianalgesic table dose of new drug}} \overset{A}{=} \frac{\text{(24-hr dose of the current drug)}}{N}$$

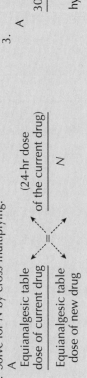

Example: 1.
Patient is taking 10 mg PO morphine q4h, 6 doses per day:
6 doses × 10 mg = 60 mg per day
Convert to oral hydromorphone:

2.

$$\frac{30 \text{ mg PO morphine}}{7.5 \text{ mg hydromorphone}} = \frac{60 \text{ mg PO morphine}}{N \text{ (24-hr dose of PO hydromorphone)}}$$

$$\frac{30 \text{ mg morphine}}{7.5 \text{ mg hydromorphone}} = \frac{4}{1} = \frac{60 \text{ mg PO morphine}}{N}$$

3. A

$$\frac{30 \text{ mg morphine}}{7.5 \text{ mg hydromorphone}} = \frac{60 \text{ mg morphine}}{N}$$

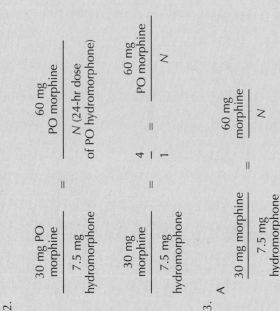

B

$$24\text{-hr dose current drug} \times \text{Equianalgesic table dose new drug} = \text{Equianalgesic table dose current drug} \times N$$

$$60 \text{ mg morphine} \times 7.5 \text{ mg hydromorphone} = 30 \text{ mg morphine} \times N$$

C

$$\frac{24\text{-hr dose current drug} \times \text{Equianalgesic table dose new drug}}{\text{Equianalgesic table dose current drug}} = N$$

$$\frac{60 \text{ mg morphine} \times 7.5 \text{ mg hydromorphone}}{30 \text{ mg morphine}} = N$$

D Answer: N will be the 24-hr dose of the new drug.

D 15 mg hydromorphone = N

E Does this answer make sense? Double-check. Plug it into the proportion in step A, and cross-multiply; the numbers should be equal.

E

$$\frac{30 \text{ mg morphine}}{7.5 \text{ mg hydromorphone}} = \frac{60 \text{ mg morphine}}{15 \text{ mg hydromorphone}}$$

4. Look up the duration of action (the dosing interval) of the new drug in the equianalgesic table and determine how many doses the patient should take each day. Divide N by the number of doses per day. This gives the amount for each scheduled dose of the new opioid.

4. Hydromorphone can be given every 4 hr, 6 doses per day. To administer 15 mg of hydromorphone in a day, divide the 24-hr dose by 6.

2.5 mg hydromorphone q4h

Because hydromorphone is available in 2-, 4-, and 8-mg tablets the dose would be rounded up or down, depending on the clinical situation.

From Gordon, D., Stevenson, K., Griffie, J., Rapp, C., Muchka, S., & Roberts, K. F. (1999). Opioid equianalgesic calculations. *Journal of Palliative Medicine, 2,* 209-218.

## Nonsteroidal Antiinflammatory Drugs

The nonsteroidal antiinflammatory drugs (NSAIDs) are believed to inhibit the production of prostaglandin syntheses, ultimately reducing the patient's pain perception. NSAIDs are considered nonopioid analgesics but when combined with opioids serve as the first line in the management of somatic pain. NSAIDs have the potential of producing gastritis, fluid retention, hypertension, renal failure, and platelet dysfunction (Levy, 1994) and thus are contraindicated in the following situations:

- Any renal impairment
- Platelet count less than 50,000 mm$^3$
- Concomitant use of corticosteroids, chemotherapy, anticoagulants
- History of gastrointestinal bleeding secondary to NSAIDs
- History of peptic ulcer disease
- Active gastrointestinal bleeding

There are multiple NSAIDs to choose from, and further discussion can be found in many existing resources; some of the more common NSAIDs and dosages are highlighted in Table 28-5.

NSAID choice is determined by availability, cost, patient convenience and adverse effects, and efficacy. The extent of gastrointestinal distress caused by NSAIDs has no relation to the severity of the gastrointestinal symptoms. Concomitant administration of misoprostol (Cytotec) or omeprazole (Prilosec) can prevent gastropathy (Twycross, Wilcock, & Thorp, 1998).

## Adjuvant Analgesics

Previous discussion has included specific pain descriptors that help the advanced practice nurse (APN) identify the distinctions among somatic, visceral, and neuropathic pain experiences. The somatic and neuropathic syndromes are discussed in the following sections. Nociceptive pain is usually responsive to nonopioid and opioid analgesics. Rarely however, do patients in the later stages of disease report only nociceptive pain; they usually have more than one pain syndrome. Therefore determining the patient's specific pain syndrome, to the extent possible, helps identify which medication is most appropriate.

Titration and sequential trials of adjuvant analgesics are important considerations for their use. Titration begins with the initiation of a low dose followed by a gradual escalation. It is important to explain to the patient that although complete pain relief will not begin immediately, finding the right dose and medication requires ongoing assessment of analgesia and adverse effects (Portenoy & Waldman, 1994). This continuous monitoring of both analgesia and side effects is an acquired skill that requires a working knowledge of the varied patient responses coupled with medication-specific pharmacokinetics.

There is no "cookbook" approach to prescribing adjuvant analgesics because patients respond differently to medications as a result of various factors (i.e., underlying pathophysiologic condition, metabolism, physical status). Box 28-1 outlines general guidelines for initiating therapy with adjuvant analgesics. It is important that the APN assess all of the symptoms that the patient is experiencing and tailor adjuvant analgesics specifically to both the pain syndrome and other symptoms. Adjuvant analgesics, also termed *coanalgesics,* are medications with primary actions other than analgesia that when combined with a nonopioid or an opioid improve pain control through a cumulative effect. The patient's description of his or her pain syndrome and underlying pathophysiologic condition are considered when choosing a specific adjuvant analgesic. Many of the adjuvant analgesics used to treat the various pain syndromes prove useful for other symptoms such as dyspnea, depression, and restlessness.

## Corticosteroids

Corticosteroids are useful because of their antiinflammatory effects. They are not only considered for treatment of somatic bone pain but also for both visceral and neuropathic pain syndromes. Corticosteroids are also used in the management of anorexia, depression, nausea, spinal cord compression, superior vena cava syndrome, organ distension, and other conditions (American Pain Society, 1999; Cherny & Portenoy, 1999; Levy, 1994). Dosing schedules vary with the disease trajectory and the underlying pathophysiologic condition. The adverse effects of corticosteroids include candidiasis, gastritis, fluid retention, hypertension, and hyperglycemia (Levy, 1994).

Corticosteroid dosage is strongly related to the underlying pathophysiologic condition; doses differ, for example, when treating pain, anorexia, intracranial edema, and spinal cord compression (see individual symptoms). When using prednisone begin 5 mg/day PO, then titrate to effect symptom control; for dexamethasone the empiric starting dose is 6 to 8 mg tid to qid PO; it may also be administered subcutaneously (Pereira & Bruera, 1997).

| BOX 28-1 | *Guidelines for the Initiation of Adjuvant Analgesics* |
|---|---|

- Perform a comprehensive patient evaluation.
- Select the drug for a specific pain syndrome and/or other symptoms.
- Maintain a working knowledge of the pharmacologic characteristics of the adjuvant analgesic selected.
- Understand individual variability.
- Identify the risks of polypharmacy.
- Consider the costs of individual adjuvant analgesics.
- Integrate adjuvant analgesics into the overall management of pain and symptoms.

From Portenoy, R., & Waldman, S. (1994). Adjuvant analgesics in pain management: Part 1. *Journal of Pain and Symptom Management, 9*(6), 390-391; Levy, M. (1994). Pharmacologic management of cancer pain. *Seminars in Oncology, 21*(6), 718-739.

## Bisphosphonates

The bisphosphonate class of medication, though costly, may be considered for the treatment of bone pain due to metastasis when other adjuvants fail. These agents inhibit osteoclast activity and are absorbed onto the bone surface, where they remain bound for weeks or months. Therefore a single infusion has a prolonged action on the osteoclasts (Twycross et al., 1998). The most widely used bisphosphonate is pamidronate disodium. Side effects include transient pyrexia, influenzalike symptoms, dyspepsia, abdominal pain, and constipation (Twycross et al., 1998). The starting dosage for pamidronate disodium is 60 to 90 mg diluted in 500 to 1000 ml normal saline solution given IV over 4 to 6 hours (Pereira & Bruera, 1997; Twycross et al., 1998).

## Radiopharmaceuticals

Under the direction of a radiation oncologist, the use of medications such as strontium 89 may be considered to relieve bone pain in the active patient with a longer prognosis. This medication is absorbed into areas of high bone turnover and can help reduce pain without interfering with marrow suppression.

## Neuropathic Pain

Numerous groups of medications, in addition to the opioids, are considered for treatment of neuropathic pain because of its complex pathophysiologic characteristics. For the purpose of drug selection it is important that the APN differentiate among continuous, lancinating, and sympathetically maintained pain. Table 28-10 highlights some of the commonly used adjuvant analgesics specific for neuropathic pain. There are several resources available to help direct sequential trial selection. Attention to intraindividual variability is important in choosing an adjuvant analgesic. Titration should proceed slowly with ongoing assessment of benefit versus harm.

# ■ DIFFICULT PAIN PROBLEMS

At times pain is difficult to treat, even with the means already suggested. As discussed, identify in advance of the need individuals who might be available for consultation about difficult pain management problems.

## Pain Management in Substance Abuse

Treating pain in patients with either a current or a past history of substance abuse presents complex psychosocial and physical issues to any clinician. These patients fall into three basic categories (Paice & Fine, 2001):
1. Persons who have used or abused drugs or other substances in the past but are no longer using them
2. Persons in methadone maintenance programs

## TABLE 28-10

*Medications Useful for the Treatment of Continuous and Lancinating Neuropathic Pain*

| Continuous neuropathic pain | **ANTIDEPRESSANTS/TRICYCLICS** |
|---|---|
| | Nortriptyline and/or desipramine: Begin 10- to 25-mg (trial 7-10 days to monitor for adverse effects) therapeutic dose 50-100 mg hs PO (amitriptyline not recommended because of its increased incidence of anticholinergic effects). Because of their long half-lives they are used once per day. Special attention should be given to their anticholinergic properties, particularly in the elderly. |
| | **LOCAL ANESTHETICS** |
| | Lidocaine 5% patch: For topical relief of postherpetic neuropathy, postthoracotomy pain, and other pain syndromes. The patches should be placed over intact skin only. Up to three patches can be used to cover the painful area and are left in place for 12 hr with 12 hr off. They may be cut to size. Adverse effects are uncommon. |
| | **OTHERS** |
| | Capsaicin cream, over-the-counter: Apply topically as directed. Caution the patient about the initial hot sensation (made of hot chili peppers) and apply with gloves. |
| | Clonidine (alpha-adrenergic agonist): Spinal doses above 300 $\mu$g/24 hr rarely improve analgesia; it is also available in oral, transdermal, and subcutaneous forms. |

From Cherny, N., & Portenoy, R. (1995). *The management of cancer pain.* Atlanta: American Cancer Society; Pereira, J., & Bruera, E. (1997). *The Edmonton aid to palliative care.* Edmonton: University of Alberta; Twycross, R., Wilcock, A., & Thorp, S. (1998). *Palliative care formulary.* Abingdon: Radcliffe Medical Press.

*Continued*

3. Persons who are actively abusing drugs

Most clinicians lack even the most basic background in and knowledge of chemical dependency and often struggle with these issues in the treatment of pain in general and certainly in the treatment of pain in patients who have a current or past history of substance abuse. Any patient in a palliative care setting may experience significant pain. The challenge is to offer those who have substance abuse histories the same compassionate, comprehensive care given any patient, with some modifications in care and use of additional resources. Many clinicians fear they will be fooled or duped into

| TABLE 28-10 | |
|---|---|
| **Medications Useful for the Treatment of Continuous and Lancinating Neuropathic Pain—cont'd** | |
| Lancinating neuropathic pain | **ANTIDEPRESSANTS, ANTIARRHYTHMICS**<br>See the section on continuous neuropathic pain in this table.<br><br>**ANTICONVULSANTS**<br>Carbamazepine: Begin 100 mg bid PO; titrate slowly to a maximum of 400 mg q8hr<br>Valproic acid: Begin 200-500 mg hs PO, titrating if necessary to 1 g qd.<br>Gabapentin: Begin 100-300 mg tid PO; titrate up as necessary; empiric data suggest effective doses greater than 3600 mg/day.<br><br>**OTHERS**<br>Baclofen (skeletal muscle relaxant): Begin with 5 mg tid PO; may increase by 5 mg every 3 days; also effective for hiccoughs at a low dosage, 5-10 mg tid. |

providing pain medications to individuals who are seeking drugs rather than pain relief. Pain is a subjective symptom, without observable physical signs, and thus in many clinicians' minds its occurrence cannot be confirmed objectively. Keep in mind that if your goal is to relieve pain, you must accept the patient's report of pain.

Although additional epidemiologic studies are needed, substance abuse is relatively rare, 3% to 5%, in tertiary care populations in which it has been studied (Gfroerer & Brodsky, 1992; Wells, Golding, & Burnam, 1989). Some researchers believe that the incidence may be a bit higher because of underreporting and institutional biases, including a lack of data from primary care centers and from persons alienated from the health care system. While the medical use of opioids has increased markedly, reports of abuse have either decreased or remained constant (Joranson, Ryan, Gilson, & Dahl, 2000). Thus treating pain aggressively with opioids does not appear to contribute to increases in the reported health consequences of opioid analgesic abuse.

Alcoholism, by many accounts America's most frequent and serious health problem, is often underdiagnosed or ignored in the assessment process (Lundberg & Passik, 1998; Maxmen & Ward, 1995). Its incidence is estimated at 20% in palliative care settings (Bruera et al., 1995). Several clinicians contend that it is a poor prognostic factor for pain control and patient and family coping (Cook & Winokur, 1993; Mansky, 1993).

Alcoholism and abuse of other substances are major public health problems that involve the persons affected as well as the families and often create a cycle that interferes with the assessment, management, and follow-up and causes the failure of the very therapies intended to improve quality of life (Passik & Portenoy, 1998). Regardless of the substance, the harmful effects of a current or past history of substance abuse are wide-ranging, including increased patient suffering, decreased quality of life and thus quality of death, reluctance to provide pain medication, masking of symptoms whose relief is important to patient comfort, questionable adherence to the therapeutic regimen, and escalating lack of trust between the patient and family and professional caregivers (Passik & Portenoy, 1998; Passik & Theobald, 2000). Refer to Chapter 7, Psychosocial Care of the Patient and Family, for discussion in greater depth.

Treating a patient with a current or past history of substance abuse requires a comprehensive approach that recognizes and considers the interaction of the biologic, chemical, social, and psychologic/psychiatric aspects of substance abuse and addiction (Passik, Portenoy, & Ricketts, 1998a). Although the principles and guidelines outlined in the discussion that follows provide a framework for treating the patient who is actively abusing a substance, they also apply to those who are substance-free but have used them in the past, and those in methadone maintenance programs (Passik, & Portenoy, 1998; Passik, Portenoy, & Ricketts, 1998a; Passik, Portenoy, & Ricketts, 1998b; Passik & Theobald, 2000).

**Involve an interdisciplinary team.**    Reflect on your expertise and identify resources that can be accessed for managing this patient and family. A team approach is essential to address the multitude of medical and psychosocial problems presented and to prevent caregiver burnout and fatigue. An ideal team includes a physician with expertise in pain management and palliative care, staff nurses, social workers, and if possible, a mental health professional versed in addiction medicine.

**Set realistic goals for care.**    Relief of pain and enhancement of quality of life are the goals of care. What is the effect of the patient's past or current history of substance abuse? Is addiction increasing patient's suffering? Are recovery programs aimed at abstinence appropriate? What should be the focus of the patient's energy and the family's and caregiver's intervention? Be mindful that patients who are seeking pain relief and do not receive it may relapse into abuse patterns to alleviate that pain (Passik & Portenoy, 1998).

**Define the problem.**    What often appears as drug-seeking behavior is, rather, pain-relief–seeking behavior. Review the definitions of addiction, tolerance, physical dependence, and pseudoaddiction. Review apparently aberrant drug-taking behaviors: Does it suggest addiction or uncontrolled pain?

**Evaluate and treat comorbid psychiatric disorders.**    Substance abuse is accompanied by a high incidence of other psychiatric disorders, including depression and personality and anxiety disorders. Being mindful of the goals of care, obtain assistance in treating these disorders. Successful treatment may enhance patient comfort and quality of life: the goal of care.

**Consider the therapeutic effect of tolerance.**    Tolerance may or not be a factor in treating the pain in persons with a current or past history of substance abuse; it is highly variable. Higher initial doses may be required along with relatively rapid dose escalation to manage pain. What appears as tolerance may indeed be rapidly advancing disease and thus worsening pain. The principle of titrating to effect applies regardless of the underlying cause of the need to increase dosage.

**Apply appropriate pharmacologic principles to treat pain.**    The principles discussed earlier apply equally to the patient with a current or past history of substance abuse. The principle of titration to effect and the individualization of therapy, including providing the right drug at the right dose, however, is often difficult in this population. Be mindful of the goals of care and the definitions of addiction, tolerance, physical dependence, and pseudoaddiction. *Remember that unrelieved pain can lead to the development of aberrant drug-related behavior, including relapse* (Passik & Portenoy, 1998).

**Select drugs and routes of administration for the symptom and setting.**    Although no data confirm this relationship, among persons with known substance abuse, long-acting medications may not contribute to aberrant drug-taking behavior as do short-acting drugs (Passik & Portenoy, 1998). Balance the medication choice with the type of pain, goals of care, and patient needs.

**Recognize specific drug abuse behavior.**    Persons with a current or past history of substance abuse, including alcohol abuse, should especially be observed for actions that suggest substance abuse. Table 28-11 outlines a spectrum of behavior that is more and less suggestive of abuse and addiction. If there is a high level of concern about aberrant behavior, the interdisciplinary team may determine and plan a higher level of monitoring, including more frequent visits, interviews with family members, and perhaps urine screening for prescribed and illicit drugs. Keep in mind the goals of care; if more monitoring is indicated, including urine drug screening, patients should be reassured that it will provide a foundation for aggressive symptom-oriented treatment (Passik & Portenoy, 1998).

**Use nonpharmacologic approaches as appropriate.**    Nonpharmacologic approaches should augment pain management, not replace the appropriate treatment of symptoms, including pain, depression, and anxiety. Include educational initiatives (e.g., methods to communicate effectively with staff members about pain and to navigate a complex medical system) and cognitive and behavioral techniques to foster relaxation and enhance coping.

## TABLE 28-11

*Spectrum of Aberrant Drug-Related Behaviors Encountered During Treatment of the Medically Ill with Prescription Drugs*

| More Suggestive of Addiction | Less Suggestive of Addiction |
|---|---|
| Selling prescription drugs | Aggressive complaining about the need for more drugs |
| Prescription forgery | |
| Stealing drugs from others | Drug hoarding during periods of reduced symptoms |
| Injecting oral formulations | |
| Obtaining prescription drugs from nonmedical sources | Requesting specific drugs |
| | Openly acquiring similar drugs from medical sources |
| Concurrent abuse of alcohol or illicit drugs | Occasional unsanctioned dose escalation or other noncompliance |
| Repeated dose escalations or similar nonadherence despite multiple warnings | Unapproved use of the drug to treat another symptom |
| Drug-related deterioration in function at work, in family, or socially | Reporting psychic effects not intended by the clinician |
| | Resistance to a change in therapy associated with tolerable adverse effects |
| Repeated resistance to changes in therapy despite evidence of adverse drug effects | Intense expressions of anxiety about recurrent symptoms |

From Passik, S. D., & Portenoy, R. K. (1998). Substance abuse issues in palliative care. In A. Berger, R. K. Portenoy, & D. E. Weissman (Eds.), *Principles and practice of supportive oncology* (pp. 513-529). Philadelphia: Lippincott-Raven.

In order to increase the quality of life, and thus the quality of death, the clinicians caring for the patient and family should focus on the reduction of suffering—whether the result of the disease process or of the patient's own acts (Passik & Theobald, 2000). Anyone who provides palliative care must either be familiar with the basic concepts of addiction treatment or have access to readily available resources in this specialty area (Passik & Portenoy, 1998). Given the effect of either a current or a past substance abuse history on patient suffering and quality of life, identification of resources in advance is essential. Unless you have a background in substance abuse disorders and are conversant with current thought in this area and treatment of pain, symptom management, and end-of-life care, you should not manage such patients and families without the appropriate assistance. The successful outcome of care and the patient and family's quality of life depends on it.

### Rapidly Escalating Pain

When pain is severe and escalating rapidly, frequent increases of the dose of opioid may lead to severe side effects. Excitatory toxicity from large opioid doses can include myoclonus, grand mal seizures, delirium, hallucinations, and hyperalgesia. Management may require dose reduction, opioid rotation, hydration, and addition of medications to control symptoms, such as midazolam, barbiturates, and baclofen. Take advantage of the resources available to you to assure patient comfort.

## ■ COMPLEMENTARY TREATMENTS

Complementary treatments such as acupuncture, acupressure, therapeutic touch, and Reiki therapy continue to grow in popularity. Although few clinical research trials document their efficacy, many patients find comfort in these treatments. Because the experience of pain is subjective, patients who experience pain relief through complementary therapies should be encouraged to continue their use.

## ■ NONPHARMACOLOGIC TREATMENTS

Nonpharmacologic intervention should be considered for all levels of pain. Mild pain may be addressed first with nonpharmacologic interventions such as heat, cold, relaxation, distraction, and positioning. In moderate to severe pain nonpharmacologic interventions must always be included with pharmacologic interventions in the plan of care. Transcutaneous electronic nerve stimulators (TENS) units may assist in pain control when the pain is musculoskeletal; however, their use for relief of pain of end-stage disease is questionable.

With our growing understanding of pain as a multidimensional experience that includes all aspects of one's life (spiritual, psychologic, social, etc.), it is critical to realize that not all pain can be relieved by medication. There are no pills, for example, that can take away loneliness or spiritual pain. We are challenged by cultural norms and constraints of language that make it easier to express physical pain than existential pain. It remains our challenge as caregivers to learn about our patients' full experience of pain and to help them understand the limits of medications and the possibilities for relief though talking, sharing, and creative expression.

## ■ PATIENT AND FAMILY EDUCATION

Potential opioid side effects should be discussed at the time of the first prescription (information should include the assurance that tolerance develops to most of the side effects of opioids except constipation). A plan for a bowel regimen appropriate to the patient should also be agreed upon.

Many patients confuse addiction with the physical dependence that occurs in all patients over time; concerns for addiction need to be addressed. The emphasis of the education must be on alleviating the fear of addiction, as it is extremely rare in patients who are adequately treated for pain. Patients should be instructed not to decrease or stop opioids suddenly except under the direction of the health care provider. Patients should be instructed on when to contact the health care provider about the frequency of use of prn medications. For example, the APN may tell a patient to call when prn medication is used more than three times a day. Provide the following in written form for the patient and family:

- A list of each medication with directions on when to take it
- Side effects and what to do if they occur
- Telephone numbers (24 hours/day, 7 days/week) of a health care professional for assistance with:
  - Problems getting or taking medications
  - New pain or unrelieved pain
  - Nausea and vomiting that prevents eating for more than 24 hours
  - No bowel movement for more than 3 days
  - Difficulty in arousing the patient
  - Confusion or other neurologic changes (Grossman, Benedetti, Payne, & Syrjala, 1999)

## ■ EVALUATION AND PLAN FOR FOLLOW-UP

Evaluation intervals are based upon the assessment and achievement of pain management goals. The frequency of follow-up is dependent upon the level of pain, planned interventions, and patient response. For example, a patient in a pain crisis may need frequent reassessment, including phone contact between visits. A patient with stable pain may need only periodic evaluations. Gather information on present pain, the worst the pain has been since the last visit, and the most relief the patient has experienced since the last visit. On the basis of the patient's underlying pathophysiologic condition you may be able to anticipate and thus assess for new pain syndromes. While caring for a patient with prostate cancer, assessing for the presence of bone pain is wise. Always be mindful of the patient- and family-related barriers to reporting pain and using analgesics discussed at the beginning of the chapter and how they might affect your plan of care.

---

✔ **CASE STUDY**

Mrs. W. is a 78-year-old woman with a history of oral pharyngeal cancer. She is known to have widespread metastatic bone disease. She enters the clinic in a wheelchair accompanied by her daughter, saying she is "absolutely miserable."

Mrs. W. reports pain in her neck that has been present for over a year and has slowly increased in intensity. It hinders her ability to turn her head. She reports it is about a 7 on a scale of 0 to 10, and is fairly constant all the time. It is described as a dull, achy pain that moves from her neck up to her head.

Her mobility has markedly decreased in the past 2 to 3 weeks. She has been taking acetaminophen 500 mg with 5 mg of hydrocodone (Vicodin), one tablet every 3 hours, with no real relief: "At first they helped; now they don't do anything." She expresses concern about becoming addicted to her pain medication.

She denies constipation. Lab values are all normal. Recent radiologic exams reveal widespread increase in disease. Mrs. W. is aware of her advancing disease and expresses a desire to be able to feed her cats, enjoy her children and grandchildren, and be as free of pain as possible. She lives alone and, overall, manages well. She is able to swallow oral medications.

**Pharmacologic Choices**
There are several options for improving the management of Mrs. W.'s pain. Because it is severe (7 on a 0 to 10 scale), it is appropriate to increase her dose of medication by 50% to 100%. (Note that Mrs. W. is already at the maximum safe dose of acetaminophen per day, or 4 grams, so instructing her to take her Vicodin, two tablets every 4 hours, is not an option.) Consider the following:

- Switch Mrs. W. to a sustained-release preparation. Presently Mrs. W. is taking a total of 40 mg of hydrocodone a day. Following the principle of increasing the opioid by 100% because of her severe pain, and using the equianalgesic conversion chart, change her medication to sustained-release morphine, 40 mg PO every 12 hours. Adequate breakthrough medication is also ordered: 10% to 20% of the 24-hour dose, or immediate-release morphine, 12 to 20 mg PO every 1 to 2 hours prn. If an increase of 50% is more appropriate, the sustained-release morphine dosage would be 30 mg PO every 12 hours with immediate-release morphine, 9 to 15 mg every 1 to 2 hours as needed.
- Add an NSAID, if not contraindicated by Mrs. W.'s history, for the pain secondary to metastatic bone disease.
- Transdermal fentanyl is not an appropriate choice at this time because her pain is not well controlled. Increases in transdermal fentanyl are only appropriate every 72 hours.

Because of the severity of her pain Mrs. W. was switched to sustained-release morphine, 40 mg PO every 12 hours, with immediate-release morphine, 12 to 20 mg PO every 1 to 2 hours as needed for breakthrough pain. Daily contact with Mrs. W. and her family was planned, and she was urged to keep a pain diary. She was a little sleepy the first day but rated her pain as 2 on a 0 to 10 scale, stating, "I can turn my head!" She reported taking no breakthrough medications. By the third day she was alert, sleeping all night, and feeding her cats and reported taking 5 mg of her breakthrough medication only once a day. She was instructed to call if she requires more than 3 doses of breakthrough medication a day.

The management of pain at end of life is essential. Uncontrolled pain robs the patient—and family—of quality of life so precious and important during these final months.

# References

AIMONE, L. D. (1992). Neurochemistry and modulation of pain. In R. S. Sinatra, A. H. Hord, B. Ginsberg, & L. M. Preble (Eds.), *Acute pain: Mechanisms and management* (pp. 29-43). St. Louis: Mosby Year Book.

AMERICAN Geriatrics Society Panel on Chronic Pain in Older Persons (1998). The management of chronic pain in older persons. *Journal of the American Geriatric Society, 46*, 635-651.

AMERICAN Pain Society. (1992). *Principles of analgesic use in the treatment of acute pain and cancer pain* (3rd ed.). Glenview, IL: Author.

AMERICAN Pain Society. (1999). *Principles of analgesic use in the treatment of acute pain and cancer pain* (4th ed.). Glenview, IL: Author.

ANDERSON, G., Vestergaard, K., Ingeman-Nielsen, M., Jensen, T. S. (1995). Incidence of central post-stroke pain. *Pain, 61*, 187-193.

BENDEBBA, M., Torgerson, W. S., & Long, D. M. (1997). Personality traits, pain duration and severity, functional impairment, and psychological distress in patients with persistent low back pain. *Pain, 72*, 115-125.

BERRY, P. H., Eagan, K., Eighmy, J. B., Kalina, K., Gallagher-Allred, C. R., Murphy, P. L., Nahman, E. J., Rooney, E. J., Smith, S. A., Volker, B. A., & Zeri, K. (1999). *Hospice and palliative nurses practice review* (3rd ed.). Dubuque, IA: Kendall/Hunt.

BOIVIE, J. (1999). Central pain. In P. D. Wall & R. Melzack (Eds.), *Textbook of pain* (4th ed.) (pp. 879-941). New York: Churchill Livingstone.

BRUERA, E., Moyano, J., Seifert, L., Fainsinger, R., Hanson, J., & Suarez-Almazor, M. (1995). The frequency of alcoholism among patients with pain due to terminal cancer. *Journal of Pain and Symptom Management, 10*, 599-603.

CASTEN, R. J., Parmalee, P. A., Kleban, M. H., Lawton, M. P., Katz, I. R. (1995). The relationships among anxiety, depression, and pain in a geriatric institutionalized sample. *Pain, 61*, 271-276.

CHERNY, N., & Portenoy, R. K. (1999). Cancer pain: Principles of assessment and syndromes. In P. D. Wall & R. Melzack (Eds.), *Textbook of pain* (4th ed.) (pp. 1017-1064). New York: Churchill Livingstone.

CODERRE, T. J., & Melzack, R. (1992). The contribution of excitatory amino acids to central sensitization and persistent nociception after formalin-induced tissue injury. *Journal of Neuroscience, 12*, 3671-3675.

COOK, B., & Winokur, G. (1993). Alcoholism as a family dysfunction. *Psychiatric Annals, 23*, 508-512.

COUSINS, M. (1994). Acute post-operative pain. In P. D. Wall & R. Melzak (Eds.), *Textbook of pain* (3rd ed.). New York: Churchill Livingstone.

COUSINS, M., & Powers, I. (1999). Acute and postoperative pain. In P. D. Wall & R. Melzack (Eds.), *Textbook of pain* (4th ed.) (pp. 474-491). New York: Churchill Livingstone.

DESBIENS, N. A., Mueller-Rizner, N., Connors, A. F., & Wenger, N. S. (1997). The relationship of nausea and dyspnea to pain in seriously ill patients. *Pain, 71*, 149-156.

FIELDS, H. L. (1987). *Pain.* New York: McGraw-Hill.

FOLEY, K. M. (1991). The relationship of pain and symptom management to patient requests for physician-assisted suicide. *Journal of Pain and Symptom Management, 6,* 289-297.

FOLEY, K. M. (1998). Pain assessment and cancer pain syndromes. In D. Doyle, G. Hanks, & N. MacDonald (Eds.), *Oxford textbook of palliative medicine* (pp. 310-331). London: Oxford Medical Publications.

GORDON, D., Stevenson, K., Griffie., J., Rapp, C., Muchka, S., Roberts, K. F. (1999). Opioid equianalgesic calculations, *Journal of Palliative Medicine, 2,* 209-218.

GFROERER, J., & Brodsky, M. (1992). The incidence of illicit drug use in the United States, 1962-1989. *British Journal of Addiction, 87,* 1385.

HEWITT, D., McDonald, M., Portenoy, R., Rosenfeld, B., Passik, S., Breitbart, W. (1997). Pain syndromes and etiologies in ambulatory AIDS patients. *Pain, 70,* 117-123.

INTERNATIONAL Association for the Study of Pain, Subcommittee on Taxonomy. (1979). Pain terms: A list with definitions and notes on usage. *Pain, 6,* 249-252.

JACOX, A., Carr, D. B., Payne, R., Berde, C. P., Breitbart., W., Cain, G., Chapman, C. R., Cleeland, C. S., Ferrell, B. R., Finley, R. S., Hester, N. O., Hill, C. S., Leak, W. D., Lipman, A. G., Logan, C. L., McGarvey, C. L., Miaskowski, C. A., Mulder, D. S., Paice, J. A., Shapiro, B. S., Smith, R. S., Stover, J., Tsou, C. V., Vecchiarelli, L., Weissman, D. E. (1994). *Management of cancer pain: Clinical practice guideline no. 9,* AHCPR Pub No. 94-0592. U.S. Department of Health and Human Services. Public Health Service. Rockville, MD: Agency for Health Care Policy and Research.

JENSEN, T. S., & Nikolajsen, L. (1999). Phantom pain and other phenomena after amputation. In P. D. Wall & R. Melzack (Eds.), *Textbook of pain* (4th ed.) (pp. 799-814). New York: Churchill Livingstone.

JORANSON, D. E., Ryan, K. M., Gilson, A. M., & Dahl, J. L. (2000). Trends in medical use and abuse of opioid analgesics. *Journal of the American Medical Association, 283,* 1710-1714.

KELLER, S. E., Weiss, J. M., Schliefer, S. J., Miller, N. E., & Stein, M. (1981). Suppression of immunity by stress: Effect of a graded series of stressors on lymphocyte stimulation in the rat. *Science, 213,* 1397-1400.

KOVACH, C., Weissman, D., Griffie, J., Matson, S., & Muchka, S. (1999). Assessment and treatment of discomfort for people with late-stage dementia. *Journal of Pain and Symptom Management, 18,* 412-419.

LEVY, M. (1994). Pharmacologic management of cancer pain. *Seminars in Oncology, 21*(6), 718-739.

LIEBESKIND, J. C. (1991). Pain *can* kill. *Pain, 44,* 3-4.

LUNDBERG, J. C., & Passik, S. D. (1998). Alcoholism and cancer. In J. C. Holland (Ed.), *Psycho-Oncology* (pp. 587-594). New York: Oxford University Press.

MANSKY, P. (1993). Reminiscence of an addictionologist: Thoughts of a researcher and clinician. *Psychiatric Quarterly, 64,* 81-106.

MAXMEN, J. S., & Ward, N. G. (1995). Substance-related disorders. In J. S. Maxmen & N. G. Ward (Eds.), *Essential psychopathology and its treatment* (2nd ed.) (pp. 132-172). New York: W. W. Norton.

MCCAFFERY, M. (1968). *Nursing practice theories related to cognition, bodily pain, and man-environment interactions.* Los Angeles: UCLA Student Store.

MCCAFFERY, M., & Pasero, C. (1999). *Pain: Clinical manual* (2nd ed.). St. Louis: Mosby.

PAICE, J. A., & Fine, P. G. (2001). Pain at the end of life. In B. R. Ferrell, & N. Coyle (Eds.), *Textbook of palliative nursing* (pp. 76-90). New York: Oxford University Press.

PASERO, C., Portenoy, R., & McCaffery M. (1999). Opioid analgesics. In M. McCaffery, & C. Pasero (Eds.), *Pain clinical manual* (2nd ed.) (pp. 161-299). St. Louis: Mosby.

PASSIK, S. D., & Portenoy, R. K. (1998). Substance abuse issues in palliative care. In A. Berger, R. K. Portenoy, & D. E. Weissman (Eds.), *Principles and practice of supportive oncology* (pp. 513-529). Philadelphia: Lippincott-Raven.

PASSIK, S. D., Portenoy, R. K., & Ricketts, P. L. (1998a). Substance abuse in cancer patients. Part 1. Prevalence and diagnosis. *Oncology, 12,* 517-521.

PASSIK, S. D., Portenoy, R. K., & Ricketts, P. L. (1998b). Substance abuse in cancer patients. Part 2. Evaluation and treatment. *Oncology, 12,* 729-734.

PASSIK, S. D., & Theobald, D. E. (2000). Managing addiction in the advanced cancer patient: Why bother? *Journal of Pain and Symptom Management, 19,* 229-234.

PAYNE, R., & Gonzales, G. R. (1998). Pathophysiology of pain in cancer and other terminal diseases. In D. Doyle, G. Hanks, & N. MacDonald (Eds.), *Oxford textbook of palliative medicine* (pp. 299-310) London: Oxford Medical Publications.

PEREIRA, J., & Bruera, E. (1997). *The Edmonton aid to palliative care.* Edmonton: University of Alberta.

PORTENOY, R. K. (1997). *Contemporary diagnosis and management of pain in oncologic and AIDS patients.* Newton, PA: Handbooks in Health Care.

PORTENOY, R. K., & Hagen, N. A. (1990). Breakthrough pain: Definition, prevalence, and characteristics. *Pain, 41,* 273-281.

PORTENOY, R., & Waldman, S. (1994). Adjuvant analgesics in pain management: Part 1. *Journal of Pain and Symptom Management, 9*(6), 390-391.

SCADDING, J. W. (1999a). Complex regional pain syndrome. In P. D. Wall & R. Melzack (Eds.), *Textbook of pain* (4th ed.) (pp. 835-849). New York: Churchill Livingstone.

SCADDING, J. W. (1999b). Peripheral neuropathies. In P. D. Wall & R. Melzack (Eds.). *Textbook of pain* (4th ed.) (pp. 815-834). New York: Churchill Livingstone.

SERLIN, R. C., Mendoza, T. R., Nakamura, Y., Edwards, K. R., & Cleeland, C. S. (1995). When is cancer pain mild, moderate or severe? Grading pain severity by its interference with function. *Pain, 61,* 277-284.

SKIDMORE-ROTH, L. (2001). *Mosby's 2001 nursing drug reference.* St. Louis: Mosby.

SKLAR L. S., & Anisman, H. (1979). Stress and coping factors influence tumor growth. *Science, 205,* 513-515.

SNELLING J. (1994). The effect of chronic pain on the family unit. *Journal of Advanced Nursing, 19,* 543-551.

STENAGER, E., Knudsen, L., Jensen, K. (1991). Acute and chronic pain syndromes in multiple sclerosis. *Acta Neurologica Scandinavica, 84,* 197-200.

SUPPORT Study Principal Investigators (1995). A controlled trial to improve care for seriously ill hospitalized patients: A study to understand prognoses and preferences for outcomes and risks of treatments (SUPPORT). *Journal of the American Medical Association, 274,* 1591-1598.

SYDOW, F. W. (1988). The influence of anesthesia and postoperative analgesic management on lung function. *Acta Chiurgica Scandinavica Supplement, 550,* 159-165.

TAYLOR, E. J., Ferrell, B. R., Grant, M., & Cheyney, L. (1993). Managing cancer pain at home: The decisions and conflicts of patients, caregivers, and their nurses. *Oncology Nursing Forum, 20,* 919-927.

Twycross, R., Wilcock, A., & Thorp, S. (1998). *Palliative care formulary*. Abingdon: Radcliffe Medical Press.

Visintainer, M. A., Volpocelli, J. R., & Seligman, M.E.P. (1982). Tumor rejection in rats after inescapable or escapable shock. *Science, 216,* 437-439.

Ward, S. E., Goldberg, N., Miller-McCauley, V., Mueller, C., Nolan, A., Pawlik-Plank, D., Robbons, A., Stormoen, D., & Weissman, D. E. (1993). Patient-related barriers to management of cancer pain. *Pain, 52,* 319-324.

Ward S. E., & Hernandez, L. (1994). Patient-related barriers to management of cancer pain in Puerto Rico. *Pain, 58,* 233-238.

Wattine M. (1988). Postoperative pain relief and gastrointestinal motility. *Acta Chirurgica Scandinavica Supplement, 550,*140-145.

Weissman, D. E., & Haddox, J. D. (1989). Opioid pseudoaddiction—an iatrogenic syndrome. *Pain, 36,* 363-366.

Wells, K. B., Golding, J. M., & Burnam, M. A. (1989). Chronic medical conditions in a sample of the general population with anxiety, affective, and substance use disorders. *American Journal of Psychiatry, 146,* 1440.

Wilke, D. J. (1995). Neural mechanisms of pain: A foundation for cancer pain assessment and management. In D. B. McGuire, C. H. Yarbro, & B. R. Ferrell (Eds.), *Cancer pain management* (2nd ed.) (pp. 61-87). Boston: Jones & Bartlett.

World Health Organization. (1990). *Cancer pain relief and palliative care* (Technical Report Series 804). Geneva: Author.

Ziegler, C., Gries, F. A., Spuler, M., & Lessmann, F. (1993). The epidemiology of diabetic neuropathy. *Diabetic Medicine, 10*(suppl. 2), 82S-86S.

# CHAPTER 29

# Palliative Care Emergencies

DEBRA E. HEIDRICH, SANDY MCKINNON

E mergency situations in palliative care differ from those typically considered classic oncologic emergencies. In acute oncology care, an oncologic emergency is often managed with the goal of treating the symptom by arresting the disease process. In palliative care emergencies, as with all of palliative care, the goals of care and the patient's place in the disease trajectory should be considered when decisions are made, whether those are to treat the symptoms alone or to treat the symptoms and the underlying cause. In addition to the syndromes and their accompanying symptoms discussed in this chapter, any acute exacerbation of a physical symptom (e.g., pain and dyspnea) should be considered an emergency and promptly treated. Likewise, psychosocial, family, spiritual, and existential crises are considered emergencies that require immediate intervention.

Palliative care emergencies are identified by some as hemorrhage, seizures, fractures, spinal cord compression, and acute confusion (Smith, 1994). With the exception of acute confusion, which is discussed in Chapter 21, all of these clinical events are discussed in this chapter. We also include superior vena cava syndrome (SVCS), hypercalcemia, and syndrome of inappropriate antidiuretic hormone (SIADH).

At times the emergency situation itself is the cause of death. It is imperative for the advanced practice nurse (APN) to prepare and plan for potential palliative care emergencies. The APN's roles include preparing the family for potential emergencies, teaching them intervention strategies to assure their loved one's comfort, and supporting the them as they cope with the relative's inevitable decline. Important conversations with the patient and family need to be reinforced with further explanations, reassurance, and support as the end draws near (Smith, 1994).

## ■ HEMORRHAGE
### Definition and Incidence

Although bleeding is a common symptom of lesions in the gastrointestinal tract, upper and lower respiratory tract, and the genitourinary tract, a hemorrhage resulting in massive bleeding is rare. Hemorrhage is a terrifying experience for patients and their families—not to mention extremely distressing for staff. It is important to identify patients at risk for a potential hemorrhage and help to develop a plan of action should this event occur (Ernst et al., 1997; Smith, 1994).

## Etiology and Pathophysiology

The mechanisms for altering the vascular integrity in the patient with an advanced illness are multiple and varied. Vessel injury, abnormal platelet and coagulation pathways, and changes in the viscosity of the blood can create a sudden hemorrhagic event (Gagnon, Mancini, Periera, & Bruera, 1998; Pruett, 1999).

- Local tumor invasion of blood vessels: This may lead to a massive bleed if the vessel is an artery (e.g., carotid) or slow loss if it is capillary oozing (e.g., GI tract).
- Invasion of the bone marrow by tumor or bone marrow failure: The malignant cells of leukemias and lymphomas can crowd out the normal hematopoietic cells, resulting in thrombocytopenia, anemia, and neutropenia due to bone marrow suppression (Pruett, 1999). Metastasis to the bone can also interfere with the functioning of the bone marrow. Bone marrow failure may occur in persons who have received extensive previous treatment with myelosuppressive chemotherapy or radiation therapy.
- Disseminated intravascular coagulation (DIC): This results from an abnormal production of high-viscosity proteins that interferes with normal blood flow. Interference with the normal blood flow disturbs the fibrinolytic system within the microvascular system. This event usually holds a very poor prognosis (Pruett, 1999) and is considered a fatal event in debilitated patients with advanced disease.
- Liver failure: Liver failure causes vitamin K deficiency, altered platelet function, and abnormal production of fibrinogen. Dietary deficiency, biliary obstruction, malabsorptive syndromes, liver disease, and warfarin therapy can all contribute to depleted vitamin K level. Chronic liver disease often leads to portal hypertension and eventual esophageal varices (Pruett, 1999).
- Medications: Numerous medications can interfere with platelet function and, when combined with an underlying pathophysiologic condition, may result in serious bleeding. Medications frequently associated with bleeding abnormalities include the following (Pruett, 1999):
  - Aspirin
  - Antibiotics
  - Nonsteroidal antiinflammatory drugs (NSAIDs)
  - Phenothiazines
  - Tricyclic antidepressants
  - Heparin
  - Cimetidine

- Thiazide diuretics
- Estrogen

## Assessment and Measurement

To assess the risk of hemorrhage from vascular rupture, identify the anatomical locations of tumors and the potential of these tumors to disturb vascular structures. Persons with head and neck tumors and GI tumors are at the greatest risk. The risk of bleeding is increased if surgical interventions have disturbed the vascular structures or removed protective layers of fat and subcutaneous tissues. Local radiation therapy after surgery further increases the risk of bleeding. Suppression of the bone marrow is also assessed. Those who received myelotoxic chemotherapy or radiation therapy to the iliac crest, sternum, or long bones and those with tumor in the bone may have poorly functioning bone marrow, leading to thrombocytopenia and increased risk for bleeding.

## History and Physical Examination

A thorough review of the patient's history identifies the potential for hemorrhage. The history includes the following:
- Bleeding from any site, including location, length of time since last occurrence, amount of blood loss, and past interventions for bleeding
- The presence of tumors in anatomical locations associated with bleeding (e.g., head and neck, GI)
- The presence of primary or metastatic malignancies in the bone marrow
- The history of antineoplastic treatments, including myelosuppressive chemotherapy and radiation therapy to the bones
- Any liver dysfunction
- Medications the patient is taking that are associated with bleeding

The presence of a small amount of bleeding may precede a more catastrophic hemorrhage. The physical examination includes observing for signs of hemoptysis, hematuria, hematemesis, melena, and nasal bleeding. The skin and mucous membranes are examined for petechiae and excessive bruising (ecchymosis). In addition, any ulcerative lesions are examined for bleeding.

## Diagnostics

Platelet count and coagulation studies identify the person at risk for bleeding and assist in identifying the cause. Liver function studies may explain abnormal coagulation times but are not necessary if the patient's history is consistent with liver dysfunction.

## Intervention and Treatment

Depending upon the patient's general condition and personal goals, the APN should consider the following:
- Prevent major bleeding by treating aggravating factors:
  - Use cough suppressants for persons with blood-tinged sputum.

- Keep the air humidified.
- Discontinue medications that contribute to bleeding potential, if possible.
- Decrease the amount of bleeding:
  - Apply pressure or compression dressings, when the underlying structures can support them.
  - Consider hemostatic agents for surface bleeding (e.g., Gelfoam, Thrombostat, collagen).
  - Consider corticosteroids to decrease the inflammation around tumors near vessels.
  - Consider a radiation therapy consultation about the advisability of shrinking tumors invading vessels.
- Evaluate the appropriateness of using medications:
  - Vitamin K may be prescribed for liver failure.
  - Hemostatic agents, such as tranexamic acid and aminocaproic acid, may be used to treat hemoptysis or gingival bleeding (Ahmedzai, 1998; Weisman, 1998).
  - Octreotide is sometimes used to treat variceal bleeding (Corley, Cello, Adkisson, Ko, & Kerlikowske, 2001; Freitas et al., 2000) but its effectiveness in treating other causes of bleeding is not clear (Archimandritis et al., 2000). Its role in the management of bleeding in palliative care is not established.
  - Platelet transfusions may be considered, depending on the patient's goals and the possibility of symptomatic benefit. In palliative care, transfusions are most appropriate if there is a temporary decrease in platelets as a result of treatments, such as in palliative chemotherapy. Repeated transfusions for disease-related bone marrow suppression often are not considered appropriate care.
- Manage the stress associated with a catastrophic bleed:
  - Gently prepare the patient and family for the potential for bleeding while providing concrete intervention strategies to use in the event that it occurs.
  - Use dark-colored towels or blankets to cover the blood and thus lessen the frightening sight of massive bleeding.
  - Have an "emergency pack" ready with a sedating drug, such as midazolam 5 to 10 mg parenterally. This short-acting benzodiazepine is effective and clears the system quickly if the bleeding is not a terminal event. Short-acting morphine is also useful for treating the dyspnea that results from significant blood loss or for providing sedation. With significant blood loss, the absorption of medications administered via the subcutaneous route may be decreased and peripheral veins may be difficult to access due to shunting of blood to the vital organs. Consider using the sublingual route or using sites on the chest or abdomen for subcutaneous injections.
- Provide support for the patient and family:
  - Arrange for a member of the interdisciplinary team to remain with the patient, if at all possible.

- Allow time for family to discuss this catastrophic event, both immediately and days or weeks after the event. This is extremely distressing for all persons involved.

### Patient and Family Education

The APN must balance the need to prepare patients and families for a potential hemorrhage with the amount of distress this information can generate. It is generally considered better to prepare patients and families at the risk of causing some fear than for the family to not be prepared and witness a massive hemorrhage. The anxiety and fear this information may cause should be addressed by providing the family with specific intervention strategies in the event a hemorrhage does occur. The teaching plan includes the following:

- Instruct the patient and family to report any signs of bleeding, including occasional nose bleeds, blood-tinged sputum, dark and tarry stools, bleeding gums, pain with urination, and easy bruising of skin.
- Instruct the family to keep emergency phone numbers for their preferred provider (e.g., APN, hospice team, palliative care team, primary physician) by the telephone.
- Teach the family to keep dark towels or blankets nearby in the event the patient starts to bleed.
- Teach the family to administer any prescribed benzodiazepine or opioid to promote comfort should hemorrhage occur.

### Evaluation and Plan for Follow-Up

All interventions to prevent a hemorrhage and to decrease the amount of bleeding are evaluated based on observation of the absence of or a decrease in bleeding. If a hemorrhage occurs, ensure that the family has support systems in place to emotionally process this traumatic experience. Witnessing a massive bleed places the family at high risk for difficulties during bereavement. The APN should facilitate referral to a counselor with knowledge and skills in supporting persons who have experienced this type of trauma.

## ■ SPINAL CORD COMPRESSION

### Definition and Incidence

Spinal cord compression (SCC) is considered a true emergency and can quickly produce neurologic defects if prompt assessment and intervention are not initiated. The degree of neurologic impairment at the time of treatment determines the patient's neurologic outcome (Pereira & Bruera, 1997). These patients often report acute, neuropathic exacerbation of pain (e.g., back pain or leg pain that may be localized or radicular in nature), leg weakness, or sensory changes. Sudden changes may also occur in bladder and bowel functions.

The incidence rate of SCC is quoted as 5% of all patients with malignancies in many texts (Caracini & Martini, 1998; Pinover & Coia, 1998) based on a 1959 report (Barron et al., 1959). The rate may actually be higher as a result of two factors: (1) patients are living longer with their malignancies, including metastatic bone disease, and (2) there is a higher incidence of the cancers associated with SCC since 1959 (Cowap, Hardy, & A'Hern, 2000; Schafer, 1997). One study showed 32% of subjects with bone metastases from prostate cancer and normal neurologic examination had occult SCC using magnetic resonance imaging (MRI) (Bayley et al., 2001). As many as 70% of persons dying from cancer have spinal metastases at autopsy (Waller & Caroline, 2000). A retrospective study of 166 subjects with documented spinal cord compression reported the median survival from date of confirmation of the SCC was 82 days, with 32% dying before discharge from the cancer center. Survival was significantly better in patients presenting with a good performance status and good neurologic status (Cowap, Hardy, & A'Hern, 2000).

## Etiology and Pathophysiology

SCC occurs when primary tumors of the spine obliterate the spinal cord, or more commonly, when a vertebra collapses as a result of lytic (malignant) destruction. The majority (85%) of lesions compressing the spinal cord are a direct result of metastatic disease (Wilkes, 1999). The most common underlying primary cancers are lung and breast cancers, followed by lymphoma, melanoma, sarcoma, prostate, and kidney (Waller & Caroline, 2000). The location of SCC is often predictable: 70% of cases are found in the thoracic spine, 20% located in the lumbosacral spine, and 10% in the cervical spine. Many patients are also diagnosed with more than one area of the spine involved (Cowap, Hardy, & A'Hern, 2000; Fuller, Heiss, & Oldfield, 1997; Waller & Caroline, 2000).

## Assessment and Measurement

The most common presenting symptom of SCC is pain (70% to 95%), which may occur days to months before diagnosis. Patients with SCC describe the pain as being constant, dull, local, aching, and progressive (becoming more intense) and radicular in nature (intermittent and/or shooting). Pain is often exacerbated by lying down, moving, sneezing, and straining (e.g., neck flexion, Valsalva maneuver). Patients often will describe pain in the cervical or lumbar area that radiates into another area, such as the shoulder or limb. Pain may be the only symptom in 10% of patients (Waller & Caroline, 2000).

Extremity weakness is a very important area of assessment. One study revealed that 95% of patients with motor weakness had a greater than 75% blockage of the spinal cord (Raney, 1991). Motor weakness accompanied with an altered sensorium should prompt the APN to seek aggressive interventions to help reverse neurologic changes. The patient may also experience sensory loss or paresthesia to the level of spinal cord compression, resulting in loss of proprioception; ataxia; urinary frequency, urgency, or retention; constipation; and impotence. Autonomic dysfunction (e.g., colon distension, large postvoid urine volumes) occurs later in SCC and indicates a poor treatment outcome. Reversing or reducing symptom severity is clearly related to prompt assessment and intervention. If treated when symptoms emerge, ambulatory patients have an 80% probability of remaining ambulatory. Of nonambulatory SCC patients who receive treatment, only 30% regain ambulation; therefore early recognition and treatment are essential to preserving and restoring optimal function.

## History and Physical Examination

A careful history and physical examination can reveal signs of pain, motor weakness, reduced muscle tone, reduced reflexes, and functional and sensory loss. Identification of changes in bowel and bladder patterns and sudden onset of these changes can help direct the APN to confirm this diagnosis.

## Diagnostics

Plain radiography findings are abnormal in most patients with spinal cord compression as a result of tumor extension. Patients with a normal radiography result and positive SCC symptoms usually have extradural metastases not secondary to vertebral involvement (Pereira & Bruera, 1997). To confirm the diagnosis, magnetic resonance imaging (MRI) is preferred. Computed tomography (CT) scanning or myelography should be used when MRI is not possible.

## Intervention and Treatment

The goals of care for the patient with SCC include preservation or recovery of neurologic function, palliation of pain, prevention of local recurrence, and preservation of spinal stability. If SCC is strongly suspected, dexamethasone should be given. Dosage recommendations vary throughout the literature. Pereira and Bruera (1997) recommend a conventional starting dose of 8 to 10 mg PO three to four times a day while Waller and Caroline (2000) suggest administering 100 mg IV immediately, followed by 24 to 96 mg PO per day; the dose is then tapered by one-third every 3 to 4 days.

Refer a patient with otherwise good functional status to an acute care center immediately to confirm the diagnosis and initiate palliative therapies, such as radiotherapy or surgery to preserve function. There appears to be no difference in effectiveness if radiation therapy is divided into 10, 5, or 2 fractions (Donato et al, 2001). The patient who was not ambulatory before the onset of SCC symptoms and who has a very limited life expectancy is not a good candidate for radiation therapy or surgery. This patient is managed with corticosteroids and analgesics as needed for good symptom control.

## Patient and Family Education

A patient identified by the APN to be at risk for SCC is taught to report any new-onset back pain, weakness in the extremities, sensory changes, or changes in bladder or bowel functioning. In the presence of these symptoms, the patient and family require information on the need for immediate evaluation and preparation for diagnostic tests. Confirmation of SCC leads to additional education needs regarding the proposed treatment plan. When more than one option is proposed for treatment (e.g., surgery or radiation therapy), assist the patient and family to gather information about the advantages and disadvantages of each treatment option. Support them in selecting the treatment plan that best fulfills their definition of quality of living.

### Evaluation and Plan for Follow-Up

The success of the intervention is based on achievement of the identified goals. For the patient with a low performance status before the onset of symptoms and for whom neither surgery nor radiation therapy is planned, the goals are to relieve pain and maximize quality of living. The APN monitors this patient's pain ratings, making adjustments in medications to assure comfort while allowing the patient to participate actively in family discussions and other activities as desired and able.

In addition to pain relief and maximizing quality of living, the goal of surgical or radiation therapy intervention is to preserve and improve physical functioning. The APN monitors the patient's ability to ambulate, bladder and bowel functioning, and sexual functioning, anticipating improvement with the intervention. As with all palliative care interventions, evaluation of the side effects of all medications is an important part of the follow-up plan.

## ■ SEIZURES
### Definition and Incidence

Seizure is defined as a paroxysmal hypersynchronous discharge of the neurons in the brain (Luckmann, 1997). The incidence of seizures in advanced cancer is approximately 1% overall, and 15% to 25% in persons with primary or metastatic brain tumors. Approximately 10% to 15% of persons with acquired immunodeficiency syndrome (AIDS) experience seizures (Caracini & Martini, 1998; Waller & Caroline, 2000). This symptom requires immediate intervention as seizures are very frightening for both the patient and family, cause profound fatigue, increase the potential for injury, and may interfere with airway clearance.

### Etiology and Pathophysiology

Seizures are often multifactorial and may be the result of brain tumors, electrolyte or metabolic disturbances, infection, drug toxicity, accumulation of drug metabolites, nonopioid drug withdrawal, or intracerebral hemorrhages (Bruera, Walker, & Lawlor, 1999; Pereira & Bruera, 1997; Smith, 1994). The most common causes in persons with advanced cancer are primary or metastatic tumors in the brain, stroke, and preexisting seizure disorder (Waller & Caroline, 2000).

Seizures occur when the basal level of excitability of the nervous system rises above a certain critical threshold. The most common types of seizures in the palliative care setting are focal seizures and tonic-clonic *(grand mal)* seizures. Focal seizures result from some localized organic lesion or functional abnormality, such as scar tissue in the brain that pulls on the adjacent tissue, a tumor that compresses an area of the brain, a destroyed area of brain tissue, or congenitally deranged local circuitry of the brain. These lesions cause rapid discharges of local neurons that may spread over adjacent cortical regions. When a wave of excitation spreads over the motor cortex, it causes a progressive march of muscle contractions throughout the opposite side of the body. A focal seizure may trigger a generalized tonic-clonic seizure (Guyton & Hall, 1996).

Tonic-clonic seizures occur when there are extreme neuronal discharges in all areas of the brain. This may be caused by strong emotional stimuli, alkalosis caused by overbreathing, drugs, fever, and loud noises or flashing lights. Discharges transmitted into the spinal cord cause generalized tonic activity, followed toward the end of the attack by alternating tonic and then spasmodic muscle contractions leading to tonic-clonic activity. Tonic-clonic seizures are followed by a postseizure depression of the central nervous system (CNS), leading to lethargy or stupor and severe fatigue (Guyton & Hall, 1996).

Medications may cause or contribute to seizure activity; this may be due to medication toxicity, use of medications that lower the seizure threshold, or abrupt withdrawal of a medication. High doses of opioids, especially morphine (related to the accumulation of morphine-3-glucuronide and phenothiazines, are cited causes of medication-related seizure activity in the palliative care setting (Caracini & Martini, 1998). Some medications that are commonly used in palliative care decrease the seizure threshold, thereby contributing to seizure activity. Of 20 drugs identified as essential in palliative medicine (Dickerson, 1999), four—amitriptyline, haloperidol, metoclopramide, and tramadol—should be used with caution in persons with seizures (Skidmore-Roth, 2001). Although not listed in the Dickerson (1999) report, chlorpromazine is also frequently used in palliative care and lowers the seizure threshold. Seizures are also possible with sudden withdrawal of alcohol, benzodiazepines, barbiturates, and baclofen.

## Assessment and Measurement

Assess the potential for seizures based on the patient's diagnosis and any previous history of seizure activity. Monitor the at-risk patient for seizure activity. If the patient has a history of seizures, assess the effectiveness of anticonvulsant therapy, as well as any untoward side effects. If a seizure does occur, a prompt referral to a neurologist is often appropriate for further diagnosis and treatment after the seizure is controlled.

## History and Physical Examination

Review the patient's history for a description of any previous seizure activity. Ask the patient if an aura is experienced before seizures or if there are signs of increased intracranial pressure (e.g., headache, nausea, projectile vomiting). Use the medical history, review of current and recently discontinued medications, and physical examination to assist in determining the underlying cause of any seizure activity.

## Diagnostics

When a brain tumor is suspected and the patient had a high performance status before the seizure, CT scanning or MRI can help determine the prognosis and help clarify treatment recommendations. It is also helpful to monitor the blood levels of anticonvulsants to ensure that the drug is within the therapeutic range.

## Intervention and Treatment

Since the incidence of seizures is relatively low, prophylaxis with anticonvulsants is not recommended unless the patient has a history of seizures. However, once the patient has experienced a seizure, anticonvulsant therapy is initiated and maintained.

Certainly the patient experiencing active seizure prompts the most urgent concern. To treat a patient who is in active seizure:

- Protect the patient from injury, using padded bedrails and a padded tongue blade or airway.
- Medicate to stop the seizure activity (Waller & Caroline, 2000):
  - If the patient does not have an intravenous (IV) line, give diazepam solution, 10 mg per rectum (PR), repeating every 5 to 10 minutes, as needed for up to three additional doses. Then begin a subcutaneous infusion of midazolam, 30 mg per 24 hours, titrating as needed.
  - If the patient has an IV line, give lorazepam, 4 mg IV over 2 to 4 minutes. Then begin an IV infusion of phenytoin, 20 mg/kg at 25 mg/min. If the seizure persists, give additional doses of phenytoin of 5 mg/kg to a maximal total dose of 30 mg/kg.
  - If seizures still persist, give phenobarbitol, 20 mg/kg IV at a rate of 100 mg/min.
  - If increased intracranial pressure is suspected, administer dexamethasone, 10 mg IV.
- Administer oxygen, if available.
  To prevent seizure activity:
- Assess for treatable or reversible causes (e.g., medications, infection, fever, substance withdrawal).
- Maintain anticonvulsant therapy:
  - Phenytoin, 300 to 400 mg PO per day.
  - Carbamazepine generally has fewer side effects than phenytoin and is considered the first-line medication for simple and complex focal seizures. Start at 50 to 100 mg PO qid and after several days change to 100 to 200 mg PO daily or bid. Maximal daily dose is 800 to 1200 mg PO bid (Twycross, Wilcock, & Thorp, 1998).

- Evaluate the interactions of other substances/medication with the serum levels of anticonvulsants. For example, chronic alcohol use, antihistamines, antacids, antineoplastics, CNS depressants, rifampin, and folic acid can decrease the effects of phenytoin; benzodiazepines, haloperidol, phenobarbital, phenytoin, and warfarin decrease the effects of carbamazepine (Skidmore-Roth, 2001).
- Determine an alternate route of administration of the anticonvulsant if the patient is not able to take oral medications and is at risk for seizures:
  - Anticonvulsants can be discontinued if the patient is comatose and seizures have not been a problem (Waller & Caroline, 2000).
  - If survival is expected for more than a few days and the patient has a definite history of seizures, identify an appropriate route of administration based on the setting as well as the abilities and preferences of the caregivers. Phenytoin is irritating to the vessels and should not be administered in peripheral veins. Its absorption rectally is highly variable and is not recommended (Burstein, Fisher, McPherson & Roby, 2000). Any of the following may be used (Waller & Caroline, 2000):
    - Phenobarbital, 100 to 200 mg IM qd or 200 to 300 mg/24 hours via continuous subcutaneous infusion
    - Valproic acid syrup, 250 to 500 mg PR tid
    - Diazepam, 10 mg PR tid

## Patient and Family Teaching

Seizures are frightening for both the patient and the family. Provide information regarding the cause of the seizure and the interventions in place to prevent further seizure activity. Reassure them that the palliative care team is monitoring the patient for any problems and is there to support them. Assist the family to identify strategies to keep the patient free from injury should a seizure occur; include instruction on how to use an airway or padded tongue blade. Teach the appropriate scheduling of anticonvulsant therapy and the importance of taking this medication as prescribed. Encourage the patient and family to report any difficulties taking the medications, such as nausea or dysphagia, so that appropriate action can be taken to maintain therapeutic drug levels of the anticonvulsant. Develop a plan for the management of an active seizure with the family. This includes knowledge of who to notify and how to initiate therapy for an active seizure with the emergency medications available.

## Evaluation and Plan for Follow-Up

The goal of intervention is to prevent future seizure activity. The APN evaluates laboratory data to ensure anticonvulsants are at therapeutic levels. Should a seizure occur despite therapeutic serum levels of the anticonvulsant, consultation with a neurologist is considered. Follow-up support is needed for the patient and family when a seizure occurs. The family whose loved one died while having a seizure is at higher risk for complicated grieving and should be referred to a bereavement counselor for evaluation and appropriate intervention.

# ■ HYPERCALCEMIA

## Definition and Incidence

Hypercalcemia is defined as a corrected serum calcium level greater than 11 mg/dl (or greater than 5.6 mEq/l). It is the most common complication of malignancy. Approximately 45% of breast cancer patients, 40% of myeloma patients, and 12% of lung cancer patients experience hypercalcemia. It is less common in lymphoma and cancers of the head and neck, esophagus, and thyroid. Hypercalcemia is rare in colon and prostate cancers. Most patients who are hypercalcemic have detectable bone metastases, but the severity of the hypercalcemia is not dependent on the extent of metastatic disease. Greater clinical difficulties may result from a sudden increase in serum calcium level than a level that has increased slowly (Krecker & Muggia, 1995; Warrell, 1997).

## Etiology and Pathophysiology

This syndrome occurs when the calcium mobilization and resorption from bone exceeds the renal threshold of calcium excretion (Krecker & Muggia, 1995). Several factors contribute to the development of hypercalcemia, including increased bone resorption due to osteoclast activity (stimulated by factors released by malignant cells) (Warrell, 1997), increased bone resorption due to direct tumor invasion of bone, decreased ability of the kidney to clear calcium, and increased calcium absorption from the GI tract. Immobility also contributes to loss of calcium from bones, increasing serum calcium level. In addition, dehydration leads to a higher concentration of calcium (and other solutes) in the serum.

Transient hypercalcemia may occur when hormone therapy is started in women with breast cancer who have widespread bone metastasis. The patient may experience a rise in the serum calcium level and an increase in bone pain within a few days of starting hormone therapy. The hormone treatment may be temporarily stopped until the hypercalcemia is corrected (Waller & Caroline, 2000).

As serum calcium levels rise, all of the major organ systems are eventually affected, including the neuromuscular, GI, cardiac, and renal systems. Early symptoms are frequently misinterpreted as the usual signs and symptoms of advanced malignancies, such as poor appetite, fatigue, nausea and vomiting, and constipation. As hypercalcemia progresses, symptoms become more prominent; they include dehydration (e.g., thirst, polyuria, poor skin hydration, dry mucous membranes), confusion, agitation, flat reflexes, and cardiac conduction changes (dysrhythmias) (Jones, 1999; Krecker & Muggia, 1995; Warrell, 1997).

## Assessment and Measurement

The APN assesses for these early signs of hypercalcemia:

- Cardiovascular: Bradycardia
- Neuromuscular: Fatigue, weakness, hyporeflexia, bone pain, lethargy, confusion
- Gastrointestinal: Anorexia, constipation, nausea
- Renal: Weight loss, polydipsia, polyuria

  If not corrected, the hypercalcemia will progress and these late signs and symptoms are seen:

- Cardiovascular: Sudden death is possible due to complete heart block
- Neuromuscular: Apathy, irritability, depression, and decreased ability to concentrate; progresses to obtundation and coma
- Gastrointestinal: Nausea and vomiting, abdominal pain, ileus
- Renal: Pruritus due to renal failure

## History and Physical Examination

The APN reviews the medical history to identify persons at high risk for hypercalcemia, keeping in mind that persons with breast cancer, lung cancer, and multiple myeloma are at the highest risk. Documentation of bone metastasis is noted. The physical examination includes assessing for any early or late symptoms of hypercalcemia.

## Diagnostics

The serum calcium level is used to verify the diagnosis of hypercalcemia when interventions to decrease the calcium in the serum will promote good quality of living. In persons clearly near the end of life for whom no interventions to correct the calcium levels are appropriate, laboratory data are not collected. Normal serum calcium levels lie within a range of 8.5 to 10.5 mg/dl (or 4.5 to 5.5 mEq/l). Approximately 50% of serum calcium is bound to serum proteins and fluctuates according to changes in serum protein concentrations. The following formula adjusts for serum concentrations of albumin and should be used to assess the severity of hypercalcemia (Waller & Caroline, 2000):

$$\text{corrected } Ca^{2+} \text{ (mg/dl)} = \text{measured } Ca^{2+} \text{ (mg/dl)} + 0.8 \text{ mg/dl} \times (4 - \text{serum albumin})$$

*or*

$$\text{corrected } Ca^{2+} \text{ (mEq/l)} = \text{measured } Ca^{2+} \text{ (mEq/l)} + 0.4 \text{ mEq/l} \times (4 - \text{serum albumin})$$

Other potentially helpful laboratory studies include BUN and creatinine levels to evaluate renal damage. An electrocardiogram may be used to monitor cardiac dysrhythmias.

## Intervention and Treatment

Patients who have symptoms of hypercalcemia or a calcium level greater than 14 mg/dl should be considered for treatment (Krecker & Muggia, 1995;

Warrell, 1997). The only long-term strategy to control hypercalcemia is to control the spread of the underlying malignancy. Because many patients have advanced malignancy and previously had acute aggressive interventions, the aim of therapy is palliative, with the goal of promoting comfort while limiting side effects (Jones, 1999). Interventions include the following:

- Prevent immobilization. A lack of weight-bearing activity increases bone resorption.
- Rehydrate the patient who is experiencing mild hypercalcemia. This may be done with encouragement of oral fluid intake but is often achieved by aggressive infusions (intravenous infusion or hypodermoclysis) of isotonic saline solution (Jones, 1999; Pereira & Bruera, 1997).
- No evidence indicates that adding furosemide is beneficial (Waller & Caroline, 2000).
- Restricting dietary calcium intake does not play an important role in decreasing serum calcium levels, except for the patient who has a diagnosis of hypercalcemia as a result of lymphoma (Jones, 1999; Mundy & Guise, 1997).
- When the corrected serum calcium level is greater than 12 mg/dl, consider treatment with bisphosphonates (e.g., pamidronate sodium, 60 to 90 mg in 500 ml normal saline solution IV over 2 to 4 hours) (Waller & Caroline, 2000).
  - Maximal effect is usually seen in 4 to 5 days; monitor for hypocalcemia.
  - Infusions may be required every 3 to 4 weeks to keep calcium levels within normal limits.
  - There may be a transient flare of bone pain after treatment with bisphosphonates, requiring an increase in NSAID and opioid dosages.
  - Although expensive, bisphosphonates have been demonstrated to be cost-effective in palliative care (Gessner, Koeberle, Thuerlimann, Bacchus, & Horisberger, 2000). Use of bisphosphonates lowers costs of treatment by reducing requirements for analgesics for bone pain, antiemetics for nausea associated with hypercalcemia, and hospitalization and related care for pathologic fractures.
  - New-generation, high-potency bisphosphonates will soon be available. One of these, zoledronic acid, has the advantage of requiring only a 5-minute infusion (Berenson et al., 2001). The appropriate use and cost effectiveness of these new medications in the palliative care setting await further evaluation.

## Patient and Family Teaching

Explain the purpose of new medications—those used to treat the hypercalcemia, as well as those prescribed to manage the unpleasant symptoms associated with it. Reinforce the importance of increasing hydration, whether oral or parenteral. Inform the patient that pain may increase initially after receiving treatment with a bisphosphonate; provide appropriate changes in orders for NSAIDs and opioids to manage this pain. Teach the patient and family to monitor for early signs of hypocalcemia after treatment with bis-phosphonates: muscle cramping and tingling of the fingertips.

In the patient for whom actively intervening to reduce the calcium level will not improve quality of living, explain the reason the patient is experiencing the symptoms associated with hypercalcemia and what is being done to control these symptoms. Provide instruction on any new medications prescribed, including appropriate administration and monitoring for side effects. Ensure the patient and family has adequate support systems in place to cope with this obvious sign of disease progression. Make referrals to the palliative care team social worker, counselor, and chaplain as appropriate.

### Evaluation and Plan for Follow-Up

The APN evaluates the patient for a lessening of uncomfortable symptoms associated with hypercalcemia regardless of the intervention plan used. When the goal is to achieve comfort by lowering the calcium level, the APN monitors the serum calcium levels to evaluate the effectiveness of the medications and to watch for hypocalcemia. Appropriate changes are made for any symptoms not managed. As the disease progresses and the patient's functional status declines, the APN evaluates when bisphosphonates should be discontinued. These medications should not be continued when they no longer improve the overall quality of living. At this time, adjustments in other medications may be required to maintain comfort.

## ■ SYNDROME OF INAPPROPRIATE ANTIDIURETIC HORMONE

### Definition and Incidence

Antidiuretic hormone (ADH) increases the permeability of the distal tubules of the kidneys to water, leading to reabsorption of water. Excessive amounts of ADH lead to water intoxication and hyponatremia. SIADH occurs in 1% to 2% of all patients with cancer; about 10% of these have small-cell lung cancer. Patients with SIADH have an increased incidence of liver and CNS metastasis and poorer survival rate than those without SIADH (Lokich, 1982).

### Etiology and Pathophysiology

SIADH can result from (1) overproduction of vasopressin in response to stimulation from tumor cells, (2) production of ectopic vasopressin by the tumor cells, or (3) stimulation of vasopressin production by medications (O'Shaughnessy & Jochen, 1998). In malignancy-related SIADH, ectopic production is the most common cause (Bower, Brazil, & Coombes, 1998). Although SIADH is most often associated with small-cell lung cancer, it also occurs with other cancers (Box 29-1).

| BOX 29-1 | *Cancers Associated with SIADH* |
|---|---|

Esophagus
Pancreas
Duodenum
Colon
Adrenal cortex
Prostate
Thymoma
Lymphoma

From O'Shaughnessy, I. M., & Jochen, A. L. (1998). Metabolic disorders in the cancer patient. In A. M. Berger, R. K. Portenoy, & D. E. Weissman (Eds.), *Principles and practice of supportive oncology* (pp. 427-433). Philadelphia: Lippincott-Raven; Bower, M., Brazil, L., & Coombes, R. C. (1998). Endocrine and metabolic complications of advanced cancer. In D. Doyle, G. W. C. Hanks, & N. MacDonald (Eds.), *Oxford textbook of palliative medicine* (2ⁿᵈ ed.) (pp. 709-725). New York: Oxford University Press

Medications may also stimulate vasopressin production as a side effect, potentially causing or contributing to the severity of SIADH. These medications include morphine, phenothiazines, tricyclic and selective serotonin reuptake inhibitor antidepressants, NSAIDs, nicotine, cyclophosphamide, and vincristine (Bower, Brazil, & Coombes, 1998; O'Shaughnessy & Jochen, 1998). Many times patients in palliative care settings are prescribed combinations of these medications, requiring a thorough evaluation.

## Assessment and Measurement

The symptoms experienced by the patient depend both on the plasma sodium level and on the rate at which the decline occurs. Persons with slowly developing SIADH may have very low serum sodium level before experiencing many symptoms. The signs and symptoms of hyponatremia include the following (Poe & Taylor, 1989):

- Early stages of SIADH (serum sodium level 115 to 130 mmol/l):
  - General: Weakness, fatigue, weight gain
  - Neurologic: Confusion, irritability, weakness, headache, altered mental status
  - GI: Nausea, vomiting, diarrhea, anorexia, thirst, abdominal cramping
  - Genitourinary (GU): Decreased urine output
  - Muscular: Myalgia, cramping
- Later stages of SIADH (serum sodium level <115 mmol/l):
  - Neurologic: Confusion, hyporeflexia, seizures, coma
  - GI: Oliguria

## History and Physical Examination

The APN must assess for the potential of developing SIADH on the basis of the disease process and medication review. The assessment includes monitoring for the signs and symptoms of hyponatremia noted previously.

## Diagnostics

Laboratory findings with SIADH include urine osmolality greater than the serum osmolality, low serum sodium level (<135 mmol/l), and high urine sodium concentration (>20 mEq/l) (O'Shaughnessy & Jochen, 1998).

## Intervention and Treatment

The APN should first consider medication as a potential cause and discontinue all offending medications whenever possible. This may be the only intervention required. For mild hyponatremia, fluid restriction may be instituted. Limiting free fluid to 800 to 1000 ml per day is not always feasible or may have a negative effect on quality of life. Considering the patient's wishes is extremely important when evaluating the appropriateness of fluid restriction.

Medications may be used to promote elimination of excessive water. Demeclocycline is an antibiotic that is used for SIADH as it inhibits the tubular reabsorption of water (Bower et al., 1998). The starting dose is 900 to 1200 mg PO per day in divided doses, followed by a maintenance dose of 600 to 900 mg PO per day. Another medication used for this purpose is urea 30 g diluted in 100 ml of orange juice. This induces osmotic diuresis. Patients need not have fluid restrictions when taking urea.

In the presence of neurologic symptoms, the APN may consider IV infusion of hypertonic (3%) saline solution, generally infused at the rate of 0.1 mg/kg/min (O'Shaughnessy & Jochen, 1998). Use this intervention only if it is anticipated that the patient's SIADH can be managed with less invasive interventions once the crisis has been treated and if the patient has the potential for good quality of life after this crisis. This intervention is rarely appropriate in the palliative care setting.

In addition to intervening to normalize the serum sodium, medications may also be prescribed to manage the nausea, diarrhea, headache, abdominal cramping, and myalgias.

## Patient and Family Teaching

Explain the purpose of the demeclocycline as well as any antiemetics, antidiarrheals, analgesics, or antispasmodics used to treat the symptoms associated with SIADH. It is helpful for the patient and family to hear that the symptoms of early stage SIADH often respond to the demeclocycline. As the disease progresses, ensure that the patient and family have adequate support systems in place to cope with this obvious sign of disease progression.

## Evaluation and Plan for Follow-Up

Monitor for improvement of symptoms after the initiation of therapy. The need for antiemetics, antidiarrheals, additional analgesics, and antispasmodics should decrease as the serum sodium level rises. If the patient continues to require these medications, consider holding the demeclocycline to evaluate for any changes in symptoms; no change in symptoms indicates the medication is not effective and should be discontinued. Continue to adjust medications to control uncomfortable symptoms as the disease progresses.

# ■ SUPERIOR VENA CAVA SYNDROME

## Definition and Incidence

The superior vena cava is a thin-walled vessel that drains venous blood from the head, neck, upper extremities, and upper thorax. Blood flow may be obstructed if this vessel is compressed, invaded, or thrombosed (Yahalom, 1997). SVCS occurs in approximately 3% to 4% of all oncology patients and is sometimes the presenting symptom (Dietz & Flaherty, 1987). Rapidly progressive SVCS may cause airway obstruction and respiratory failure. Slowly progressive SVCS has fewer symptoms, as there is time for development of collateral circulation.

## Etiology and Pathophysiology

Most often, SVCS is due to tumors involving the mediastinum. The large majority (75%) of cases are seen in patients with lung cancer (Jones, 1987), followed by non-Hodgkin's lymphoma, metastatic breast cancer, Kaposi's sarcoma, and germ-cell tumors. In addition, patients who have central venous access devices and pacemakers may be at increased risk for SVCS. Treatment of the underlying disease process, which is often possible with newly diagnosed cancer, relieves the symptoms of SVCS. But this syndrome can recur, most often in patients with small-cell lung cancer (Dietz & Flaherty, 1987).

## Assessment and Measurement

The early signs and symptoms of SVCS include the following (Dietz & Flaherty, 1987; Hunter, 1998; Yahalom, 1997):
- Dyspnea
- Facial swelling, especially upon arising in the morning
- Neck and arm swelling
- Neck vein distention
- Pronounced veins on trunk
- Nonproductive cough
    The later signs and symptoms of SVCS include the following:
- Stridor
- Hoarseness
- Periorbital and conjunctival redness and edema
- Neurologic changes (due to increased ICP):
    - Headache
    - Irritability
    - Blurry vision and other visual disturbances
    - Vertigo
    - Changes in mental status

## History and Physical Examination

The presence of the symptoms associated with SVCS leads to a review of the medical history to identify the presence of any disease process or medical intervention (e.g., central venous catheter, pacemaker) that may cause compression of the superior vena cava. Dyspnea is the most common presenting symptom of SVCS. Dyspnea has many potential causes; however, the combination of dyspnea and facial swelling are hallmark signs of SVCS. The presence of the additional symptoms noted in the physical examination are further evidence of this syndrome.

## Diagnostics

A chest radiograph showing a mass, mediastinal widening or pleural effusion may confirm the suspicion of SVCS. Before ordering the chest radiograph, the APN should evaluate the effect of verifying the diagnosis on the treatment plan. In persons who are not candidates for radiation or chemotherapy and who will be treated symptomatically, there is no need for a radiograph. When SVCS is the presenting symptom of advanced cancer, other diagnostic procedures to determine the underlying malignancy may be required, such as bronchoscopy or mediastinoscopy. These procedures are not necessary when the cell type is known or if chemotherapy is not an option.

## Intervention and Treatment

The goal of the treatment is to relieve the symptoms. Chemotherapy is appropriate in persons with previously untreated small-cell lung cancer or lymphoma. Patients who have been heavily treated with chemotherapy in the past are less likely to have a favorable response to additional chemotherapy. SVCS is usually very responsive to a single dose of radiation, regardless of tumor type. Thus a referral to a radiation oncologist is appropriate (Ahmedzai, 1998). Dexamethasone (6 to 10 mg PO q6h) may decrease inflammation that is caused by tumor or radiation. Symptoms, in particular dyspnea, should be treated aggressively (see Chapter 24).

## Patient and Family Education

The educational plan includes teaching the patient and family to manage the distressing symptoms associated with SVCS, especially dyspnea. When diagnostic procedures are needed to confirm the diagnosis for treatment planning, the patient is taught the rationale for the procedure and prepared for what to expect during testing. Should radiation therapy or chemotherapy be prescribed, appropriate information is provided to ensure that the patient and family are aware of the benefits and risks of the treatment and that they know how to manage any side effects. In persons with far advanced disease, SVCS may be a terminal event. Ensure that the patient and family have adequate support systems in place to manage symptoms and address psychologic, emotional, and spiritual needs.

## Evaluation and Plan for Follow-Up

The goal of care is patient comfort. When the uncomfortable symptoms associated with SVCS are controlled, the intervention plan is effective and maintained. The patient whose SVCS was successfully treated with radiation therapy or chemotherapy may live in fear of a recurrence of this distressing syndrome. Provide reassurance that the palliative care team will continue to monitor for any uncomfortable symptoms and intervene to treat them.

# ■ PATHOLOGIC BONE FRACTURE

## Definition and Incidence

Pathologic bone fracture is a fracture that occurs secondary to destruction of the bone by malignancies. Any patient with primary bone cancer or bone metastases is at risk for pathologic fractures. It is estimated that 30% to 70% of persons with cancer develop bone metastasis at some time; pathologic fractures occur in about 9% of persons with bone metastasis (Waller & Caroline, 2000). Metastatic breast cancer is responsible for about 50% of all pathologic fractures, followed by multiple myeloma, lung cancer, and prostate cancer (Galasko, 1998). Any person with metastasis to the bone is potentially at risk for fracture. The most common site of fracture is in the femur, although any bone can be affected.

## Etiology and Pathophysiology

Pathologic fractures occur when malignant cells invade the bone, creating lytic lesions. These lesions reduce the cortical strength of the bone. By the time a lytic lesion is evident on radiograph, the cortex is generally involved. There is a direct correlation between the amount of cortex involvement and the incidence of fracture. With 25% to 50% of the cortex involved, the risk of fracture is 3.7%; with 50% to 75% of the cortex involved, the risk of fracture increases dramatically to 61%; and with more than 75% of the cortex involved, the risk of fracture is 79% (Fidler, 1981). Although most pathologic fractures occur when there is a large lytic lesion, the bone may also be weakened by multiple small, permeative metastases (Galasko, 1998). The trauma of a fall may lead to the fracture of a weakened bone, but the bone may spontaneously fracture with no precipitating event.

## Assessment and Measurement

The hallmark symptom of bone metastasis is pain. Symptoms of a pathologic fracture include increase in pain, deformity, local swelling, abnormal mobility, and shock. There may or may not be a precipitating injury (Smith, 1994).

## History and Physical Examination

The presence of a bone metastasis identifies the individual at potential risk for pathologic fracture. Ask the patient about any documented bone metastasis and the presence of bone pain. Sometimes the patient and family hear a crack or snap when the fracture occurs; ask if anyone heard this sound. Identify if there was a precipitating event, such as a fall; if the fracture occurred during routine caregiving; or if the fracture was spontaneous. The physical examination involves examining the site of reported increased pain for deformity, edema, and ecchymosis.

## Diagnostics

Plain radiographs more clearly delineate lytic changes and fracture than do bone scans. It may be prudent to obtain radiographs for persons with significant bone pain in weight-bearing bones to identify the risk of fracture (Janjan & Weissman, 1998). Those at high risk may be candidates for primary internal fixation to prevent fracture. Magnetic resonance imaging (MRI) is preferred for the evaluation of vertebral fracture.

## Intervention and Treatment

Prophylactic interventions may prevent fracture. Persons with lytic bone lesions of 2.5 cm or larger in weight-bearing bones or with more than 50% cortical bone loss are at high risk for fracture. Persons with a life expectancy of greater than 1 to 2 months, a good performance status, and no hypercalcemia should be referred to an orthopedic surgeon for primary internal fixation of the lytic area. This procedure may be followed with radiation therapy to prevent further bone destruction (Waller & Caroline, 2000). Surgery has been shown to relieve pain and improve mobility for both persons with impending fracture and those with fractures (Ampil & Sadasivan, 2001).

Consider using bisphosphonates to reduce the risk of pathologic fracture in persons at high risk. These medications have been demonstrated to reduce the incidence of skeletal complications, including pathologic fracture, in persons with breast cancer and multiple myeloma (Berenson et al., 2001; McCloskey, Guest, & Kanis, 2001). Also, evidence is mounting that bisphosphonates are helpful for persons with prostate cancer (Lee, Fong, Singer, & Guenette, 2001).

A fracture is generally not a terminal event. Immediate treatment should include adequate analgesia with opioids and NSAIDs or corticosteroids, followed by splinting or immobilization of the affected area. Radiograph examinations should be obtained and orthopedic or surgical consultation is advised. Follow-up treatment with radiation or chemotherapy may also be considered, depending on the patient's overall condition, functional status, and the underlying disease processes.

## Patient and Family Teaching

Patient acceptance of diagnostic studies and interventions to prevent pathologic fracture is improved when the rationale is explained. Identify the alternatives for treating potential fractures with patients and discuss the benefits and burdens of each so that the patient can make an informed choice when more than one treatment option is available.

For patients with pathologic fracture, provide information on all changes in medications. If corticosteroids are included in the plan, discuss the schedule for decreasing doses. Encourage the patient to report pain and the effectiveness of interventions to treat the pain. Inform the patient that there may be a flare of bone pain when initiating bisphosphonates and discuss the plan for managing this increase in pain.

If a pathologic fracture occurs while a family member is providing care, reassure the person that he or she did not cause the fracture. Reinforce that the bone was weakened from the cancer and that it is likely the fracture would have occurred even without moving the patient. This information may need to be reinforced many times to assist the caregiver in coping with this event.

### Evaluation and Plan for Follow-Up

The effectiveness of interventions to prevent fracture is evaluated by the absence of this complication. With a pathologic fracture the goals of care are to manage pain and preserve mobility. Changes in the plan of care are made to maximize comfort and quality of living.

## ■ SUMMARY

Palliative care emergencies do not occur frequently. When one of these emergencies does occur, it causes physical discomfort and emotional distress and negatively affects quality of life. The APN must prepare and plan for potential palliative care emergencies in order to prevent those that can be prevented. Interventions are planned to maximize physical, psychologic, emotional, and spiritual comfort, promoting optimal quality of life for the individual.

---

**✔ CASE STUDY**

A home care hospice nurse has requested a joint home visit with an APN to evaluate her patient's new complaints and sudden onset of distressing symptoms described as unrelieved pain, weakness, and urinary incontinence. The patient, Mrs. M, is a 54-year-old woman with metastatic breast cancer who has been followed by hospice services for the past 2 weeks. Early this morning, she called her nurse with a surprising and sudden complaint of unrelenting shooting pain in both of her legs, difficulty ambulating, and the presence of urinary incontinence. The APN arrives at Mrs. M's home and reviews the patient's history and recent plan of care with the hospice nurse, including all of the patient's recent diagnostic tests and current medications. Mrs. M's recent bone scan revealed that she has extensive bone metastasis and her last laboratory analysis of her serum calcium was slightly elevated.

After a thorough physical examination, the APN identifies that Mrs. M has extreme neurologic deficits on both of her lower extremities; she is unable to detect pressure and/or pain on her bilateral lower extremities. The APN learns that Mrs. M has had progressive changes in ambulation in the last 12 hours, accompanied with urinary incontinence. Prior to this time, Mrs. M had been actively caring for herself and capable of maintaining her activities of daily living. She is very frightened by this sudden change in her physical condition and has been planning to attend her niece's wedding the following weekend. Mrs. M's medications include: sustained-release morphine 30 mg PO bid, ibuprofen 600 mg PO tid, baclofen 5 mg PO tid, and Peri-Colace PO as needed for constipation.

The APN is certain that Mrs. M is experiencing SCC and immediately sets up an emergency transfer to the local hospital for an MRI, immediate serum calcium level test, and immediate radiation therapy to relieve her symptoms. The APN also discontinues the ibuprofen and immediately orders dexamethasone 24 mg PO for relief of her offensive symptoms. Mrs. M is transferred to the acute care setting and is found to be positive for SCC. The prompt assessment and intervention allows Mrs. M to attend her niece's wedding as she had planned. Since Mrs. M's functional status had been good, the APN made the decision to send her into the acute care setting for aggressive interventions—knowing that prolonging treatment would eventually lead to plegia. Should Mrs. M have been less functional, the APN could have initiated aggressive corticosteroid interventions in her home.

## References

AHMEDZAI, S. (1998). Palliation of respiratory symptoms. In D. Doyle, G. W. C. Hanks, & N. MacDonald (Eds.), *Oxford textbook of palliative medicine* (2nd ed.) (pp. 583-616). New York: Oxford University Press.

AMPIL, F. L., & Sadasivan, K. K. (2001). Prophylactic and therapeutic fixation of weight-bearing long bones with metastatic cancer. *Southern Medical Journal, 94,* 394-396.

ARCHIMANDRITIS, A., Tsirantonaki, M., Tryphonos, M., Kourtesas, D., Sougioultzis, S., Papageorgiou, A., & Tzivras, M. (2000). Ranitidine versus ranitidine plus octreotide in the treatment of acute non-variceal upper gastrointestinal bleeding: A prospective randomized study. *Current Medical Research and Opinion, 16,* 178-183.

BARRON, K., Hirano, A., Araki, S., & Terry, R. (1959). Experiences with metastatic neoplasms involving the spinal cord. *Neurology, 9,* 91-100.

BAYLEY, A., Milosevic, M., Blend, R., Logue, J., Gospodarowicz, M., Boxen, I., Warde, P., McLean, M., Catton, C., & Catton, P. (2001). A prospective study of factors predicting clinically occult spinal cord compression in patients with metastatic prostate carcinoma. *Cancer, 92,* 303-310.

BERENSON, J. R., Rosen, L. S., Howell, A., Porter, L., Coleman, R. E., Morley, W., Dreicer, R., Kuross, S. A., Lipton, A., & Seaman, J. J. (2001). Zoledronic acid reduces skeletal-related events in patients with osteolytic metastases. *Cancer, 91,* 1191-1200.

BOWER, M., Brazil, L., & Coombes, R. C. (1998). Endocrine and metabolic complications of advanced cancer. In D. Doyle, G. W. C. Hanks, & N. MacDonald (Eds.), *Oxford textbook of palliative medicine* (2nd ed.) (pp. 709-725). New York: Oxford University Press.

BRUERA, E., Walker, P., & Lawlor, P. (1999). Opioids in cancer pain. In C. Stein (Ed.), *Opioids in pain control: Basic and clinical aspects* (pp. 309-324). New York: Cambridge University Press.

BURSTEIN, A., Fisher, K., McPherson, M., & Roby, C. (2000). Absorption of phenytoin from rectal suppositories formulated with polyethylene glycol base. *Pharmacotherapy, 20,* 562-567.

CARACINI, A., & Martini, C. (1998). Neurological problems. In D. Doyle, G. W. C. Hanks, & N. MacDonald (Eds.), *Oxford textbook of palliative medicine* (2nd ed.) (pp. 727-749). New York: Oxford University Press.

CORLEY, D. A., Cello, J. P., Adkisson, W., Ko, W. F., & Kerlikowske, K. (2001). Octreotide for acute esophageal variceal bleeding: A meta-analysis. *Gastroenterology, 120,* 946-954.

COWAP, J., Hardy, J. R., & A'Hern, R. (2000). Outcome of malignant spinal cord compression at a cancer center: Implications for palliative care services. *Journal of Pain and Symptom Management, 19,* 257-264.

DICKERSON, D. (1999). Global investigation of the 20 essential drugs in palliative care. *European Journal of Palliative Medicine, 6*(4), 130-135.

DIETZ, K. A., & Flaherty, A. M. (1987). Oncologic emergencies. In S. L. Groenwald, M. H. Frogge, M. Goodman, & C. H. Yarbro (Eds.), *Cancer nursing principles and practice* (3rd ed.) (pp. 800-839). Boston: Jones & Bartlett Publishers.

DONATO, V., Bonfili, P., Bulzonetti, N., Santarelli, M., Osti, M., Tombolini, V., Banelli, E., & Enrici, R. (2001). Radiation therapy for oncologic emergencies. *Anticancer Research, 21*(3C), 2219-2224.

ERNST, S., Brasher, P., Hagen, N., Paterson, A., MacDonald, N., & Bruera, E. (1997). A randomized, controlled trial of intravenous clodronate in patients with metastatic bone disease and pain. *Journal of Pain and Symptom Management, 13,* 319-326.

FIDLER, M. (1981). Incidence of fracture through metastasis in long bones. *Acta Orthopaedia Scandinavia, 52,* 623-627.

FREITAS, D. S., Sofia, C. Pontes, J. M., Gregorio, C., Cabral, J. P., Andrade, P., Ross, A., Camacho, E., Ferreira, M., Portela, F., Romaozinho, J. M., Tome, L., Gouveia, H., Leitao, M., Pimenta, I., & Donato, A. (2000). Octreotide in acute bleeding esophageal varices: A prospective randomized study. *Hepatogastroenterology, 47,* 1310-1314.

FULLER, B. G., Heiss, J., & Oldfield, E.H. (1997). Spinal cord compression. In V.T. DeVita, S. Hellman, & S. A. Rosenberg (Eds.), *Cancer: Principles and practice of oncology,* Vol. 2 (5th ed.) (pp. 2476-2486). Philadelphia: Lippincott-Raven.

GAGNON, B., Mancini, I., Periera, J., & Bruera, E. (1998). Palliative management of bleeding events in advanced cancer patients. *Journal of Palliative Care, 14,* 50-54.

GALASKO, C.S.B. (1998). Orthopaedic principles and management. In D. Doyle, G. W. C. Hanks, & N. MacDonald (Eds.), *Oxford textbook of palliative medicine* (2nd ed.) (pp. 477-487). New York: Oxford University Press.

GESSNER, W., Koeberle, D., Thuerlimann, B., Bacchus, L., & Horisberger, B. (2000). Economic analysis of terminal care for patients with malignant osteolytic bone disease and pain treated with pamidronate. *Supportive Care in Cancer, 8,* 115-122.

GUYTON, A. D., & Hall, J. E. (1996). States of brain activity—sleep; brain waves; epilepsy; psychoses. In A. D. Guyton & J. E. Hall (Eds.), *Textbook of medical physiology* (9th ed.) (pp. 761-768). Philadelphia: W. B. Saunders.

HUNTER, J. C. (1998). Structural emergencies. In J. K. Itano & K. N. Taoka (Eds.), *Core curriculum for oncology nursing* (3rd ed.) (pp. 340-354). Philadelphia: W. B. Saunders.

JANJAN, N. A., & Weissman, D. E. (1998). Primary cancer treatment: Antineoplastic. In A. M. Berger, R. K. Portenoy, & D. E. Weissman (Eds.), *Principles and practice of supportive oncology* (pp. 43-59). Philadelphia: Lippincott-Raven.

JONES, L. A. (1987). Superior vena cava syndrome: An oncologic complication. *Seminars in Oncology Nursing, 3,* 211-215.

JONES, L. (1999). Electrolyte imbalances. In C. Yarbro, M. Frogge, M., & M. Goodman (Eds.), *Cancer symptom management* (2nd ed.) (pp. 438-456). Sudbury, MA: Jones & Bartlett.

KRECKER, E., & Muggia, F. M. (1995). Oncologic emergencies. In M. C. Brain & P. P. Carbone (Eds.), *Current therapy in hematology-oncology* (5th ed.) (pp. 600-609). St. Louis: Mosby.

LEE, M. V., Fong, E. M., Singer, F. R., & Guenette, R. S. (2001). Bisphosphonate treatment inhibits the growth of prostate cancer cells. *Cancer Research, 61,* 2602-2608.

LOKICH, J. J. (1982). The frequency and clinical biology of the ectopic hormone syndromes of small-cell carcinoma. *Cancer, 50,* 2111-2114.

LUCKMANN, J. (1997). Caring for people with neurologic disorders. In J. Luckmann (Ed.), *Saunder's manual of nursing care* (pp. 651-741). Philadelphia: W. B. Saunders.

MCCLOSKEY, E. V., Guest, J. F., & Kanis, J. A. (2001). The clinical and cost considerations of bisphosphonates in preventing bone complications in patients with metastatic breast cancer or multiple myeloma. *Drugs, 61,* 1253-1274.

MUNDY, G., & Guise, T. (1997). Hypercalcemia of malignancy. *American Journal of Medicine, 103,* 134-145.

O'SHAUGHNESSY, I. M., & Jochen, A. L. (1998). Metabolic disorders in the cancer patient. In A. M. Berger, R. K. Portenoy, & D. E. Weissman (Eds.), *Principles and practice of supportive oncology* (pp. 427-433). Philadelphia: Lippincott-Raven.

PEREIRA, J., & Bruera, E. (1997). Emergencies in palliative care. In J. Pereira & E. Bruera (Eds.), *The Edmonton aid to palliative care* (pp. 66-78). Edmonton: University of Alberta, Division of Palliative Care.

PINOVER, W., & Coia, A. (1998). Palliative radiation therapy. In A. M. Berger, R. K. Portenoy, & D. E. Weissman (Eds.), *Principles and practice of supportive oncology* (pp. 603-626). Philadelphia: Lippincott-Raven.

POE, C. M., & Taylor, L. M. (1989). Syndrome of inappropriate antidiuretic hormone: Assessment and nursing implications. *Oncology Nursing Forum, 16,* 373-382.

PRUETT, J. (1999). Bleeding. In C. Yarbro, M. Frogge, & M. Goodman (Eds.), *Cancer symptom management* (2nd ed.) (pp. 285-303). Sudbury, MA: Jones & Bartlett.

RANEY, D. (1991). Malignant spinal cord tumors: A review and case presentation. *Journal of Neuroscience Nurse, 23,* 44-49.

SCHAFER, S. (1997). Oncologic complications. In S. Otto (Ed.), *Oncology nursing* (3rd ed.) (pp. 406-474). St Louis: Mosby.

SKIDMORE-ROTH, L. (2001). *2001 Nursing Drug Reference.* St Louis: Mosby.

SMITH, A. M. (1994). Emergencies in palliative care. *Annals of the Academy of Medicine Singapore, 23,* 186-190.

TWYCROSS, R., Wilcock, A., & Thorp, S. (1998). *Palliative care formulary.* Oxon, UK: Radcliffe Medical Press.

WALLER, A., & Caroline, N. L. (2000). *Handbook of palliative care in cancer* (2nd ed.). Boston: Butterworth-Heinemann.

WARRELL, R. P. (1997). Metabolic emergencies. In V. T. DeVita, S. Hellman, & S. A. Rosenberg (Eds), *Cancer: Principles and practice of oncology* (Vol. 2) (5th ed.) (pp. 2486-2500). Philadelphia: Lippincott-Raven.

WEISMAN, S. J. (1998). Supportive care in children with cancer. In A. M. Berger, R. K. Portenoy, & D. E. Weissman (Eds.), *Principles and practice of supportive oncology* (pp. 845-852). Philadelphia: Lippincott-Raven.

WILKES, G. (1999). Neurological disturbances. In C. Yarbro, M. Frogge, & M. Goodman. (Eds.), *Cancer symptom management* (2nd ed.) (pp. 344-381). Sudbury, MA: Jones & Bartlett.

YAHALOM, J. (1997). Superior vena cava syndrome. In V. T. DeVita, S. Hellman, & S. A. Rosenberg (Eds.), *Cancer: Principles and practice of oncology,* (Vol. 2) (5th ed.) (pp. 2469-2476). Philadelphia: Lippincott-Raven.

CHAPTER **30**

# *Pruritus*

CAROL L. SCOT

## ■ DEFINITION AND INCIDENCE

Pruritus (itching) can best be defined indirectly as a sensation that leads to a desire to scratch (Greaves & Wall, 1999). Pruritus may be generalized or localized, constant or intermittent, and occurring in apparently normal skin or obviously inflamed skin. The incidence of pruritus varies with disease and age.

Patients with advanced diseases can suffer every type of pruritus: some may have long-standing pruritic conditions; others may have pruritus of recent onset, associated with drug reactions, infections, advanced systemic disease, advanced age, or other conditions.

Itching is often seen as a minor social or even humorous disability, but it can be severe and intractable enough to cause abject misery (Greaves & Wall, 1999).

### Pruritus in Inflamed Skin

Itch is the dominant symptom of skin disease (Greaves & Wall, 1996). Any inflammatory skin condition, such as candidiasis, lichen planus, scabies, psoriasis, or eczema, is usually pruritic. An increase in the temperature of the skin lowers the threshold for itching. In inflammation the blood flow to the skin is increased, raising the skin temperature and therefore intensifying itching. Drug reactions can produce pruritus alone or with inflammation and rash. Scratching can further complicate inflammation by causing tissue damage. Itchy wheals (scratch prurigo) and chronic lichenified patches (prurigo nodularis) may develop (Greaves & Wall, 1996).

### Pruritus in Noninflamed Skin

Biliary obstruction and elevated plasma bile salt level are associated with highly distressing and persistent pruritus. This complication of cholestasis can be so difficult to manage that it can lead to severe sleep deprivation and become an indication for liver transplantation (Bergasa et al., 1995). Hepatic and pancreatic malignancies are often associated with pruritus. Elevated bile salt levels and pruritus also occur in advanced chronic hepatitis C, which is not a cholestatic condition (Lebovics et al., 1997).

The only malignancy strongly associated with pruritus (other than those that cause bile obstruction) is Hodgkin's disease. Itch is a presenting symptom in 5% to 10% of cases, and occurs at some time in about a third of patients (Ende et al., 1998).

Pruritus affects 80% of renal dialysis patients and is one of the most distressing symptoms of renal insufficiency.

General intractable itching is a common symptom of thyrotoxicosis. As in inflammation the raised temperature of the skin that results from increased blood flow with hyperthyroidism lowers the threshold to itch.

A lifelong cause of pruritus may be aquagenic pruritus, in which wetting the skin with water of any temperature causes severe itching with a pricking sensation, lasting about an hour after a shower or bath, with no apparent change in the skin. In some patients the same attacks can occur with change of ambient temperature (Greaves & Wall, 1999). A group of symptoms identical to those of aquagenic pruritus can also occur in 50% of patients with polycythemia vera.

Patients with human immunodeficiency virus (HIV) may suffer pruritus generated by any of the usual causes discussed. They also can have a pruritic papular eruption that shows histologic evidence of eosinophilic folliculitis.

At least 50% of persons older than 70 suffer extensive pruritus at some time. If none of the other causes of itch is present, xerosis—dryness of the skin—is the most likely cause, because senescent skin holds less water than younger skin. Ironically the dry skin may also lead to water-induced itching.

Persistent localized itching in normal skin is an uncommon condition. It can occur on the outer surface of the elbows *(brachioradial pruritus)*, and is thought to be due to chronic sun exposure; it also occurs in the condition of *meralgia paresthesias,* in which there is persistent itching in the center of the back (Greaves & Wall, 1996).

Itching also can be a symptom of anxiety, with or without associated depression. If scratch excoriation is limited to accessible areas and other causes have been eliminated, this is a likely diagnosis. Although the itch is reported as constant, observation of the patient shows infrequent brief episodes of itching, which can nevertheless cause extensive excoriation. Complaints not just of itch, but of formication—the sensation of something like ants crawling on the skin—are usually symptoms of psychotic or severe psychoneurotic problems, for which adjunctive psychiatric treatment is required.

## ■ ETIOLOGY AND PATHOPHYSIOLOGY

Even though much of the physiologic process of itch has been described, it is still not completely understood, with the consequence that no specific effective antiitch drug is available (Greaves & Wall, 1999).

Itch occurs only in skin and cornea, and itch sensitivity is unevenly distributed in the skin. The skin needs to be neurologically intact for pruritus to occur. Itch shares many molecular and neurophysiologic mechanisms with pain, including transmission by the slow, small, unmyelinated C fibers.

The classic model for itch was that itch-causing substances stimulated specific itch fibers. Such fibers have not been found, and there is now doubt that they exist. The current theory is that itch occurs when local groups of the small fibers in the skin are intermittently excited. If a large area of skin is then stimulated by scratching, rubbing, or transdermal electrical nerve stimulation, central surround inhibition which overwhelms the weak stimulus and suppresses the itch, is generated (Greaves & Wall, 1996).

Another itch phenomenon is very similar to pain perception in skin. A well-localized area of itch is surrounded by an area of heightened sensitivity that responds with intense itch to light touch or other minor stimulus (allokinesis); it is similar to allodynia, in which pain is induced by light stimuli in an area surrounding a localized focus of pain (Greaves & Wall, 1996).

Unraveling the mysteries of the mechanisms of itching is complicated by evidence of a central nervous system contribution. Some patients experience itching with opioid medications: pruritus of central origin (Bergasa et al., 1995). There are also the problem of "social itch," as well as itching caused by expectation and emotional states (Greaves & Wall, 1996). It is not known why reading or talking about itch or being in the presence of someone who is scratching can generate itch. There is also no explanation why anxiety can lead to itching.

A long list of substances, including amines, lipids, peptides, and proteins, has been found to be associated with pruritus. Histamine plays a major role. Inflamed skin contains increased amounts of histamine, and many other substances associated with itch act by releasing histamine from the mast cells in skin. If histamine is injected into the skin superficially, it causes itching; injected more deeply, it causes pain. The histamine produces itch by the H1 receptor, not the H2 receptor.

The tissue fluid from many inflammatory dermatoses, such as psoriasis and contact allergic dermatitis, contains increased amounts of prostaglandin E2. Prostaglandin E2 contributes to itch by lowering the threshold of the skin to the itching provoked by histamine and other mediators (Greaves & Wall, 1996).

Tachykinins, such as substance P and vasoactive internal peptide (VIP) are found with others in pruritic skin. They can cause inflammation and contribute to histamine release.

In psoriasis abnormal arachidonic acid metabolism appears to play a part. Greatly increased amounts of arachidonic acid metabolites have been found in psoriatic plaques. A study that used dietary polyunsaturated ethyl ester lipids to act as competitive inhibitors of arachidonic acid showed a reduction in pruritus and healing in a majority of patients, especially those with mild to moderate disease (Lassus, Dahlgren, Halpern, Santalahti, & Happonen, 1990).

Atopic dermatitis is a common inflammatory skin condition characterized by severe pruritus and associated with a number of immunologic abnormalities. Treatment with the medication thymopentin, which stimulates the immune system, reduces pruritus and erythema in a significant number of patients (Lueng et al., 1990).

Endogenous opioid peptides may contribute to itch in both inflamed and noninflamed skin and operate centrally to regulate the extent of intensity and quality of perceived itch (Greaves & Wall, 1996).

## ■ ASSESSMENT AND MEASUREMENT

When pruritus is associated with inflamed skin, the condition is often easy to characterize and measure. Contact allergy can be diagnosed by the pattern of redness or rash, as, for instance, when redness surrounds and underlies tape or jewelry. The locations and appearances of rashes can be virtually diagnostic, as in the typical linear scabies rash between fingers and in axillary folds and the scaling rash of psoriasis on elbows and knees.

In normal skin pruritus, like pain, is a purely subjective sensation, which the clinician evaluates on the patient's report or on the evidence of scratching. The patient's description of itching therefore is the starting point of the assessment. The timing of symptoms and the circumstances surrounding them may be helpful, even diagnostic, for conditions such as aquagenic pruritus or food or drug allergies.

## ■ HISTORY AND PHYSICAL EXAMINATION

In the ideal medical interview the patient describes his or her symptoms freely and spontaneously and stops when what needs to be communicated has been expressed. The clinician then repeats any information that needs clarification and asks any indicated further questions. When the current problems have been discussed, the clinician may ask other questions to uncover any other problems.

A person suffering from itch may fail to communicate the fact. A patient with intermittent itch may forget to mention it, and even a patient with constant itch may have more urgent matters to discuss that put it out of mind. If a patient is observed scratching, questions about itch obviously need to be asked. For a patient without obvious clues the symptom of itch may be uncovered in more wide-ranging questions, such as whether the patient has any skin problems, such as lumps, bumps, rashes, or itching?

When the symptom of pruritus has been identified, it needs to be characterized. Is it localized or general, constant or intermittent? When did it start? When does it occur, or when is it worst? (It would make little sense to prescribe morning treatment for a patient who is bothered by itch only at night.) What makes the itching better, what makes it worse? What measures have been tried, and with what effect?

For all patients with itch a careful and complete drug history, to include prescription, over-the-counter, and recreational drugs, needs to be taken. The drug history may reveal medications associated with pruritus, such as opiates, amphetamines, quinidine, salicylates, B vitamins, niacinamide, barbiturates, oxycodone, and tramadol (Goolsby, 1998). The drug history also should include any medications currently being used to control the pruritus.

The physical examination should include a survey of the entire skin surface, with special attention to areas identified as itchy. All skin abnormalities should be noted, including areas of excoriation, dryness, and lichenification.

# ■ DIAGNOSTICS

## Localized Pruritus

No diagnostics other than the history and physical may be needed for localized pruritus, especially if the inflammation has the classic features of a known cause and responds well to treatment. For instance, a contact dermatitis that resolves with avoidance of the inciting substance and short-term use of systemic antihistamines, topical antihistamine, or steroid cream needs no further attention.

In other typical rashes, as with candidiasis, tinea corporis, or lice infestations, microscopic identification of the cause may be desirable. Rashes that are not easily diagnosed and do not respond to treatment should be referred to a dermatologist and may require a skin biopsy.

## Generalized Pruritus

A patient with known renal failure or bile duct obstruction probably needs no further investigation into the cause of generalized pruritus. But those with no obvious explanation need first a careful history, including a drug history; followed by a full physical examination, with pelvic and rectal examination; chest radiograph; blood count, thyroid, renal, and liver function testing; and stool examination for occult blood and parasites. A skin biopsy from pruritic skin to rule out pemphigus may be indicated if no other cause is found (Greaves & Wall, 1999).

# ■ INTERVENTION AND TREATMENT

An earlier statement warrants repetition: "Even though much of the physiologic process of itch has been described, it is still not completely understood, with the consequence that *no specific effective antiitch drug is available.*" All of the following measures may or may not be effective, to varying degrees.

## Preventive Measures

Because aging skin is more susceptible than younger skin to drying and itching, aging patients and their caregivers should limit patients' exposure to soap and water, and use emollients liberally. Exposure to water and evaporation should be followed by heavy water-barrier substances such as petroleum jelly, olive oil, or mineral oil preparations. Soaps used should be mild, like glycerin or Dove or Basis. Waterless cleansers, such as Cetaphil are also available. Ambient air should also be adequately humidified.

## Pharmacologic Interventions

Antihistamines are the mainstay of antipruritic treatment. In some conditions, such as atopic dermatitis, the older sedating antihistamines, such as diphenhydramine (Benadryl) and hydroxyzine (Atarax), appear to be more effective than the newer nonsedating drugs. Whether part of the relief of pruritus is due to the sedation is not known (Greaves & Wall, 1999).

This pruritus is associated with high plasma levels of bile salts, even though there is little or no correlation between concentrations of bile salts and severity of itching. In spite of this, measures to lower bile salt concentration often significantly relieve pruritus. This may mean that other substances that exist with bile salts and are eliminated with them actually cause the itching (Greaves & Wall, 1999).

The most readily available means to lower bile salt concentration is cholestyramine resin, a bile acid sequestrant. The regimen begins with one packet or scoop mixed with food or liquid once or twice a day. The usual maintenance dose is two to four scoops or packets a day. Side effects, which are principally gastrointestinal, can include bloating, constipation, and aggravation of hemorrhoids. As with other constipating drugs bowel problems should be anticipated and treated aggressively. Ursodeoxycholic acid therapy or ultraviolet B (UVB) radiation may also help alleviate bile-salt–associated pruritus (Ende et al., 1998).

Patients who experience renal failure and severe pruritus usually gain temporary relief with dialysis. Although the population of mast cells in their skin is higher than normal and the histamine level is also often higher, antihistamines rarely give effective relief. For patients with pruritus and hyperparathyroidism parathyroidectomy has provided relief. But for most of these patients relief often is partial. At the end of life, when dialysis and surgery are not appropriate options, interventions may include emollients for dry skin, sedating antihistamines, and use of high-potency steroid creams. Phototherapy by UVB may also be effective.

Some research in the pruritus of two conditions, renal failure and cholestasis, has focused on the increased levels of endogenous opioids that occur with advanced renal and hepatic disease. Because opioids can be a source of pruritus, researchers have attempted to control pruritus with antiopioid drugs, such as naloxone, with some success (Bergasa et al., 1995; Peer et al., 1996).

Application of capsaicin cream can stop severe localized itching in normal skin. Capsaicin is toxic to C fibers and causes a painful burning sensation when applied. Some patients find it tolerable and useful, but others consider the treatment worse than the pruritus (Greaves & Wall, 1999).

Because many pruritic conditions are associated with allergic reactions, steroid creams and oral steroids are often used to control the reaction and the itching. Steroids must be used cautiously. The dangers associated with short-term or long-term steroid use must be kept in mind, especially for oral steroids. A misdiagnosed skin rash, for example, herpes zoster, treated with an oral steroid preparation can produce a fulminating lethal disease. Oral steroids used as briefly as 1 or 2 weeks have been known to cause psychologic problems and aseptic necrosis, and long-term steroid use can cause muscle weakness, osteoporosis, and susceptibility to infection.

### Nonpharmacologic Interventions

Because itching is intensified with warmth, every effort should be made to keep the skin cool. Light clothing, air conditioning, fans, tepid showers, and cooling lotions may help. Over-the-counter preparations such as menthol lotion, calamine lotion, or aqueous cream may provide relief. Distraction during the day, through pleasant companions, games, videos, fragrances, and music, and sedation at night may help.

## ■ PATIENT AND FAMILY EDUCATION

Patients and families need to be aware of the preceding information, including the fact that no specific effective antiitch drug is yet available.

Patients and families should always be reassured that the patient's complaints will be taken seriously and attended to; that there are many measures available with some hope of lessening of pruritus; but that it would be unrealistic to promise complete suppression of itching.

Patients and families also need to be educated about how heat intensifies itch and cooling alleviates it. An elderly patient needs to be informed of the need for aging skin to be kept well hydrated and of the methods for providing adequate hydration. Finally, patients and families always need to be educated about the possible side effects of medications and techniques to handle them.

## ■ EVALUATION AND PLAN FOR FOLLOW-UP

The frequency of follow-up depends on the severity of the pruritus and the degree of the patient's distress. If an inflammatory condition has been complicated by cellulitis of the underlying tissues, the patient may need hospitalization or daily examinations until improvement is confirmed.

In severe allergic reactions the allergen may be cleared from the body very slowly, and follow-up may continue for weeks or months. Follow-up must be planned carefully with the patient. Any deterioration or worsening of symptoms should be reported immediately.

If the treatment measures prescribed are effective and the pruritic condition improves, reevaluation and follow-up are necessary to confirm the improvements and to encourage continuing use of a successful regimen, if needed.

✔ **CASE**

**STUDY**    F. S. is a 77-year-old man admitted for home hospice care. His terminal diagnosis is liver and kidney failure, with ascites. He also has peripheral vascular disease and lower extremity edema. He complains of itching of his feet and legs.

Physical examination reveals blood pressure of 100/58, respiratory rate of 18, pulse rate of 60, and temperature of 98.0° F. He has extensive edema and stasis changes in his legs and feet, an open 2-cm area on the left outer thigh, and toes that are dark purple. His toenails are thickened.

His medications include bumetanide (Bumex), 2 mg PO 2/day; isosorbide mononitrate (Imdur) 60 mg PO ½/day; verapamil, 40 mg PO tid; isosorbide, 60 mg PO ½/day; pentoxifylline (Trental), 400 mg PO tid; spironolactone (Aldactone), 100 mg PO bid; propoxyphene napsylate, 100 mg with acetaminophen 650 mg (Darvocet-N 100) PO q4h prn for pain; digoxin (Lanoxin), 0.125 mg PO qd; nitroglycerin, 0.4 mg SL prn for chest pain; oxygen, 2 to 3 L per nasal cannula prn for dyspnea; hydroxyzine HCl (Atarax), 25 mg PO tid; and diphenhydramine (Benadryl), 25 mg PO q6h prn for itching. For skin care of the lower extremities, three times a week his legs and feet are soaked in warm water with ¼ cup pHisoHex, rinsed with normal saline solution, followed by 10% urea, 2.5% curea (Aquaphor), and Eucerin cream applied to the legs and feet (but not the toes), which are then wrapped (Kerlex, Ace).

Over the next 3 months, he continues to have severe itching, and more open areas develop. About 3 months later, his physician changes the leg care to daily plain-water soaks with saline solution rinse and application of Bag Balm with triple antibiotic ointment to open areas, as well as aloe vera gel. The hydroxyzine is discontinued and replaced with cetirizine HCl (Zyrtec), 10 mg PO qd.

Within another month his legs have not improved, and generalized itching of the arms, chest, back, and flanks has developed. His physician refers him to a dermatologist.

At the first dermatology appointment, the dermatologist orders injections of methylprednisolone (Depo-Medrol), 40 mg, and triamcinolone acetonide (Kenalog), 20 mg. He also prescribes a 2-week course of amoxicillin/potassium clavulanate potassium (Augmentin) and increases the Zyrtec dosage to 20 mg/day. He changes the skin care to washing his legs twice a week with his regular shower, applying silver sulfadiazine (Silvadene) to open areas three times a week, and applying triamcinolone acetonide 0.1% cream to the legs three times a week and to all other pruritic areas twice a day.

At follow-up with the dermatologist 2 weeks later, F. S. again receives an injection of triamcinolone acetonide, 20 mg. F. S. experiences noticeable immediate relief with the injections and the application of triamcinolone acetonide cream. The upper body cream was reduced to daily or alternate-day application.

On this regimen his itching is controlled and he is much more comfortable. The dermatologist continues to follow up with him and 2 months later adds econazole nitrate (Spectazole) cream, applied to the feet and toes twice daily, and itraconazole (Sporanox), two capsules PO qd.

A month later, F. S. again has a course of amoxicillin/potassium clavulanate, and the following month the econazole nitrate and itraconazole are discontinued. Nystatin polyene antifungal powder is added to the regimen for the feet.

The patient died peacefully at home 9 months after entering hospice care.

## References

BERGASA, N. V., Alling, D. W., Talbot, T. L., Swain, M. G., Yurdaydin, C., Turner, M. L., Schmitt, J. M., Walker, E. C., & Jones, E. A. (1995). Effects of naloxone infusions in patients with the pruritus of cholestasis. *Annals of Internal Medicine, 123,* 161-167.

ENDE, J., Epstein, P. E., Branch, W. T., Hatem, C. J., Henrich, J. B., Kroenke, K., Lofgren, R. P., Mackler, S. A., Merli, G. J., Milan, F. B., Novack, D. H., Osheroff, J. A., Paauw, D. S., Simel, D. L., Sullivan, G. M., & Young, M. J. (1998). Primary care internal medicine. In J. H. Holbrook (Ed.), *Medical knowledge self-assessment program* (pp. 1-164). Philadelphia: American College of Physicians.

GOOLSBY, M. J. (1998). The elusive itch. *ADVANCE for Nurse Practitioners, 6,* 61-64.

GREAVES, M. W., & Wall, P. D. (1996). Pathophysiology of itching. *Lancet, 348,* 938-940.

GREAVES, M. W., & Wall, P. D. (1999). Pathophysiology and clinical aspects of pruritus. In I. M. Freedberg, A. Z. Eisen, K. Wolff, K. F. Austen, L. A. Goldsmith, S. I. Katz, & T. B. Fitzpatrick (Eds.), *Fitzpatrick's dermatology in general medicine* (5th ed.) (pp. 487-494). Hightstown, NJ: McGraw-Hill.

LASSUS, A., Dahlgren, A. L., Halpern, M. J., Santalahti, J., & Happonen, H. P. (1990). Effects of dietary supplementation with polyunsaturated ethyl ester lipids (Angiosan) in patients with psoriasis and psoriatic arthritis. *Journal of International Medical Research, 18,* 68-73.

LEBOVICS, E., Seif, F., Kim, D., Elhosseiny, A., Dworkin, B. M., Casellas, A., Clark, S., & Rosenthal, W. S. (1997). Pruritus in chronic hepatitis C. *Digestive Diseases and Sciences, 42,* 1094-1099.

LUENG, D. Y. M., Hirsch, R. L., Schneider, L., Moody, C., Takaoka, R., Li, S. H., Meyerson, L. A., Mariam, S. G., Goldstein, G., & Hanifan, J. M. (1990). Thymopentin therapy reduces the clinical severity of atopic dermatitis. *Journal of Allergy and Clinical Immunology, 85,* 927-933.

PEER, G., Kivity, S., Agami, O., Fireman, E., Silverberg, D., Blum, M., & Iaina, A. (1996). Randomized crossover trial of naltrexone in uremic pruritus. *Lancet, 348,* 1552-1554.

# Ulcerative Lesions

DEBRA E. HEIDRICH

## ■ DEFINITION AND INCIDENCE

Persons at the end of life are at risk for development of skin ulcerations that are the effects of weakness, immobility, and inadequate nutrition and of the underlying disease processes. In particular, pressure ulcers and malignant cutaneous wounds (MCWs) create physical and psychoemotional challenges for patients.

Pressure ulcers are wounds characterized by cellular necrosis due to pressure or shearing force. The incidence in any particular practice setting is somewhat difficult to determine as study designs vary significantly. For example, some studies include stage I pressure ulcers and some do not, and as a result study outcomes vary greatly. In the acute care setting the incidence of pressure ulcers ranges from 2.7% to 29.5%, with increased incidence in higher-risk groups, such as the elderly and persons with paralysis. The incidence of pressure ulcers in the nursing home setting is 2.4% to 23%. There are no good data from home care studies (AHRQ, 1992).

MCWs are ulcerating skin lesions that develop when malignant cells infiltrate the epithelium (Foltz, 1980). MCWs may occur as single lesions or in groups (Haisfield-Wolfe & Baxendale-Cox, 1999). Approximately 5% to 10% of persons with metastatic malignancies have MCWs, usually during the last 3 to 6 months of life (Crosby, 1998; Foltz, 1980; Thiers, 1986; Waller & Caroline, 2000). The malignant processes associated with the development of cutaneous metastases include breast cancer, malignant melanoma, lung cancer, and colorectal cancer (Crosby, 1998). These wounds are sometimes called fungating tumor wounds. This term refers to the tendency of these wounds both to ulcerate and to proliferate (Mortimer, 1998).

Both pressure ulcers and MCWs can have devastating physical and psychosocial effects. These wounds can be a source of pain, anemia, and infection, and these sometimes unsightly and foul-smelling lesions can cause self-concept disturbance, social isolation due to shame or embarrassment, anxiety, fear, and depression (Foltz, 1980; Goodman, Ladd, & Purl, 1993; Miller, 1998; Waller & Caroline, 2000).

# ■ ETIOLOGY AND PATHOPHYSIOLOGY

## Pressure Ulcers

Pressure ulcers develop when the soft tissue is compressed between a bony prominence and an external surface, disrupting the blood supply. The results are local ischemia, hypoxia, edema, and inflammation, followed by cell death (Hess, 1999). The risk factors for the development of pressure ulcers include immobility, incontinence, inadequate nutrition, and altered level of consciousness (AHRQ, 1992).

## Malignant Cutaneous Wounds

MCWs may result from primary skin lesions or metastasis from other malignant processes. As mentioned, breast cancer is the most common cause of MCWs. Up to 25% of persons with breast cancer experience skin metastasis (Waller & Caroline, 2000). The malignancies associated with the development of MCWs are listed in Box 31-1.

The initial appearance of a primary skin malignancy may be a sore that does not heal. Metastatic MCWs may begin as hard dermal or subcutaneous nodules and may be fixed to underlying tissue (Crosby, 1998; Thiers, 1986). These lesions are most commonly in the vicinity of the primary tumor (Crosby, 1998). However, MCWs are also seen at a secondary site related to metastatic disease (Goodman et al., 1993; Miller, 1998). They may vary in color from flesh toned to red and are usually asymptomatic at early stages (Crosby, 1998).

---

| BOX 31-1 | *Tumors Associated with Malignant Cutaneous Wounds* |
|---|---|

**PRIMARY SKIN MALIGNANCIES**
Untreated basal cell carcinoma
Untreated squamous cell carcinoma
Malignant melanoma

**METASTASTIC SPREAD FROM PRIMARY MALIGNANCY**
Breast
Head and neck
Lung
Stomach
Kidney
Uterine
Ovarian
Colon
Bladder
Lymphoma
Melanoma

From Mortimer, P. S. (1998). Management of skin problems: Medical aspects. In D. Doyle, G. W. C. Hanks, & N. MacDonald (Eds.), *Oxford textbook of palliative medicine* (2nd ed.) (pp. 617-627). New York: Oxford University Press; Crosby, D. L. (1998). Treatment and tumor-related skin disorders. In A. M. Berger, R. K. Portenoy, & D. E. Weissman (Eds.), *Principles and practice of supportive oncology* (pp. 251-264). Philadelphia: Lippincott-Raven; Waller, A., & Caroline, N. L. (2000). *Handbook of palliative care in cancer.* Boston: Butterworth-Heinemann.

Malignancies spread to the cutaneous tissues via direct extension or embolization into the vascular or lymph channels (Goodman et al., 1993; Mortimer, 1998). Eventually these lesions infiltrate the epithelium and supporting lymph and blood vessels, interfering with blood flow and the supply of oxygen and nutrients to the tissues and leading to ulceration (Haisfield-Wolfe, & Baxendale-Cox, 1999; Mortimer, 1998). Capillary rupture, necrosis, and infection are common, leading to a purulent, friable, and malodorous ulceration (Foltz, 1980; Mortimer, 1998).

Infections in MCWs may be caused by both anaerobic and aerobic pathogens. Anaerobic organisms proliferate in necrotic tissue. The foul-smelling odor of many of the MCWs is due to the release of malodorous volatile fatty acids as metabolic end products of anaerobic activity (Mortimer, 1998). These wounds can readily become infected with aerobic organisms and produce yellow to green purulent discharge.

## Wound Healing

Many local and systemic factors that influence wound healing must be considered when planning preventive interventions for pressure ulcers and treatment strategies for both pressure ulcers and MCWs (Hess, 1999):

- Local factors:
  - Pressure disrupting the blood supply to the capillary bed—Pressure must be eliminated to allow tissues to receive the oxygen and nutrients required for maintenance and healing.
  - Dry environment—Moisture enhances epidermal cell migration and increases speed of healing three- to fivefold.
  - Edema—Any edema can increase the pressure in the tissues and interfere with blood supply, oxygen transport, and cellular nutrition.
  - Infection—Wounds cannot heal in the presence of infections.
  - Necrosis—Healthy tissue cannot grow where there is necrotic tissue. This dead tissue must be removed before healing can occur. Necrosis may appear as slough, which is moist, loose, and stringy necrotic tissue that is typically yellow, or eschar, which appears as dry, thick, leathery tissue and may be black.
  - Incontinence—The irritation and moisture produced by urinary or fecal incontinence can cause additional skin breakdown and certainly impede healing.
- Systemic factors:
  - Age—The elderly tend to have compromised immune, circulatory, and respiratory systems as well as inadequate nutrition and hydration, which challenge healing.
  - Body build—Persons who have extensive adipose tissue tend to have a poor blood supply, which impedes healing and increases the destructive potential of pressure ulcers. Emaciated patients often lack the oxygen and nutritional stores required for wound healing.
  - Chronic disease—Several chronic diseases are associated with poor wound healing. Persons who have coronary artery disease and

peripheral vascular disease tend to have vascular insufficiency, which leads to inadequate oxygen supply and nutrition to the tissues. Granulation tissue production depends on insulin. Thus persons with diabetes mellitus generally experience impaired wound healing.

- Nutritional status—Wound healing requires proteins; carbohydrates; fats; vitamins A, C, and K; pyridoxine; riboflavin; thiamine; copper; zinc; and iron. Persons with impaired nutrition will certainly be at greater risk for skin breakdown and poor wound healing.
- Immunosuppression—Persons who do not have an intact immune system in general experience delay in wound healing. They are also at risk for development of infections that further interfere with healing.

# ■ ASSESSMENT AND MEASUREMENT

There are two validated risk assessment tools for identifying those persons at greatest risk for development of pressure ulcers, the Braden Scale and the Norton Scale (AHRQ, 1992). Both scales produce risk scores based on known risk factors, such as mobility, mental status, and moisture. These scales are readily available in the published guidelines from the Agency for Healthcare Research and Quality (AHRQ). It is important to reassess risk at intervals, especially in the palliative care setting, where declining functional status and nutritional impairment are anticipated.

When any type of ulceration is present, documentation of the degree of tissue destruction is an important aspect of assessment. Pressure ulcers and MCWs each have a staging system. Staging of pressure ulcers is well defined in the literature and summarized in the AHRQ (1992) guidelines:

- Stage I: Nonblanchable erythema of intact skin.
- Stage II: Partial-thickness skin loss involving epidermis and/or dermis. These lesions appear as superficial abrasions, blisters, or shallow craters.
- Stage III: Full-thickness skin loss involving damage or necrosis of subcutaneous tissue. These lesions appear as deep craters and may or may not entail undermining of adjacent tissues.
- Stage IV: Full-thickness skin loss with extensive destruction, tissue necrosis or damage to muscle, bone, or supporting structures. These, too, are deep craters. Undermining and sinus tracts are common.

## Staging of Malignant Cutaneous Wounds

Recognizing that the staging system for pressure ulcers does not necessarily apply to assessment of MCWs, Haisfield-Wolfe & Baxendale-Cox (1999) developed and tested a specific staging system for these lesions, which is presented in Table 31-1. The purpose of this scale is to clarify communication among health care professionals to improve patient care, consultation, and comparison of research results.

Photographic documentation may be helpful in assessing and monitoring all types of ulcerative lesions (Miller, 1998). Haisfield-Wolfe &

## TABLE 31-1

### Malignant Cutaneous Wound Staging System

| Staging Classification | Stage 1 | Stage 1N | Stage 2 | Stage 3 | Stage 4 |
|---|---|---|---|---|---|
| **WOUND** | | | | | |
| Closed wound/intact skin | X | | | | |
| Closed wound/superficially open to drain then close/hard and fibrous | | X | | | |
| Open wound/dermis and epidermis tissue involved | | | X | | |
| | | | | X | |
| Open wound/full thickness skin loss involving subcutaneous tissue | | | | | X |
| Open wound/invasive to deep anatomic tissues and structures | | | | | |
| **PREDOMINANT COLOR** | | | | | |
| Red/pink | X | X | X | | |
| Red/pink/yellow | | | | X | X |
| **HYDRATION** | | | | | |
| Dry | X | | | | |
| Both moist and dry | | X | | | |
| Moist | | | X | X | X |
| **DRAINAGE** | | | | | |
| None | X | | | | |
| Clear/purulent | | X | | | |
| Serosanguineous/bleeding | | | X | | |
| Purulent/serosanguineous | | | | X | |
| Serosanguineous/bleeding/purulent | | | | | X |
| **PAIN** | | | | | |
| No | X | | | | |
| Pain possible | | X | X | X | |
| Yes | | | | | X |
| **ODOR** | | | | | |
| No | X | X | | | |
| Yes | | | X | X | X |
| **TUNNELING/UNDERMINING** | | | | | |
| No | X | X | X | X | |
| Yes | | | | | X |

From Haisfield-Wolfe, M. E., & Baxendale-Cox, L. M. (1999). Staging of malignant cutaneous wounds: A pilot study. *Oncology Nursing Forum, 26,* 1055-1064.

Baxendale-Cox (1999) used digital photography as an adjunct to observation to assess and record the MCW accurately on initial assessment and follow-up.

## Wound Assessment Variables

In addition to the stage of the wound the following information is documented for all ulcerative lesions:

- Color of the wound (Hess, 1999):
  - Red or pink color generally indicates clean, healthy granulation tissue.
  - Yellow may be the result of infection-related exudate or necrotic slough.
  - Black tissue indicates eschar from necrosis.
  - Some wounds have mixed colors. Clinicians use one of two approaches in documenting the color of mixed wounds: (1) use the least desirable color or (2) estimate the percentage of each color within the wound (Hess, 1999). For clear communication, the palliative care team should adopt one of these two approaches as a standard.
- Size of the wound (Hess, 1999):
  - The length and width are measured, using established landmarks for measurement.
  - The depth is noted at the deepest point. This is measured by inserting a sterile applicator into the deepest area, holding or marking the applicator stick at the skin surface level, and measuring from the tip of the stick to the mark.
  - Tunneling, which is tissue destruction under intact skin, is also noted and measured. It is measured by inserting a sterile applicator into tunneled areas, holding or marking the applicator stick at the wound edge, and measuring from the tip of the stick to the mark.
- Appearance is assessed. The moisture content of the wound bed and the color and condition of the skin surrounding the pressure ulcer are noted (Hess, 1999).
- Drainage (Hess, 1999):
  - The amount of drainage is noted. It may be described (1) verbally, as scant, moderate, large, or copious; (2) in terms of the number of soaked dressings; or (3) by weight of the dressings.
  - The color and consistency of the drainage are documented. Drainage may be serous, sanguineous, serosanguineous, or purulent.
- Odor is also noted. Wound odor may be described as pungent, strong, foul, fecal, or musty.
- Pain at the site may indicate infection, tissue destruction, or vascular insufficiency. The absence of pain may indicate nerve damage (Hess, 1999).
- Temperature of the intact skin is also noted. Heat is a sign of pressure ulcer formation and can also indicate an underlying infection (Hess, 1999).

# ■ HISTORY AND PHYSICAL EXAMINATION

Medical history identifies those persons who have diseases that create skin integrity risks, such as heart disease, peripheral vascular disease, diabetes, and cancer. Past treatments that may affect skin integrity and wound healing, such as radiation therapy or extensive surgery, are also important aspects of the patient's history. In addition, the advanced practice nurse (APN) assesses the patient's activity level, mobility, level of consciousness, nutritional status, and hydration status. Many of these factors are included in the risk assessment tools described.

The routine skin inspection includes observing for any areas of discomfort, redness, edema, or ulceration, paying special attention to bony prominences, heels, and elbows. In addition, for persons at risk for MCWs the skin is inspected for the presence of any new nodules, especially in the same general region as the primary tumor. The presence of incontinence or excessive diaphoresis must also be noted for all patients.

When an ulcerative lesion are present at initial assessment a history of the lesion is important, including how long it has been present, previous treatments for the lesion, the effectiveness of these treatments, and the psychosocial effect of the lesion on the patient and family (Miller, 1998).

# ■ DIAGNOSTICS

On occasion wound cultures may be appropriate to determine the exact organism causing an infection, to guide subsequent more specific interventions. Orders must be written to obtain cultures for both aerobic and anaerobic organisms. It is often appropriate to forgo cultures and treat the likely infection on the basis of the appearance and odor of the exudate.

# ■ INTERVENTION AND TREATMENT
## Prevention of Pressure Ulcers

- Document the risk assessment.
- Assess skin routinely. The frequency depends on the risk assessment. For persons who are relatively inactive daily inspection by the nurse and/or primary caregiver is recommended.
- Keep the skin clean and free of excessive external moisture:
  - Use mild cleansers that minimize irritation and dryness.
  - Treat dry skin with moisturizers.
  - If there is incontinence, perspiration, or drainage, use padding or dressing materials that wick moisture away from skin.
  - There are no research studies on which to base the practice of using moisture barriers to protect skin, and no studies on these products have tested for statistical significance (AHRQ, 1992). However use of a moisture barrier to protect skin is part of the practice standards of many agencies.

- Prevent friction and shear injuries:
  - Use proper positioning and careful transfer and turning techniques. Two-person lifts using the bed sheets or a pad for turning and lifting are very helpful.
  - Friction can also be reduced by using lubricants, such as corn starch or petroleum jelly, polyurethane thin film dressings over heels and elbows, or protective padding, such as heel or elbow protectors.
- Encourage a high-protein, high-calorie diet and provide vitamin C and zinc supplements when the patient's condition is such that healing can be anticipated and when the patient does not experience discomfort in ingesting food or supplements. When healing is not likely, focusing on nutrition is not in the patient's best interest.
- Encourage mobility or range of motion exercise as appropriate for the patient's physical condition.
- Reduce pressure on tissues:
  - Teach the patient and caregiver the importance of turning and repositioning at least every 2 hours.
  - Active or passive range of motion exercises can also be used to relieve pressure and to maintain muscle tone.
  - Prevent positioning on the trochanter.
  - Use supports, such as wedges, pillows, and heel supports.
  - Persons who are at high risk may benefit from using a special pressure-reducing device, such as air-filled overlays, alternating air-filled mattress overlays, gel- or water-filled mattress overlays, and specialty mattresses and beds (AHRQ, 1992; Hess, 1999).
  - Prevent the pressure of chair sitting by teaching patients to shift their weight every 15 minutes, if they are able, or by instructing caregivers to reposition the patient in the chair at least every hour. Pressure-reducing devices, such as foam, gel, or air chair pads, may also be used.
  - Instruct caregivers not to use doughnut-type devices.
- Prevent other mechanical tissue damage. Evidence suggests that massage over bony prominences may actually lead to deep tissue trauma and increase the risk of pressure ulcers (AHRQ, 1992). All caregivers need to be instructed not to massage any reddened areas.

### Treatment of Malignant Cutaneous Wounds

An ulceration that is confined to local recurrence may be treated by one or a combination of the following: surgery, radiation therapy, chemotherapy, or hyperthermia. However lesions that only recur locally are rare in end-of-life care as most skin ulcerations are a manifestation of a disseminated disease. Hormonal manipulation may shrink some lesions associated with metastatic breast cancer. Most often the care is directed to minimizing infection, bleeding, and odor (Foltz, 1980; Goodman et al., 1993; Miller, 1998).

## Care and Dressing of Ulcerations

All ulcerative lesion treatment plans include instructions for the cleansing solution, frequency of cleansing, type of dressing materials, and frequency of dressing changes. In addition each includes a time frame for reevaluation (Hess, 1999). Consultation with an enterostomal therapist is helpful when treating particularly challenging wounds.

- Irrigate the wound to flush out cellular debris and drainage. Wounds are irrigated between dressing changes. The type of dressing often guides the frequency. For example, hydrocolloid dressings may be changed only once a week. Infected or draining wounds require more frequent dressing changes.
  - Use normal saline solution or water for a wound with no signs of infection. A bulb syringe, gravity drip through intravenous (IV) tubing, or piston syringe with rubber catheter attached may be used.
  - Use one of the following for short-term treatment of infected and foul-smelling wounds. All of these solutions are toxic to fibroblasts, inhibiting wound healing (Hess, 1999). The solutions must be rinsed from the wound with normal saline solution. Use these solutions for infected wounds only and discontinue after infection is adequately treated:
    - Acetic acid solution is effective for Pseudomonas infection (Hess, 1999). This solution can be made from equal parts of vinegar and water (Foltz, 1980).
    - Hydrogen peroxide works for mechanical cleansing, helping to dissolve and remove crusted exudate.
    - Povidone-iodine can be used for its broad-spectrum antimicrobial action (Hess, 1999).
    - Sodium hypochlorite solution (Dakin solution) is effective for staphylococcal and streptococcal infections (Hess, 1999). It may also be helpful for managing odor. This solution can be made by using one part of household bleach to nine parts of water (Foltz, 1980).
- Débridement is performed to remove necrotic tissue and promote healing (Walker, 1996; Hess, 1999). When healing is anticipated, this is a necessary step. In the palliative care setting complete healing of a pressure ulcer is not always possible and healing of a MCW is next to impossible. Thus the APN must consider the purpose and potential outcomes of débridement for each individual. When removal of necrotic tissue will decrease infection, reduce inflammation, and improve comfort, débridement is appropriate. If the débridement procedure itself causes significant discomfort, the removal of the "protective" layer of eschar causes prolonged pain or active bleeding, or the patient is not likely to live long enough to derive benefit, débridement is inappropriate.
  - Surgical débridement is the fastest method, but also the most uncomfortable. It may require general anesthesia. As complete wound healing is rarely possible in wounds with necrotic tissue in end-of-life care, surgical débridement is rarely appropriate.

- Mechanical débridement is the use of wet-to-dry dressings to pull necrotic tissue from the wound. It may be helpful for removing encrusted, purulent materials. The disadvantage of this method is that it is nonselective: healthy tissue is also removed with the dry dressings.
- Enzymatic débridement is the use of topical enzymes to digest necrotic tissue. These products must be used cautiously to prevent the breakdown of healthy tissue, but they can be very effective. Because of the negative effect on healthy tissue topical enzymes should be discontinued when more than half of the wound bed is clean (Walker, 1996). These medications tend to be expensive, so the ability of the family to pay for the prescription may be a consideration. Enzymes that have been used for this purpose include collagenase (Santyl), fibrinolysin (Elase), papain (as in Accuzyme Papain-Urea Debriding Ointment), and streptokinase (Rao, Sane, & Georgiev, 1975; Walker, 1996; Waller & Caroline, 2000).
- Autolytic débridement is the use of the body's own enzymes and white blood cells to remove the necrotic tissue. Many dressings are designed to promote this process (Walker, 1996; Hess, 1999), including transparent films, hydrocolloids, semipermeable polyurethane foams, and hydrogels.
- Clean the skin around the wound with normal saline solution or plain water.
- Pack deep wounds; dressing needs to be flexible enough to touch all wound surfaces:
  - Any solution used on the packing materials must be nontoxic to cells. A possible exception is the use of wet-to-dry dressings moistened with Dakin solution for débridement and odor control. However, as mentioned, both the procedure and the solution are cytotoxic and should be discontinued as soon as the wound bed is reasonably clean.
  - Many companies manufacture wound fillers. They are available in pastes, granules, powders, beads, and gels. They provide a moist healing environment, promote autolytic débridement, and absorb exudate (Hess, 1999). They may also promote comfort. Cost of these products should be considered.
  - Wounds that require packing/fillers of any kind generally require a secondary dressing.
- Select a dressing that promotes a moist, but not wet environment. The stage of the wound and the amount of drainage guide the selection of the appropriate dressing:
  - Use moisture-retentive dressings for wounds that have light to moderate drainage. Examples include polyurethane transparent film dressings for Stage I/II ulcers and hydrocolloid dressings for Stage II/III ulcers.
  - Use absorbent dressings for wounds with moderate to heavy drainage. There are many excellent products on the market, both absorbent wound fillers and absorbent dressings:
    - If wound drainage is less than 50 ml/day an absorbent dressing may be sufficient.

- If wound drainage is greater than 50 ml/day, a wound drainage bag or pouch may be helpful. Using a drainage collection system allows accurate measurement of drainage, decreases dressing changes, decreases contamination, improves comfort, and protects surrounding skin (Hess, 1999). A good seal around any appliance used to collect drainage is important. Stomahesive paste or a similar product may be helpful to fill in creases or indentations in the skin and improve the seal (Miller, 1998). An enterostomal therapist can provide insight about the most cost-effective type of drainage bag and sealant to use.
- Keep in mind that sterile absorbent dressings are more expensive than clean absorbent materials. Sanitary pads and disposable diapers are made to be absorbent and may be used as secondary dressings when the APN determines that a clean dressing is sufficient (Goodman et al., 1993).
- Dry wounds may benefit from use of one of the many hydrogels available. Most are ointments, and some are combined with other dressing materials.
- Protect surrounding skin.
  - Remove all dressings carefully to prevent damage to surrounding tissue. An acetone-free adhesive remover or baby oil may be helpful in removing old dressings.
  - When significant drainage necessitates frequent dressing changes, avoid using tape to secure dressings if possible. Options include gauze wrap bandages, flexible netting or stretch elastic bands (e.g., tube tops), and Montgomery straps.
  - Skin sealants, petroleum-based products, and other water-resistant products may be used to protect the surrounding skin from wound drainage. As noted, no research findings support this practice (AHQR, 1992), but many clinicians have seen benefits from using these products.
- Control bleeding. MCWs are especially prone to bleeding as a result of the disruption of the capillary bed. The selection of an intervention depends on the degree of oozing and patient tolerance.
  - Reduce any trauma to the tissue by keeping the wound moist and using nonadherent dressings. If dressings become too dry, it may be helpful to moisten with saline solution before removal (Goodman et al., 1993). Wet-to-dry dressings should be avoided.
  - Pressure may be applied to visible bleeding vessels, but only if the underlying structures can support the force (Foltz, 1980; Waller & Caroline, 2000).
  - Silver nitrate sticks can be used for pinpoint capillary oozing (Foltz, 1980).
  - Gauze soaked in 1:1000 epinephrine can be applied over areas of bleeding (Waller & Caroline, 2000).
  - Coagulant dressings, such as absorbable gelatin (Gelfoam), are helpful for multiple areas of oozing.

- Sucralfate paste is another option for widespread oozing. Crush a 1-g sucralfate tablet and mix with 2 to 3 ml water-soluble gel (Waller & Caroline, 2000).
- Radiation therapy is also an option for some patients (Mortimer, 1998).
- Control odor. Odor is often a problem with MCWs. This is most likely caused by infection in necrotic tissue and can be minimized if the lesion can be adequately cleansed and débrided or the infection treated with a bacteriostatic agent. Additional measures that filter or mask the odor are beneficial when other interventions do not eliminate it:
  - Topical metronidazole is active against anaerobic bacterial infections and has been demonstrated to be helpful in controlling wound odor (Rice, 1992; Poteete, 1993; Finlay, Bowszyc, Ramlau, & Gwiezdzinski, 1996). Most studies use metronidazole 0.75% to 0.8% gel. Some practitioners report that use of metronidazole (parenteral) solution to irrigate wounds controls odor well. Metronidazole irrigation has not been studied to compare its effectiveness or cost to those of topical gel.
  - Sodium hypochlorite solution can be used for its débriding and bacteriostatic properties, either in irrigation or on wet-to-dry dressings (Foltz, 1980; Hess, 1999). Use with caution, however, as it is very irritating to healthy tissues (both in and around the wound) and interferes with blood clotting.
  - A chlorophyll-containing ointment applied to the wound or chlorophyll tablets taken orally may be helpful (Goodman et al., 1993). However no studies have compared the effectiveness of this intervention with that of the others discussed.
  - Some dressings are designed to filter odors by a carbon/charcoal layer. Some products on the market are combination dressings, with both absorptive and carbon-filtering layers. Until comparative studies are available, the APN must determine the best product with respect to amount of drainage, size of wound, ease of use, and cost. The following are dressings with carbon layers (Hess, 1999):
    - Lyofoam C Polyurethane Foam Dressing with Activated Carbon (ConvacTec) is designed to neutralize odors on wounds with light or moderate exudate.
    - CarboFlex Odor Control (ConvaTec) is designed for odor control on wounds with light exudate.
    - Odor-Absorbent Dressing (Hollister) is designed for odor control on dry wounds or as a secondary dressing over an absorbent dressing if there is exudate.
  - Home remedies for controlling odor include honey, sugar, yogurt, or buttermilk in wounds (Goodman et al., 1993; Miller, 1998). No studies have evaluated the effectiveness of these treatments.
  - Deodorizers can be used to mask odors. These often have odors of their own, which may or may not be desirable to the patient:
    - Some deodorizers (e.g., Banish, Hexon) can be used sparingly on dressings.

- Room deodorizers, including commercial products, scented candles, and scented oils (e.g., spirit of wintergreen), may be used.
- Some clinicians report using pans of charcoal briquettes under the bed to assist in absorbing room odor. No studies have reported on the effectiveness of this approach.
- Treat pain. Depending on the severity of the pain the APN may select a local treatment, a systemic analgesic, or a combination of several interventions.
  - Aluminum hydroxide/magnesium hydroxide suspension (Maalox) or yogurt applied to the wound may relieve burning sensations (Waller & Caroline, 2000). However, Maalox can be drying and yogurt can be messy and require frequent dressing and linen changes. The reports of using these interventions are anecdotal; no research has documented their effectiveness.
  - Topical morphine made with 5 mg morphine solution in 5 ml neutral gel is an option for severe wound pain (Waller & Caroline, 2000).
  - As some of the pain is due to inflammation, systemic nonsteroidal antiinflammatory drugs (NSAIDs) are appropriate. For moderate to severe pain an opioid analgesic may be required.

## ■ PATIENT AND FAMILY EDUCATION

The patient and family require instruction in the prevention and management of ulcerative lesions. A comprehensive teaching plan includes the following:
- Teach general assessment and skin care measures:
  - Inspect the skin daily for redness, irritation, or breakdown.
  - Keep the skin clean and prevent excessive dryness:
    - Avoid hot water, use a mild cleanser, and minimize force and friction on skin (AHRQ, 1992).
    - Keep air humidified.
    - Use a moisturizer on the skin.
    - Clean the patient as soon as possible if there is urinary or bowel incontinence.
  - Avoid massage over bony prominences.
  - Keep the bed and bed clothing clean and dry. Use incontinence pads as necessary.
- Teach measures to reduce pressure and friction:
  - Use heel and elbow protectors.
  - Use a recommended special mattress/overlay.
  - Position the patient to prevent pressure, using pillows, wedges, or other padding. Prevent positioning of the patient on the trochanter.
  - Keep the head of the bed at its lowest comfortable position to prevent shearing that can occur when the patient slides down in bed.
  - Use good technique when lifting, using two-person lifts whenever possible. Use lift pads instead of dragging the patient.

- Teach appropriate wound cleansing and dressing techniques for those situations in which the family will be providing some of the wound care. Teaching should include demonstration, verbal instruction, and return demonstration. Ensure that the caregiver is comfortable with the procedure. Issues to be addressed in the teaching plan include the following:
  - Preparation and storage of cleansing solution
  - Cleansing techniques for wound and surrounding skin
  - Use of all dressing products, including fillers and secondary dressings
  - Appropriate disposal of soiled dressing materials
- Teach the patient and family to report any changes to their health care team:
  - Changes in wound size, color, drainage, or odor
  - Changes in the appearance of surrounding skin
  - Signs of discomfort

## ■ EVALUATION AND PLAN FOR FOLLOW-UP

The APN monitors for changes in any of the wound assessment variables from the baseline and changes the intervention plan accordingly. The goal of care is determined by the underlying cause and the patient's overall condition. Even for pressure ulcers it may not be appropriate to expect wound healing because of the poor nutritional status and impaired circulation many patients have at the end of life. Under these circumstances the goal may be to prevent or minimize progression and prevent infection. For MCWs in end-of-life care, the goal is to promote physical and psychoemotional comfort by managing pain, drainage, infection, and odor.

The entire team is involved in the planning, intervention, and evaluation process. Support from social workers/counselors, home health aides, clergy, and volunteers is required to address the many needs of the patient and family. Consultation with an enterostomal therapist is extremely helpful when facing particularly challenging wounds.

---

✔ **CASE STUDY** Mrs. Jones is 83 years old and has a diagnosis of metastatic breast cancer. She has an extensive fungating tumor wound covering most of the right side of her chest. The skin is reddish purple from the clavicle to the bottom of the rib cage and from the axilla to the sternum, and there are multiple raised, hard nodules across the chest. There are multiple areas where the skin appears to have surface abrasions, and there is an open wound located about 5 cm from the sternum and 15 cm from the clavicle that measures 10 cm across and 8 cm down. The wound bed is light red around the edges, but about 60% of the wound is covered by a yellowish, stringy, purulent material. The wound is deepest at the sternal margin and measures 1.5 cm. No tunneling is observed and there is no bleeding. The patient reports that the wound is not painful, but the foul odor is "driving her and her family crazy." She has been cleaning the wound with soap and water using a gauze pad and covering it with a gauze dressing. There is a moderate amount of serosanguineous drainage noted. Mrs. Jones reports the gauze gets soaked and needs to be changed four or five times each day. She also says that the surface abrasions surrounding the wound were caused by the tape.

The APN determines that this is a stage III MCW. She recommends using Dakin solution to cleanse and débride the slough from the wound three times daily, followed by rinsing with normal saline solution for 3 days. After the first 3 days, saline solution only is to be used for wound cleansing. Bulb syringes are used for both the Dakin and saline solutions. The surrounding skin is cleaned with normal saline solution and a thin layer of petroletum jelly is applied around the wound to protect the skin from drainage. Metronidazole 0.75% gel is applied topically to the wound bed. A wet-to-damp gauze dressing is selected, and saline solution is used to wet the gauze, which is then fluffed to fill the wound lightly. This dressing is covered with a gauze pad, which is reinforced with a sanitary napkin. An elastic "tube top" is used to secure the dressing in place to prevent tape from touching the sensitive skin.

After 1 week the APN reassesses the wound and finds that only about 20% of it shows signs of slough and the odor has decreased. The padding has been sufficient to control the drainage during the day, but the dressing is sometimes soaked through by morning. The cleansing and dressing procedures are continued and additional padding by sanitary napkins used at night. After another week the metronidazole gel is discontinued as the wound odor is no longer a problem. The APN changes the dressing procedure to cleansing with normal saline solution, filling the wound bed with an alginate, covering the alginate with a gauze pad to fit the wound, and covering the gauze with a pad (telfa). The dressing is secured with the tube top, and the caregiver is instructed to change the dressing every 3 days or when there are signs of moisture on the pad. (If the surrounding tissue were healthy and could tolerate the adhesive, a hydrocolloid wound filler and dressing might have been selected at this point. This dressing might allow for more time between dressing changes.)

A month later the wound is larger, now measuring 11 cm by 8.5 cm. The wound bed is 90% pink and drainage is moderate. The dressing requires changing every 2 days, but these procedures are becoming more difficult because Mrs. Jones is weaker and maneuvering the tube top for dressing changes requires much effort by both Mrs. Jones and her caregiver. To make securing the dressing easier, the APN applies four 2- by 5-cm strips of hydrocolloid dressing wafers to the healthy skin at the four corners of the wound and tapes the dressing in place, using the hydrocolloid wafer as the tape anchor.

# References

AGENCY for Healthcare Research and Quality (AHRQ) (formerly the AHCPR) (1992). *Pressure ulcers in adults: Prediction and prevention: Clinical practice guideline number 3.* Rockville, MD: Author.

CROSBY, D. L. (1998). Treatment and tumor-related skin disorders. In A. M. Berger, R. K. Portenoy, & D. E. Weissman (Eds.), *Principles and practice of supportive oncology* (pp. 251-264). Philadelphia: Lippincott-Raven.

FINLAY, I. G., Bowszyc, J., Ramlau, C., & Gwiezdzinski, Z. (1996). The effect of topical 0.75% metronidazole gel on malodorous cutaneous ulcers. *Journal of Pain and Symptom Management, 22,* 158-162.

FOLTZ, A. T. (1980). Nursing care of ulcerating metastatic lesions. *Oncology Nursing Forum, 7*(2), 8-13.

GOODMAN, M., Ladd, L. A., & Purl, S. (1993). Integumentary and mucous membrane alterations. In S. L. Groenwald, M. H. Frogge, M. Goodman, & C. H. Yarbro (Eds.), *Cancer nursing principles and practice.* Boston: Jones & Bartlett.

HAISFIELD-WOLFE, M. E., & Baxendale-Cox, L. M. (1999). Staging of malignant cutaneous wounds: A pilot study. *Oncology Nursing Forum, 26,* 1055-1064.

HESS, C. T. (1999). *Clinical guide: Wound care* (3rd ed.). Springhouse, PA: Springhouse Corporation.

MILLER, C. (1998). Skin problems in palliative care: Nursing aspects. In D. Doyle, G. W. C. Hanks, & N. MacDonald (Eds.), *Oxford textbook of palliative medicine* (2nd ed.) (pp. 642-656). New York: Oxford University Press.

MORTIMER, P. S. (1998). Management of skin problems: Medical aspects. In D. Doyle, G. W. C. Hanks, & N. MacDonald (Eds.), *Oxford textbook of palliative medicine* (2nd ed.) (pp. 617-627). New York: Oxford University Press.

POTEETE, V. (1993). Case study: Eliminating odors from wounds. *Decubitus, 6*(4), 43-46.

RAO, D. B., Sane, P. G., & Georgiev, E. L. (1975). Collagenase in the treatment of dermal and decubitus ulcers. *Journal of the American Geriatric Society, 23,* 22-30.

RICE, T. T. (1992). Metronidazole use in malodorous skin lesions. *Rehabilitation Nursing, 17,* 244-245, 255.

THIERS, B. H. (1986). Dermatologic manifestations of cancer. *CA: A Cancer Journal for Clinicians, 36,* 130-148.

WALKER, D. (1996). Choosing the correct wound dressing. *American Journal of Nursing, 96*(9), 35-39.

WALLER, A., & Caroline, N. L. (2000). *Handbook of palliative care in cancer.* Boston: Butterworth-Heinemann.

# Prognostic Guidelines for the Noncancer Diagnoses

T he following prognostic guidelines for the noncancer diagnoses of heart disease, pulmonary disease, dementia, HIV disease, liver disease, renal disease, stroke and coma, and amyotrophic lateral sclerosis serve as a starting point in determining a patient's eligibility for hospice or palliative care services. These guidelines are by no means absolute but they represent, in general, disease markers that indicate a significantly decreased prognosis, should the disease run its usual course. These guidelines may be helpful in considering when referral to a hospice or palliative care program may be appropriate and also as a basis for discussing care options with care providers and the patient and family.

You may obtain the complete version of these guidelines, including extensive references, by contacting the National Hospice and Palliative Care Organization (NHPCO). We appreciate the NHPCO's willingness to allow us to reprint portions of them. The NHPCO is also a valuable resource for other information regarding hospice, palliative care, and grief and bereavement. Refer to Appendix B for contact information.

## ■ MEDICAL GUIDELINES FOR DETERMINING PROGNOSIS: HEART DISEASE

I. Symptoms of recurrent congestive heart failure (CHF) at rest.

    A. These patients are classified as New York Heart Association (NYHA) Class IV (see Appendix III).

    B. *Ejection fraction of 20% or less* is helpful supplemental objective evidence, but should not be required if not already available.

II. Patients should already be *optimally treated* with diuretics and vasodilators, preferably angiotensin-converting enzyme (ACE) inhibitors.

    A. The patient experiences persistent symptoms of congestive heart failure despite attempts at maximal medical management with diuretics and vasodilators.

    B. "Optimally treated" means that patients who are not on vasodilators have a medical reason for refusing these drugs, e.g. hypotension or renal disease.

    C. Although newer beta blockers with vasodilator activity, e.g. carvedilol, have recently been shown to decrease morbidity and mortality in chronic CHF, they are not included in the definition of "optimal treatment" at this time.

III. In patients with refractory, optimally treated CHF as defined above, each of the following factors have been shown to decrease survival further, and thus may help in educating medical personnel as to the appropriateness of hospice for cardiac patients.

    A. Symptomatic supraventricular or ventricular arrhythmias that are resistant to antiarrhythmic therapy.

    B. History of cardiac arrest and resuscitation in any setting.

    C. History of unexplained syncope.

    D. Cardiogenic brain embolism, i.e., embolic CVA of cardiac origin.

    E. Concomitant HIV disease.

# ■ MEDICAL GUIDELINES FOR DETERMINING PROGNOSIS: PULMONARY DISEASE

I. Severity of chronic lung disease documented by:

A. Disabling dyspnea at rest, poorly or unresponsive to bronchodilators, resulting in decreased functional activity, e.g., bed-to-chair existence, often exacerbated by other debilitating symptoms such as fatigue and cough.

Forced Expiratory Volume in One Second (FEV1), after bronchodilator, less than 30% of predicted, is helpful supplemental objective evidence, but should not be required if not already available.

B. Progressive pulmonary disease.

1. Increasing visits to Emergency Department or hospitalizations for pulmonary infections and/or respiratory failure.

2. Decrease in FEV1 on serial testing of greater than 40 ml per year is helpful supplemental objective evidence, but should not be required if not already available.

II. Presence of cor pulmonale or right heart failure (RHF).

A. These should be due to advanced pulmonary disease, not primary or secondary to left heart disease or valvulopathy.

B. Cor pulmonale may be documented by:

1. Echocardiography.

2. Electrocardiogram.

3. Chest x-ray.

4. Physical signs of RHF.

III. Hypoxemia at rest on supplemental oxygen.

A. pO2 less than or equal to 55 mm Hg on supplemental oxygen.

B. Oxygen saturation less than or equal to 88% on supplemental oxygen.

IV. Hypercapnia

   A. pCO2 equal to or greater than 50 mm Hg.

V. Unintentional progressive weight loss of greater than 10% of body weight over the preceding six months.

VI. Resting tachycardia greater than 100/minute in a patient with known severe chronic obstructive pulmonary disease.

## ■ MEDICAL GUIDELINES FOR DETERMINING PROGNOSIS: DEMENTIA

I. Functional Assessment Staging

   A. Even severely demented patients may have a prognosis of up to two years. Survival time depends on variables such as the incidence of comorbidities and the comprehensiveness of care.

   B. The patient should show *all* of the following characteristics:

      1. Unable to ambulate without assistance.

        *This is a critical factor.* Recent data indicate that patients who retain the ability to ambulate independently do not tend to die within six months, even if all other criteria for advance dementia are present.

      2. Unable to dress without assistance.

      3. Unable to bathe properly.

      4. Urinary and fecal incontinence.

        a. Occasionally or more frequently, over the past weeks.

        b. Reported by knowledgeable informant or caregiver.

      5. Unable to speak or communicate meaningfully.

        a. Ability to speak is limited to approximately a *half dozen or fewer intelligible and different words,* in the course of an average day or in the course of an intensive interview.

II. Presence of Medical Complications.

    A. The presence of medical comorbid conditions of sufficient severity to warrant medical treatment, documented within the past year, *whether or not the decision was made to treat the condition,* decrease survival in advanced dementia.

    B. Comorbid Conditions associated with dementia:

        1. Aspiration pneumonia.

        2. Pyelonephritis or other upper urinary tract infection.

        3. Septicemia.

        4. Decubitus ulcers, multiple, stage 3-4.

        5. Fever recurrent after antibiotics

    C. Difficulty swallowing food or refusal to eat, sufficiently severe that patient cannot maintain sufficient fluid and calorie intake to sustain life, with patient or surrogate refusing tube feedings or parenteral nutrition.

        1. Patients who are receiving tube feedings must have documented impaired nutritional status as indicated by:

            a. Unintentional, progressive weight loss of greater than 10% over the prior six months.

            b. Serum albumin less than 2.5 gm/dl may be a helpful prognostic indicator, but should not be used by itself.

## ■ MEDICAL GUIDELINES FOR DETERMINING PROGNOSIS: HIV DISEASE

I. CD4+ Count

    A. Patients whose CD4+ count is below 25 cells/mcL, measured during a period when patient is relatively free of acute illness, may have a prognosis less than six months, but should be followed clinically and observed for disease progression and decline in recent functional status.

B. Patients with CD4+ count above 50 cells/mcL who are followed by an experienced AIDS practitioner probably have a prognosis longer than six months unless there is a non–HIV-related co-existing life-threatening disease. In one study of CD4+ counts and mortality, median survival of the entire population of patients with CD4+ >50 was 11.9 months.

II. Viral Load

A. Patients with a persistent HIV RNA (viral load) of >100,000 copies/ml may have a prognosis less than six months.

B. Patients with lower viral loads may have a prognosis of less than six months if:

1. They have elected to forego antiretroviral and prophylactic medication.

2. Their functional status is declining.

3. They are experiencing complications listed in IV below.

III. Life-threatening complications with median survival:

The following HIV-related opportunistic diseases all are associated with prognosis less than six months. Note that prognosis may be longer for certain conditions if patient elects treatment:

| | |
|---|---|
| A.  CNS lymphoma | 2.5 months |
| B.  Progressive multifocal leukoencephalopathy | 4 months |
| C.  Cryptosporidiosis | 5 months |
| D.  Wasting (loss of 33% lean body mass) | <6 months |
| E.  MAC bacteremia, untreated | <6 months |
| F.  Visceral Kaposi's sarcoma unresponsive to therapy | 6 month mortality 50% |
| G.  Renal failure, refuses or fails dialysis | < 6 months |
| H.  Advanced AIDS dementia complex | 6 months |
| I.  Toxoplasmosis | 6 months |

IV. The following factors have been shown to decrease survival significantly and should be documented if present:

A. Chronic persistent diarrhea for one year, regardless of etiology.

B. Persistent serum albumin <2.5 gm/dl.

C. Concomitant substance abuse.

D. Age greater than 50.

E. Decisions to forego antiretroviral, chemotherapeutic and prophylactic drug therapy related specifically to HIV disease.

F. Congestive heart failure, symptomatic at rest.

# ■ MEDICAL GUIDELINES FOR DETERMINING PROGNOSIS: LIVER DISEASE

I. Laboratory indicators of severely impaired liver function:

Patients with this degree of impairment have a poor prognosis. The patient should show both of the following:

A. Prothrombin time prolonged more than 5 sec. over control.

B. Serum albumin <2.5 gm/dl.

II. Clinical indicators of end-stage liver disease:

The patient should show *at least* one of the following:

A. Ascites, refractory to sodium restriction and diuretics, or patient non-compliant.

1. Maximal diuretics generally used: Spironolactone 75-150 mg/day plus furosemide de ≥40 mg/day.

B. Spontaneous bacterial peritonitis.

1. Median survival 30% at one year; high mortality even when infection cured initially if liver disease is severe or accompanied by renal disease.

C. Hepatorenal syndrome.

1. In patient with cirrhosis and ascites, elevated creatinine and BUN with oliguria (400 ml/da) and urine sodium concentration <10 mEq/l.

2. Usually occurs during hospitalization; survival generally days to weeks.

D. Hepatic encephalopathy, refractory to protein restriction and lactulose or neomycin, or patient non-compliant.

  1. Manifested by: decreased awareness of environment, sleep disturbance, depression, emotional lability, somnolence, slurred speech, obtundation.

  2. Physical exam may show flapping tremor of asterixis, although this finding may be absent in later stages.

  3. Stupor and coma are extremely late-stage findings.

E. Recurrent variceal bleeding.

  1. Following initial variceal hemorrhage, one third died in hospital, one third rebled within six weeks; two thirds survived less than 12 months.

  2. Patient should have rebled *despite therapy,* or refused further therapy, which currently includes:

    a. Injection sclerotherapy or band ligation, if available.

    b. Oral beta blockers.

    c. Transjugular intrahepatic portosystemic shunt (TIPS).

F. Not a candidate for a liver transplant.

III. The following factors have been shown to worsen prognosis and should be documented if present:

A. Progressive malnutrition

B. Muscle wasting with reduced strength and endurance.

C. Continued active alcoholism, i.e. >80 g ethanol per day

D. Hepatocellular carcinoma

E. HBsAg positivity

# ■ MEDICAL GUIDELINES FOR DETERMINING PROGNOSIS: RENAL DISEASE

I. Laboratory criteria for renal failure.

These values may be used to assess patients with renal failure who are not dialyzed, as well as those who survive more than a week or two after dialysis is discontinued. Patients with this degree of renal failure can be expected to die shortly without dialysis.

    A. Creatinine clearance of less than 10cc/min (less than 15 cc/min for diabetics) AND

    B. Serum creatinine greater than 8.0 mg/dl (greater than 6.0 mg/dl for diabetics).

*Notes:* 1. Creatinine clearance may be estimated by using the following formula, thus avoiding a 24-hour urine collection:

$$\text{Ccreat} = \frac{(140 - \text{age in yrs.})\,(\text{body wt. in kg});}{(72)\,(\text{serum creat in mg/dl})} \quad \text{multiply by 0.85 for women.}$$

    2. Blood urea nitrogen (BUN) values are not used in the determination of critical renal failure, since they can be extremely elevated from prerenal azotemia due to dehydration, hypovolemia or other causes.

II. Clinical signs and syndromes associated with renal failure.

The following clinical signs are used as criteria for beginning dialysis. For patients with end-stage renal disease who are not to be dialyzed, the following may help define hospice appropriateness:

    A. Uremia: clinical manifestations of renal failure.

        1. Confusion, obtundation

        2. Intractable nausea and vomiting

        3. Generalized pruritis

        4. Restlessness, "restless legs"

    B. Oliguria: Urine output less than 400cc/24 hrs.

    C. Intractable hyperkalemia: persistent serum potassium >7.0 not responsive to medical management.

    D. Uremic pericarditis.

    E. Hepatorenal syndrome.

    F. Intractable fluid overload.

III. In hospitalized patients with ARF, these comorbid conditions predict early mortality:

    A. Mechanical ventilation.
    B. Malignancy—other organ systems.
    C. Chronic lung disease.
    D. Advanced cardiac disease.
    E. Advanced liver disease.
    F. Sepsis.
    G. Immunosupression/AIDS.
    H. Albumin <3.5 gm/dl.
    I. Cachexia.
    J. Platelet count <25,000.
    K. Age >75.
    L. Disseminated intravascular coagulation.
    M. Gastrointestinal bleeding.

# ■ MEDICAL GUIDELINES FOR DETERMINING PROGNOSIS: STROKE AND COMA

I. *During the acute phase immediately following a hemorrhagic or ischemic stroke,* any of the following are strong predictors of early mortality:

    A. Coma or persistent vegetative state secondary to stroke, beyond three days' duration.

    B. In post-anoxic stroke, coma or severe obtundation, accompanied by severe myoclonus, persisting beyond three days past the anoxic event.

    C. Comatose patients with any 4 of the following on day 3 of coma had 97% mortality by two months:

    1. Abnormal brain stem response

    2. Absent verbal response

    3. Absent withdrawal response to pain

    4. Serum creatinine >1.5 mg/dl

    5. Age >70

D. Dysphagia severe enough to prevent the patient from receiving food and fluids necessary to sustain life, in a patient who declines, or is not a candidate for, artificial nutrition and hydration.

E. If computed tomographic (CT) or magnetic resonance imaging (MRI) scans are available, certain specific findings may indicate decreased likelihood of survival, or at least poor prognosis for recovery of function even with vigorous rehabilitation efforts, which may influence decisions concerning life support or hospice. It should be borne in mind that clinical variables, not imaging studies, are the primary criteria for hospice referral.

II. *Once the patient has entered the chronic phase,* the following clinical factors may correlate with poor survival in the setting of severe stroke, and should be documented. The referenced factors have been studied in relation to prognosis in stroke, whereas others may be found elsewhere in these Guidelines where they relate to declining patients in general, or to comparable conditions such as dementia.

A. Age greater than 70.

B. Poor functional status, as evidenced by Karnofsky score of <50%. See Appendix II.

C. Post-stroke dementia, as evidenced by a FAST score of greater than 7. See Appendix IV.

D. Poor nutritional status, whether on artificial nutrition or not:

    1. Unintentional progressive weight loss of greater than 10% over past six months.

    2. Serum albumin less than 2.5 gm/dl, may be a helpful prognostic indicator, but should not be used by itself.

E. Medical complications related to debility and progressive clinical decline. It is assumed that these patients are in chronic care situations similar to those with end-stage dementia. Although studies are not available to relate these directly to six-month prognosis in stroke, their presence should be documented.

1. Aspiration pneumonia.

2. Upper urinary tract infection (pyelonephritis).

3. Sepsis.

4. Refractory stage 3-4 decubitus ulcers.

5. Fever recurrent after antibiotics.

# ■ MEDICAL GUIDELINES FOR DETERMINING PROGNOSIS: AMYOTROPHIC LATERAL SCLEROSIS (ALS)

The following factors may define those ALS patients with expected survival of approximately six months. These patients generally fit one of the following categories

1. *Both* rapid progression of ALS *and* critically impaired ventilatory capacity.
2. *Both* rapid progression of ALS *and* critical nutritional impairment, with a decision not to receive artificial feeding.
3. *Both* rapid progression of ALS and life-threatening complications.

I. Rapid progression of disease and critically impaired ventilatory capacity.

A. Rapid progression of ALS.
*The patient should have developed most of their disability within the past 12 months.* Patients with slow progression may survive for longer periods, although clinical judgment may still indicate they may be within six months of death.
Examples would include, within the past year:

1. Progressing from independent ambulation to wheelchair- or bed-bound.

2. Progressing from normal to barely intelligible or unintelligible speech.

3. Progressing from normal to blenderized diet.

4. Progressing from independence in most or all Activities of Daily Living (ADL's) to needing major assist by caretaker in all ADL's.

B. Critically impaired ventilatory capacity.
   The patient should have, within the past 12 months, developed extremely severe breathing disability. Examples include:

   1. Vital Capacity (VC) less than 30% of predicted.

   2. Significant dyspnea at rest.

   3. Requiring supplemental oxygen at rest.

   4. Patient declines intubation or tracheostomy and mechanical ventilation.
   Note: Patients who are already on assisted ventilation, whether by negative-pressure external means (e.g. Cuirass) or positive-pressure through tracheostomy, may survive for periods considerably longer than six months unless there is a life-threatening comorbid condition, e.g. recurrent aspiration pneumonia.

II. Rapid progression of ALS *and* critical nutritional impairment.

   A. Rapid progression of ALS. Please see I.A. above.

   B. Critical nutritional impairment.

      Most ALS patients develop swallowing difficulties early in the illness, so that gastrostomy feeding is reasonable.

      However, some patients with end-stage or rapidly-advancing ALS may choose not to undergo artificial feeding.

      These patients may have a prognosis of less than six months if their oral intake of nutrients and fluids is insufficient to sustain life.

      Nutritional impairment may be documented by:

      1. Continued weight loss.

      2. Dehydration or hypovolemia.

III. Rapid progression of ALS and life-threatening complications.

   A. Rapid progression of ALS. Please see I.A. above.

B. Life-threatening complications.

   1. Recurrent aspiration pneumonia.

      This may occur whether or not the patient is receiving tube feedings.

   2. Decubitus ulcers, multiple, Stage 3-4, particularly if infected.

   3. Upper urinary tract infection, e.g. pyelonephritis.

   4. Sepsis.

   5. Fever recurrent after antibiotics.

## References

Excerpted with permission from: Standards and Accreditation Committee, Medical Guidelines Task Force (1996). Medical guidelines for determining prognosis in selected noncancer diseases (2nd ed.). Virginia: National Hospice and Palliative Care Organization.

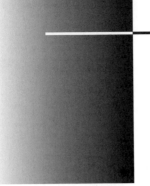

# Internet Resources

Aging with Dignity
http://www.agingwithdignity.org
888-5-WISHES
National nonprofit organization that promotes human dignity as America ages, with emphasis on improved care for those near the end of life; distributes *Five Wishes,* an easy to use advance directive that over 1 million American families have used to discuss how they want to be treated during times of serious illness; has new project to promote *Five Wishes* in the workplace.

American Academy of Hospice and Palliative Medicine
http://www.aahpm.org
An organization of physicians and other health professionals dedicated to the advancement of the practice, research, and education of hospice and palliative medicine.

American Alliance of Cancer Pain Initiatives
http://www.aacpi.org
State-based initiatives and their participants provide education, training, information, and organizational support to health care providers, cancer patients, and their families. The site includes links to all state initiatives, information, e-mail addresses, and a list of professional and patient educational materials available from AACPI and other organizations.

American Hospice Foundation
http://www.americanhospice.org
202-223-0204
Educational and training materials for schools, the workplace, faith communities, and hospices, including Grief-at-School, Grief-at-Work, Talking about Hospice: Tips for Physicians, Tips for Nurses, and Hospice & Alzheimer's Disease; offers on-site, full-day training workshops for managers, employee assistance professionals, educators, bereavement counselors, and mental health professionals.

American Pain Foundation
http://www.painfoundation.org
A nonprofit organization representing patients with pain; includes
extensive resources for patients, families, and health care professionals
regarding pain management and current issues.

American Pain Society
http://www.ampainsoc.org
847-375-4715
Advances pain-related research, education, treatment, and professional
practice; maintains database of pain treatment centers and an internet
resource list for pain professionals.

Americans for Better Care of the Dying
http://www.abcd-caring.org
202-895-9485
Dedicated to social, professional, and policy reform to improve care for
patients with serious illness and their families.

Beth Israel Medical Center: MAYDAY Resource Center for Pain Medicine
    and Palliative Care
http://www.stoppain.org
877-620-9999
Serves as a clearinghouse for the dissemination of educational materials in
pain medicine and palliative care and as a nucleus of scholarship for
physicians, nurses, pharmacists, psychosocial professionals, patients, and
family caregivers.

Center to Advance Palliative Care
http://www.capcmssm.org
212-241-7885
Provides technical assistance to hospital and health systems interested in
planning and establishing palliative care services.

City of Hope Pain/Palliative Care Resource Center
http://www.prc.coh.org
626-359-8111 x63829
Serves as a clearinghouse for the dissemination of information on
resources that enable individuals and institutions to improve the quality of
pain management. The center is a central source for collecting a variety of
materials, including pain assessment tools, patient education materials,
quality assurance materials, research instruments, and other resources.

Community-State Partnerships Program
http://www.midbio.org/npo-about.htm
816-842-7110
Promotes broad-based policy reform at the state and community level.
Publications include: *Making Our Voices Heard: A Guide to Public Engagement,*
an 85-page manual; *State Initiatives in End-of-Life Care,* a policy brief series
on various topics; and *Media Tactics,* a newsletter. See also the "Pathways
Project" on this site.

Compassion Sabbath
http://www.midbio.org/cs/index.htm
816-221-1100
Interfaith initiative to provide clergy and religious leaders with tools for
addressing the spiritual needs of dying people and their families. Resources
include the *Compassion Sabbath Resource Kit,* consultation, faculty,
networking, and peer contact information.

Decisions Near the End of Life at the Education Development Center
    (EDC), Inc.
http://www.edc.org/CAE/Decisions/dnel.html
617-969-7100 x2388
An institution-based, multidisciplinary quality improvement program in
use in over 225 U.S. health care institutions; includes extensive curriculum
resources, a needs assessment survey tool, and annotated bibliographies on
major topics in end-of-life care. National leadership conferences are held
annually for new teams.

Edmonton Regional Palliative Care Program
Edmonton, Alberta, Canada
http://www.palliative.org
Clinical information including reviews on palliative care topics, listings of
publications, a journal watch, palliative care tips for primary care
physicians and nurses, and tools for clinical assessment. A patient and
family section provides basic information on death, dying, grief, and
bereavement.

Education for Physicians on End-of-Life Care
http://www.epec.net
877-524-EPEC (toll free)
Educates physicians and other members of the interdisciplinary team
through its core curriculum on essential clinical competencies required to
provide quality end-of-life care. The core curriculum teaches fundamental
skills in communication, ethical decision making, palliative care,
psychosocial considerations, and pain and symptom management.

End-of-Life Nursing Education Consortium
http://www.aacn.nche.edu/elnec
202-463-6930
A comprehensive national education program instituted to develop a core of expert nursing educators and to coordinate national nursing efforts in end-of-life care.

End-of-Life Physician Education Resource Center
http://www.eperc.mcw.edu
414-805-4607
Assists physician educators and others in locating high-quality, peer-reviewed training materials. Search materials are indexed by end-of-life care topics and educational formats.

Family Caregiver Alliance
http://www.caregiver.org
A nonprofit organization providing support and information for caregivers, including an online support group and specialized information on Alzheimer's disease, stroke, traumatic brain injury, Parkinson's disease, ALS, and similar illnesses. Extensive information is also available on every conceivable aspect of caregiving including end-of-life decision making conservatorship, and evaluation of research findings. Many resources are available in Spanish and Chinese.

Growth House
http://www.growthhouse.org
Includes a search engine that offers access to the net's most comprehensive collection of reviewed resources for end-of-life care. The Inter-Institutional Collaborating Network (IICN) on end-of-life care links health care organizations through a shared network.

Hospice Foundation of America
http://www.hospicefoundation.org
202-638-5419
A nonprofit, grassroots foundation promoting the hospice philosophy of care, informing the public about end-of-life options, and training health care workers and the families they serve in issues related to loss, spirituality, and psychosocial issues, including the annual National Living with Grief Teleconference.

Hospice & Palliative Nurses Association
http://www.hpna.org
412-361-2470
Provides convenient access to current information in the areas of hospice and palliative nursing, including information on conferences and certification of hospice and palliative nurses.

Innovations in End-of-Life Care
http://www.edc.org/lastacts
An international online journal featuring peer-reviewed examples of promising practices in end-of-life care. Each bimonthly issue focuses on a different theme.

Institute for Healthcare Improvement
http://www.ihi.org
An independent, nonprofit organization offering resources and services to help health care organizations make long-lasting improvements that enhance clinical outcomes and reduce cost.

International Association for Hospice and Palliative Care
http://www.hospicecare.com
A nonprofit organization whose mission is to increase the availability and access to high quality hospice and palliative care worldwide through promoting communication; facilitating and providing education; and providing information for patients, professionals, healthcare providers, and policy makers.

Last Acts
http://www.lastacts.org
A national coalition to improve care and caring near the end of life. The goal of the coalition is to bring death-related issues out in the open and help individuals and organizations pursue better ways of caring for the dying.

Mayday Pain Project
http://www.painandhealth.org
906-343-6545
Increases awareness and provides objective information concerning the treatment of pain. The website is set up as an index for visitors and contains carefully chosen internet links and resources.

National Hospice and Palliative Care Organization (NHPCO)
http://www.nhpco.org
703-837-1500
The largest nonprofit membership organization representing U.S. hospice and palliative care programs and professionals. The NHPCO develops public and professional educational programs and materials, convenes meetings and symposia on emerging issues, provides technical informational resources to members, conducts research, monitors congressional and regulatory activities, and works closely with other organizations interested in end-of-life care.

National Institute for Healthcare Research (NIHR)
http://www.nihr.org
Encourages professional collaboration to advance the understanding of spirituality and health. As an educational, medical, and social science research organization, the NIHR develops world-class educational programs, conducts research on the spirituality-health interface, and reviews and disseminates research findings.

Pain and Policy Studies Group (PPSG)
http://www.medsch.wisc.edu/painpolicy
608-263-7662
Facilitates public access to domestic and international information about pain relief and public policy. Intended audiences include patients, the public, and professionals in medicine, pharmacy, nursing, palliative care, cancer care, law, and other related disciplines.

Partnership for Caring: America's Voices for the Dying
http://www.partnershipforcaring.org
pfc@partnershipforcaring.org
800-989-9455
A national nonprofit organization devoted to raising consumer expectations and demand for excellent end-of-life care; offers resources for talking about end-of-life choices, the process of health care, and state-specific advance directives.

Project on Death in America (PDIA)
http://www.soros.org/death
212-548-0600
PDIA's mission is to understand and transform the culture and experience of dying and bereavement through initiatives in research, scholarship, humanities, and arts and to foster innovations in the provision of care, public education, professional education, and public policy.

Promoting Excellence in End-of-Life Care
http://www.promotingexcellence.org
406-243-6668
Manages 22 grant-funded projects designed to demonstrate excellence in end-of-life care in institutional settings. Promoting Excellence in End-of-Life Care also facilitates a network of peer workgroups that comprise innovators and emerging leaders across the spectrum of palliative care.

Safe Crossings
http://www.providence.org/safecrossings
Designed to meet the needs of children up to age 18 facing the loss of a loved one. The website is designed to provide activities and resources for kids, families, and professionals.

Supportive Care of the Dying
http://www.careofdying.org
503-215-5053
Develops and tests innovative projects with individuals and organizations working to improve delivery of care to those facing the end of life. Print and video products are available on many end-of-life issues, including the improvement of physician communication with patients and families.

# Index

## A

**Abandonment**
fears of terminally ill, 99-100
**Abdomen**
assessment of
in advanced cancer patients, 173
bloated
with ascites, 191-196
cramping
with constipation, 224-225
with diarrhea, 281
extended
with ascites, 191-192
increased girth of
with ascites, 191-192
with end-stage heart disease, 132
pain
with colorectal cancer, 168
with constipation, 224-225
diagram illustrating sites of, 351f
**Abdominal lymphadenopathy**
with non-Hodgkin's lymphoma, 170
**Aberrant drug-related behaviors**
recognizing, 375t
unrelieved pain causing, 374-376
**Abnormal respiratory reflex**, 327
**Absent-mindedness**
behavior with normal grief, 59
**Abuse**
alcohol, 130, 201, 256b, 257t, 262-263,
271, 327-328, 370, 372-373,
375t
drugs
and pain management, 370,
372-373
**Acceptance**
stage of Kübler-Ross' theories, 57
**ACE inhibitors**, 128, 133
**Acetylcholine**, 158, 167
**Acetylcholinesterase**, 159
**Acid-base signs**
signaling chronic renal failure, 150t
**Acidosis**
and renal failure, 148t, 149

**Acquired immunodeficiency syndrome (AIDS)**
causing acute pain, 350t
assessment and measurement of,
182-184
cachexia and anorexia with, 213-218
definition of, 181
delirium with, 255
diarrhea associated with, 281, 290
diseases related to, 181-187
end-stage symptoms management,
185-186
etiology and pathophysiology, 182
and fatigue, 318
intervention and treatment, 184-185
nausea and vomiting with, 333
severe pain with, 349
**Active euthanasia**
*versus* assisted suicide, 100
definition of, 100
**Activities of daily living (ADLs)**
assessing
with fatigue, 321
with pain management, 357
issues
and pain management, 346
**Activity tolerance**, 131
**Acupressure**
for pain, 371
to treat nausea and vomiting, 338
**Acupuncture**
to help dyspnea, 312
for pain, 371
to treat nausea and vomiting, 338
**Acute heart failure**
associated with atherosclerosis, 130
**Acute infarction**
definition of, 127
survival rates, 128
**Acute pain**
causes of, 350t
**Acute somatic pain**, 347t
**Acute traumatic grief**
Lindemann on, 55-56
**Acute visceral pain**, 347t
**Addiction**
definition of, 355
fears with pain medications, 354-356
and pain management, 370, 372-373